Therapeutics and Control of Sheep and Goat Diseases

Guest Editors

GEORGE C. FTHENAKIS, DVM, MSc, PhD
PAULA I. MENZIES, DVM, MPVM

VETERINARY CLINICS
OF NORTH AMERICA:
FOOD ANIMAL PRACTICE

www.vetfood.theclinics.com

Consulting Editor
ROBERT A. SMITH, DVM, MS

March 2011 • Volume 27 • Number 1

SAUNDERS an imprint of ELSEVIER, Inc.

W.B. SAUNDERS COMPANY
A Division of Elsevier Inc.

1600 John F. Kennedy Boulevard • Suite 1800 • Philadelphia, PA 19103-2899

http://www.vetfood.theclinics.com

VETERINARY CLINICS OF NORTH AMERICA: FOOD ANIMAL PRACTICE Volume 27, Number 1
March 2011 ISSN 0749-0720, ISBN-13: 978-1-4557-0522-1

Editor: John Vassallo; j.vassallo@elsevier.com

Veterinary Clinics of North America: Food Animal Practice (ISSN 0749-0720) is published in March, July, and November by Elsevier Inc., 360 Park Avenue South, New York, NY 10010-1710. Subscription prices are $199.00 per year (domestic individuals), $278.00 per year (domestic institutions), $93.00 per year (domestic students/residents), $225.00 per year (Canadian individuals), $363.00 per year (Canadian institutions), $284.00 per year (international individuals), $363.00 per year (international institutions), and $142.00 per year (international and Canadian students/residents). To receive student/resident rate, orders must be accompanied by name of affiliated institution, date of term, and the signature of program/residency coordinator on institution letterhead. *Clinics* subscription prices. All prices are subject to change without notice. **POSTMASTER:** Send address changes to *Veterinary Clinics of North America: Food Animal Practice*, Elsevier Health Sciences Division, Subscription Customer Service, 3251 Riverport Lane, Maryland Heights, MO 63043. Customer Service (orders, claims, online, change of address): Elsevier Health Sciences Division, Subscription Customer Service, 3251 Riverport Lane, Maryland Heights, MO 63043. Tel: 1-800-654-2452 (U.S. and Canada); 314-447-8871 (ouside U.S. and Canada). Fax: 314-447-8029. E-mail: journalscustomerservice-usa@elsevier.com (for print support); journalsonlinesupport-usa@elsevier.com (for online support).

Reprints. For copies of 100 or more, of articles in this publication, please contact the Commercial Reprints Department, Elsevier Inc., 360 Park Avenue South, New York, NY 10010-1710. Tel.: 212-633-3812; Fax: 212-462-1935; E-mail: reprints@elsevier.com.

Veterinary Clinics of North America: Food Animal Practice is covered in *Current Contents/Agriculture, Biology and Environmental Sciences, MEDLINE/PubMed (Index Medicus), and Excerpta Medica.*

Printed and bound in the United Kingdom

Transferred to Digital Print 2011

Contributors

CONSULTING EDITOR

ROBERT A. SMITH, DVM, MS
Diplomate, American Board of Veterinary Practitioners; Veterinary Research
and Consulting Services, LLC, Greeley, Colorado

GUEST EDITORS

GEORGE C. FTHENAKIS, DVM, MSc, PhD
Diplomate, European College of Animal Reproduction; Diplomate, European College
of Small Ruminant Health Management; European Veterinary Specialist in Small Ruminant
Health Management; Veterinary Faculty, University of Thessaly, Karditsa, Greece

PAULA I. MENZIES, DVM, MPVM
Diplomate, European College of Small Ruminant Health Management; Associate
Professor, Population Medicine Department, Ontario Veterinary College, University
of Guelph, Guelph, Ontario, Canada

AUTHORS

JOSÉ A. ABECIA, DVM, PhD
Diplomate, European College of Small Ruminant Health Management; European
Veterinary Specialist in Small Ruminant Health Management; Dept de Producción,
Animal y Ciencia de los Alimentos, Facultad de Veterinaria, Universidad de Zaragoza,
Zaragoza, Spain

GARETH F. BATH, BVSc
Diplomat, European College of Small Ruminant Health Management; European Veterinary
Specialist in Small Ruminant Health Management; Professor, Department of Production
Animal Studies, Faculty of Veterinary Science, Onderstepoort, University of Pretoria,
Gauteng, South Africa

JOSÉ M. BLASCO, DVM, PhD
Unidad de Sanidad Animal, CITA/Gobierno de Aragón, Zaragoza, Spain

CHRISTOS BROZOS, DVM, PhD
School of Veterinary Medicine, Aristotle University of Thessaloniki, Thessaloniki, Greece

JUAN FELIPE DE JESÚS TORRES-ACOSTA, DVM, PhD
Facultad de Medicina Veterinaria y Zootecnia, Universidad Autónoma de Yucatán, Mérida,
Yucatán, México

ELISA M. ERMILIO, DVM
Associate, Country Companions Veterinary Services, Bethany, Connecticut

VIRGINIA R. FAJT, DVM, PhD
Diplomate, American College of Veterinary Clinical Pharmacology; Clinical Assistant Professor, Department of Veterinary Physiology and Pharmacology, College of Veterinary Medicine and Biomedical Sciences, Texas A&M University, College Station, Texas

FERNANDO FORCADA, DVM, PhD
Dept de Producción, Animal y Ciencia de los Alimentos, Facultad de Veterinaria, Universidad de Zaragoza, Zaragoza, Spain

ILEKTRA A. FRAGKOU, DVM, PhD
Veterinary Faculty, University of Thessaly, Karditsa, Greece

GEORGE C. FTHENAKIS, DVM, MSc, PhD
Diplomate, European College of Animal Reproduction; Diplomate, European College of Small Ruminant Health Management; European Veterinary Specialist in Small Ruminant Health Management; Veterinary Faculty, University of Thessaly, Karditsa, Greece

APOSTOLOS D. GALATOS, DVM, PhD
Diplomate, European College of Veterinary Anaesthesia and Analgesia; European Veterinary Specialist in Anesthesia; Associate Professor, Department of Surgery, Faculty of Veterinary Medicine, University of Thessaly, Karditsa, Greece

ANTONIO GONZÁLEZ-BULNES, DVM, PhD
Dept de Reproducción, Instituto Nacional de Investigación y Tecnología Agraria y Alimentaria, Ctra de la Coruña, Madrid, Spain

HERVÉ HOSTE, DVM, PhD
Diplomate, European Veterinary Parasitology College; Institut National de la Recherche Agronomique/ENVT, Ecole Nationale Vétérinaire de Toulouse, Toulouse, France

RAMON A. JUSTE, DVM, PhD
Diplomate, European College of Small Ruminant Health Management; Department of Animal Health, NEIKER -Tecnalia, Bizkaia, Spain

CHRISTOPHER J. LEWIS, BVetMed, DSHP, MRCVS
Diplomate, European College of Small Ruminant Health Management; European Veterinary Specialist in Small Ruminant Health Management; Sheep Veterinary Services, Audlem, Cheshire, United Kingdom

DAVID LONGBOTTOM, PhD
Pentlands Science Park, Moredun Research Institute, International Research Centre, Bush Loan, Penicuik, Midlothian, Scotland, United Kingdom

VASIA S. MAVROGIANNI, DVM, PhD
Diplomate, European College of Small Ruminant Health Management; European Veterinary Specialist in Small Ruminant Health Management; Veterinary Faculty, University of Thessaly, Karditsa, Greece

PAULA I. MENZIES, DVM, MPVM
Diplomate, European College of Small Ruminant Health Management; Associate Professor, Population Medicine Department, Ontario Veterinary College, University of Guelph, Guelph, Ontario, Canada

BALDOMERO MOLINA-FLORES, DVM, MSc
The Emergency Center for Transboundary Animal Disease Operations Unit for North Africa, Food and Agriculture Organization of the United Nations, Tunis, Tunisia

VALENTIN PEREZ, DVM, PhD
Professor, Department of Animal Health, Faculty of Veterinary Medicine, University of León, León, Spain

JOHN W. PLANT, BVSc
Veterinary Specialist (Sheep Medicine), North Rocks, New South Wales, Australia

ANNE L. RIDLER, BVSc, PhD
Diplomate, European College of Small Ruminant Health Management; European Veterinary Specialist in Small Ruminant Health Management; Department of Veterinary Clinical Sciences, The Royal Veterinary College, North Mymms, Hertfordshire, United Kingdom

NEIL D. SARGISON, BA, VetMB, PhD, DSHP, FRCVS
Diplomate, European College of Small Ruminant Health Management; European Veterinary Specialist in Small Ruminant Health Management; Professor, University of Edinburgh, Royal (Dick) School of Veterinary Studies, Large Animal Practice, Easter Bush Veterinary Centre, Roslin, Midlothian, Scotland, United Kingdom

LISA C. SCOTT, MSc
Ontario Veterinary College, University of Guelph, Guelph, Ontario, Canada

PHILIP R. SCOTT, DVMS, MPhil, FRCVS
Diplomate, European College of Bovine Health Management; Diplomate, European College of Small Ruminant Health Management; European Veterinary Specialist in Bovine Health Management; Reader, Division of Veterinary Clinical Sciences, Royal (Dick) School of Veterinary Studies, University of Edinburgh, Roslin, Midlothian, Scotland, United Kingdom

MARY C. SMITH, DVM
Diplomate, American College of Theriogenologists; Professor, Department of Population Medicine and Diagnostic Sciences, College of Veterinary Medicine, Cornell University, Ithaca, New York

SMARAGDA SOTIRAKI, DVM, PhD
Diplomate, European Veterinary Parasitology College; National Agricultural Research Foundation, VRI NAGREF Campus, Thermi Thessaloniki, Greece

SNORRE STUEN, DVM, PhD, DrPhilos
Diplomate, European College of Small Ruminant Health Management; European Veterinary Specialist in Small Ruminant Health Management; Department of Production Animal Clinical Sciences, Norwegian School of Veterinary Science, Sandnes, Norway

DAVID M. WEST, BVSc, PhD
Institute of Veterinary, Animal and Biomedical Sciences, Massey University, Palmerston North, New Zealand

PETER A. WINDSOR, DVSc, PhD, GradCertEdStud
Diplomate, European College of Small Ruminant Health Management; European Veterinary Specialist in Small Ruminant Health Management; Specialist Veterinary Surgeon (Pathobiology); Farm Animal and Veterinary Public Health Group, Faculty of Veterinary Science, University of Sydney, Camden, New South Wales, Australia

AGNES C. WINTER, BVSc, PhD, DSHP, MRCVS, FRAgS
Diplomate, European College of Small Ruminant Health Management; European Veterinary Specialist in Small Ruminant Health Management; Walmgate York, North Yorkshire; Honorary Professor, School of Veterinary Science, University of Liverpool, Liverpool, United Kingdom

Contents

be performed. Apart from improving animal welfare standards, anesthesia and analgesia are essential to make the procedures easier and improve both animal and personnel safety. This article provides an overview of the anesthetic and analgesic agents and techniques commonly used in sheep and goats.

Control of *Brucella ovis* Infection in Sheep

Anne L. Ridler and David M. West

Approach to control of *Brucella ovis* would vary in different countries and areas depending on farm and flock characteristics and economic factors. Eradication by a test-and-slaughter approach is the most desirable option in areas where it is logistically and financially feasible. Vaccination is used in areas with a high incidence of infection where eradication would be difficult. Voluntary accreditation programs have been established in some countries and are of particular benefit to pedigree ram breeders.

Pharmaceutical Control of Reproduction in Sheep and Goats

José A. Abecia, Fernando Forcada, and Antonio González-Bulnes

Small ruminant species such as sheep and goats are short-day breeders, which is a crucial factor affecting the offer of lambs and kids throughout the year. An appropriate management of reproduction allows ewes and does to breed in the spring to increase the supply of product to the marketplace on a year-round basis. Pharmaceutical control of reproduction is possible, usually through administration of hormones or analogues related to the natural estrous cycle, such as progesterone, prostaglandins, and/or melatonin.

Control of Important Causes of Infectious Abortion in Sheep and Goats

Paula I. Menzies

This article summarizes control measures for the most common causes of abortion in North America, New Zealand, the United Kingdom, and Europe. When dealing with an abortion outbreak in a flock or herd, diagnostic investigation is critical to assuring that any future control measures are effective and worthwhile. Biosecurity is an important consideration for any abortion control program, and should be promoted regardless of whether an abortion problem exists in the flock. Many of the infectious agents that cause abortion in small ruminants are also zoonotic pathogens, and producers should be educated to avoid risk to themselves and their families.

Control and Eradication of *Brucella melitensis* Infection in Sheep and Goats

José M. Blasco and Baldomero Molina-Flores

Brucella melitensis is the main etiological agent of brucellosis in sheep and goats, and is also the main agent responsible for human brucellosis, a predominantly occupational disease related to professions in direct contact with livestock. As there is currently no viable method of preventing human brucellosis to safeguard people attention must be directed toward effectively controlling the disease in sheep and goats. This review focuses on the different strategies in different socioeconomic and epidemiologic situations that can be applied to either control or eradicate brucellosis in sheep and goats.

The paper reviews treatment and control of pregnancy toxaemia, hypocalcaemia, hypomagnesaemia, the important peri-parturient diseases of small ruminants. Treatment of pregnancy toxemia benefits from early instigation, ie, upon timely diagnosis and is based on administration of energy sources to sick animals. Removal of fetuses, by induced parturition or caesarean section, should also be carried out. Individual cases within a farm require close monitoring of other animals and measures to avoid development of further clinical cases. Treatment of hypocalcemia is based on administration of calcium solution. Finally, hypomagnesemic animals need urgent treatment with calcium and magnesium solutions.

This article indicates the principles for treatment of mastitis in ewes/does and explains the reasons why treatment may occasionally fail. It presents the principles for administration of antimicrobial agents at drying off of the animals. Finally, it addresses the risk of antimicrobials present in milk when improper withdrawal periods are used and the issues around testing for inhibitors before putting the milk into in a farm's tank.

Clostridia cause many different diseases, all characterized by sudden death, most occurring worldwide. Diseases caused by clostridia can be divided into 4 groups: those affecting the alimentary system (the enterotoxemias), those affecting the parenchymatous organs, those causing myonecrosis and toxemia, and those causing neurologic disorders. Their mode of action is to produce one or more potent toxins when multiplying under favorable conditions. Considerable variation exists between different strains of the same organism. Specific trigger factors are required to induce toxin production. Excellent control is obtained by the use of toxoid vaccines. Protection is passed to the lamb via the colostrum.

Control of paratuberculosis in small ruminants can be easily achieved by vaccination. Vaccination prevents clinical cases and thus may lead to increased production at a highly profitable benefit-to-cost ratio. Because bacterial shedding is greatly reduced, vaccination can help control the general contamination risks. There are no restrictions to vaccination in sheep, but potential interference with diagnosis of tuberculosis must be taken into account in goats. Other control strategies have failed, because of either high costs or lack of efficacy on a large scale.

THE CLINICS ARE NOW AVAILABLE ONLINE!

Access your subscription at:
www.theclinics.com

Preface

Therapeutics and Control of Sheep and Goat Diseases

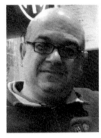 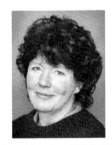

George C. Fthenakis, DVM, MSc, PhD   Paula I. Menzies, DVM, MPVM
Guest Editors

Therapeutics is the branch of medicine that is concerned with the remedial treatment of disease.[1] The word derives etymologically from the Greek word '$\theta\varepsilon\rho\alpha\pi\varepsilon\dot{\upsilon}\varepsilon\iota\nu$' (ie, to treat medically, heal) and describes an entire scientific field dedicated to the art of healing. In small ruminants, treatment of the individual animal is very often coupled with the decision to take action within the flock/herd, in order to prevent introduction or spread of the disease. Hence, the broader term "control" may be used interchangeably with "treatment" to denote actions taken to maintain the health of the population. Appropriate treatment is based on and follows an accurate diagnosis; similarly, this issue follows the publication, in Elsevier's *Small Ruminant Research*, of a special volume on "Sheep Diagnostic Medicine."[2]

In flocks/herds of small ruminants, consideration of only the individual patient for treatment may lead to recrudescence and further spread of the disease within the population. However, treatment of the individual animal that is ill does help to protect the rest of the flock, as it may reduce spread of disease. Treatment is also essential to the welfare of animals with disease. So, this volume on therapeutics of sheep and goats includes content that addresses not only the treatment of animals that show evidence of clinical disease, but also describes strategic administration of pharmaceutical agents to those that are at risk, ie, could become ill, as well as to those that could be a source of infection to healthy animals. The volume also addresses the issue of antimicrobial resistance in pathogens of sheep and goats, which is of particular importance when considering the health of humans working with small ruminants or consuming their products. The volume also outlines issues concerning drug use in small ruminants, which are considered to be minor species in much of the world and, therefore, often lacking in approved medicines in many jurisdictions.

Vet Clin Food Anim 27 (2011) xiii–xiv
doi:10.1016/j.cvfa.2010.11.001
vetfood.theclinics.com

The 20 articles in this issue present clinical aspects of treatment and control of the most important diseases of small ruminants. The articles have been authored or coauthored by American, Australian, or European veterinary specialists. The articles by international contributors provide a global perspective of small ruminant diseases. Among the contributors, there are 13 Diplomates of the European College of Small Ruminant Health Management (ECSRHM), which is, worldwide, the highest transnational body of veterinary specialization in the discipline.

Many thanks go to all the authors for accepting the invitation to contribute and for accommodating a tight schedule in meeting deadlines. Acknowledgements are also due to the editors of the series, Dr Robert A. Smith and Mr John Vassallo, for their support and solutions during the editorial process.

George C. Fthenakis, DVM, MSc, PhD
Veterinary Faculty
University of Thessaly
43100 Karditsa, Greece

Paula I. Menzies, DVM, MPVM
Population Medicine Department
Ontario Veterinary College
University of Guelph
Guelph N1G 2W1, Ontario, Canada

E-mail addresses:
gcf@vet.uth.gr (G.C. Fthenakis)
pmenzies@uoguelph.ca (P.I. Menzies)

REFERENCES

1. Shorter Oxford. In: The Shorter Oxford English dictionary on historical principles. 3rd edition. Brighton: Guild Publishing; 1983. p. 2281.
2. Fthenakis GC, Gouletsou PG, Mavrogianni VS, et al. Introduction to special SRR issue 'Sheep diagnostic medicine'. Small Rumin Res 2010;92:1.

Drug Laws and Regulations for Sheep and Goats

Virginia R. Fajt, DVM, PhD

KEYWORDS

- Antimicrobial resistance • Extralabel drug use
- Food animal residue avoidance databank (FARAD)
- Goat • Minor species • Sheep • Tissue residue
- Withdrawal period

Although the process of pharmacotherapeutic decision making seems intuitive to the experienced veterinary clinician, it is important to periodically assess the process, to ensure that appropriate decisions are being made. Decision making for drug use and selection involves the following steps:

1. Identification of the physiologic or pathophysiologic process requiring alteration in the patient (eg, increased gastrointestinal parasite load, hypovolemia, bacterial infection of the lungs)
2. Decision whether use of a drug would affect the pathophysiologic changes
3. Identification of potential drugs that may produce the desired effect (this implies knowledge of mechanisms of action and therapeutic effects of drugs)
4. For each drug identified, establishing whether there are any of the following obstacles to its use; (a) undesirable adverse effects, (b) contra-indications in the patient, (c) concurrent disease states, (d) inability to monitor efficacy or (e) legal implications for its use
5. Selection of drug and drug regimen for administration.

This article focuses on step 4(e) by reviewing the legal obligations and potential regulatory obstacles to use of drugs, in the United States in particular, with other countries mentioned as appropriate. To set the stage for defining legal drug use, a review of the drug approval process is provided, as well as a discussion of drugs currently approved for use in sheep and goats in the United States.

The author has nothing to disclose.
Department of Veterinary Physiology and Pharmacology, College of Veterinary Medicine and Biomedical Sciences, Texas A&M University, MS 4466, College Station, TX 77843-4466, USA
E-mail address: vfajt@cvm.tamu.edu

The author is not nor has ever been an employee of a regulatory or legal agency; therefore, all interpretations are the author's alone. The respective agency should be contacted with questions regarding any information contained herein.

LABELED/LICENSED DRUGS
Approval of New Veterinary Drugs

Drugs are defined by US federal laws as articles intended for use in the diagnosis, cure, mitigation, treatment, or prevention of diseases and articles (other than food) intended to affect the structure or any function of the body.[1] Therefore, a drug is defined not by whether it is termed a drug or not, but rather its intended use. If water were used for treatment of disease, that water would be a drug and would be subject to laws and regulations; if that water is not approved for that specific use, such use is a violation of the Federal Food Drug and Cosmetic Act. Similar definitions are also legally used by Health Canada.

The process for approval or so-called labeling or licensing of drugs for sheep and goats involves collection of data on safety and efficacy.[2] This approval process differs from country to country. Safety of drugs includes safety of the target animal, safety of humans exposed to the drug during administration and use, safety of humans consuming animal products after the animal has been treated with the drug, and safety for the environment of animals treated with the drug. The evidence required to document efficacy of a drug in the United States is outlined in Guidance #61[2] (**Table 1**) and includes recommendations for parasiticides, antimicrobials, and production drugs, with suggested options when appropriate for use of data from other species (in particular cattle) to document efficacy.

Tables 2–5 list veterinary drugs currently approved for sheep and goats in the United States and Canada. Experienced veterinarians are aware that there is a paucity of drugs licensed for these animal species, resulting in either inability to treat particular conditions or requiring the use of drugs in an extralabel manner, in particular the use of drugs approved in other species of animals. The European Medicines Agency approves veterinary drugs for the European Union, although individual European countries also have national agencies that license drugs at country level (see **Table 1**).

Office of Minor Use and Minor Species at the US Food and Drug Administration Center for Veterinary Medicine

Within the US Food and Drug Administration (FDA) Center for Veterinary Medicine (CVM), the Office of Minor Use and Minor Species (MUMS) supports the development of these drugs. MUMS can designate a new animal drug as one for a minor use or minor species, in which case grants may be available to support drug approval and a period of exclusivity applies to that approval (designation does not imply that the drug may be marketed; drug approval must first be granted). MUMS also maintains a list of so-called indexed drugs; these are drugs that may be marketed before collection of safety and efficacy data. Indexing is not available for drugs for food animals.

The list of designated drugs at the time of writing (2010) includes, for sheep, moxidectin and the progesterone EAZI-BREED CIDR, with both now approved for use. For goats, albendazole and the progesterone EAZI-BREED CIDR have been designated, but neither has yet been approved for use. Their designation allows a drug sponsor to apply for grants for data development that would lead to approval. Drug sponsors for drugs for minor species are not always pharmaceutical companies, but may be university or extension personnel with an interest in minor species. Approvals of drugs for minor species may use data published in Public Master Files, which may include safety or efficacy data generated by companies or other sponsors, or these approvals may use data acquired via requesting permission from a pharmaceutical company to share proprietary data from previous drug approvals in other species.

Historically, the NRSP-7 (National Research Support Project No. 7) of the US Department of Agriculture has provided support for the development of data for minor species, including sheep and goats. This project continues to operate in the United States, in cooperation with the FDA MUMS office, to provide support and funding that will lead to the approval of new animal drugs for small ruminants.

EXTRALABEL USE OF VETERINARY DRUGS
Legal Basis for Extralabel Use of Veterinary Drugs in the United States

The Animal Medicinal Drug Use Clarification Act (AMDUCA) of 1994 authorized veterinarians in the United States to use drugs in an extralabel manner under particular circumstances.[3] Extralabel use is the use in any manner not included on the label (ie, not licensed), and may include nonlicensed route of administration, indications, animal species, dose, or frequency. This authorization for extralabel use applies only to drugs approved by the FDA and does not include authorization for extralabel use of other products used in animals that are approved by other agencies, such as pesticides (approved by the US Environmental Protection Agency) or vaccines and other biologic or immunologic products (approved by the US Department of Agriculture). There is no legal provision for using these products in any manner not included on the label, and the veterinarian may incur liability should these products be used in a nonlabeled manner.

Extralabel use may be permissible under AMDUCA, when the health of the animal is threatened and death or suffering may result if the animal is not treated. Extralabel use is not permitted for production drugs, including drugs that manipulate the estrus cycle, drugs that enhance growth, or drugs that induce lactation. Extralabel use of drugs must be performed by or on the order of a licensed veterinarian, within the context of a veterinarian-client-patient relationship (VCPR). A VCPR is present under the following circumstances: (1) the veterinarian has assumed responsibility for making clinical judgments regarding the health of the animal(s) and the need for medical treatment, and the client has agreed to follow the veterinarian's instructions; (2) the veterinarian has sufficient knowledge of the animal(s) to initiate at least a general or preliminary diagnosis of the medical condition of the animal(s); this means that the veterinarian has recently seen and is personally acquainted with the keeping and care of the animal(s) by virtue of an examination of the animal(s), or by medically appropriate and timely visits to the premises where the animal(s) are kept; (3) the veterinarian is readily available or has arranged for emergency coverage, for follow-up evaluation in the event of adverse reactions or the failure of the treatment regime.

The law does not define exactly what timely visits are, under the assumption that this may differ for different types of animals and types of operations. Species groups are encouraged to develop their own definitions of timely to give guidance to veterinarians working with those species.

Permissible Extralabel Use of Veterinary Drugs in the United States

To determine if a particular extralabel use being contemplated is legal, the American Veterinary Medical Association (AVMA) has developed an algorithm (see **Table 1**). As stated earlier, the first requirements are the presence of a VCPR and at least a preliminary diagnosis, as well as the therapeutic (ie, nonproduction use) need for the use. If the animal is a food animal, which includes all sheep and goats, if a drug exists that is

Table 1
Recommended Web sites for information about drug regulation

Topic	Description	Electronic Address
US-based Web Sites		
American Veterinary Medical Association (AVMA) Animal Medicinal Drug Use Clarification Act Flowchart	Hierarchy and algorithm for determining acceptability of extralabel drug use	http://www.avma.org/reference/amduca/amduca1.asp
AVMA Guidance on Internet pharmacies	—	http://www.avma.org/issues/prescribing/default.asp
AVMA Guidance on prescribing and dispensing drugs	—	http://www.avma.org/issues/prescribing/prescribing_faq.asp
AVMA Guidelines for judicious antimicrobial use	General guidelines; some species groups have expanded these into more comprehensive and specific guidelines	http://www.avma.org/issues/policy/jtua.asp
Food and Drug Administration Center for Veterinary Medicine (FDA CVM)	Home page for the CVM	http://www.fda.gov/AnimalVeterinary/default.htm
FDA CVM Compliance Policy Guide on compounding	Outlines FDA policy on acceptable and unacceptable compounding	http://www.fda.gov/downloads/ICECI/ComplianceManuals/CompliancePolicyGuidanceManual/UCM200461.pdf
FDA CVM Form FDA 1932a for Adverse Drug Event Reporting	Veterinary Adverse Experience, Lack of Effectiveness or Product Defect Report	http://www.fda.gov/downloads/AboutFDA/ReportsManualsForms/Forms/AnimalDrugForms/ucm048817.pdf
FDA CVM Guidance #61	Guidance for Industry: FDA Approval of New Animal Drugs for Minor Uses and for Minor Species	http://www.fda.gov/downloads/AnimalVeterinary/GuidanceComplianceEnforcement/GuidanceforIndustry/UCM052375.pdf
Food Animal Residue Avoidance Databank (FARAD)	Provides recommended withdrawal times for drugs and chemicals	http://www.farad.org
Food Safety and Inspection Service, US Department of Agriculture	The Blue Book outlines the National Residue Program (ie, the plan for sampling for drug and chemical residues in meat in the United States)	http://www.fsis.usda.gov/PDF/2009_Blue_Book.pdf

Name	Description	URL
Food Safety and Inspection Service, US Department of Agriculture	The Red Book present results from scheduled and inspector-generated sampling for drug and chemical residues in meat in the United States	http://www.fsis.usda.gov/PDF/2008_Red_Book.pdf
Minor Species/Minor Use Program	US program for increasing approval for minor species and minor uses of drugs	http://www.nrsp-7.org/introduction.htm
National Association of Boards of Pharmacy	To find contact information for state board of pharmacy	http://www.nabp.net/boards-of-pharmacy/
National Association of Boards of Pharmacy Vet-VIPPS (Verified Internet Pharmacy Practice Sites)	Accreditation program for Internet pharmacies; refers to nonfood and companion animals only	http://www.nabp.net/programs/accreditation/vet-vipps/
National Organic Program	Regulations related to organic production in the United States	http://www.ams.usda.gov/nop/indexIE.htm
Pasteurized Milk Ordinance	All regulations related to producing milk	http://www.fda.gov/Food/FoodSafety/Product-SpecificInformation/MilkSafety/NationalConferenceonInterstateMilkShipments NCIMSModelDocumentsPasteurizedMilkOrdinance2007/default.htm
Canada-based Web sites		
Canadian Food Inspection Agency	Regulations regarding livestock feeds including medicated feeds in Canada	http://www.inspection.gc.ca/english/anima/feebet/feebete.shtml
Canadian global FARAD (gFARAD)	One branch of gFARAD that provides Canadian-specific recommendations for withdrawal times	http://www.cgfarad.usask.ca/
Canadian Veterinary Medical Association policy on extralabel drug use	—	http://canadianveterinarians.net/ShowText.aspx?ResourceID=63
Health Canada Veterinary Drug Directorate	Home page for veterinary drugs in Canada	http://www.hc-sc.gc.ca/dhp-mps/vet/index-eng.php
European Union-based Web site		
European Medicines Agency Committee for Medicinal Products for Veterinary Use	European agency responsible for drug regulations and drug approval in the European Union	http://www.ema.europa.eu/index/indexv1.htm

Table 2
Drugs approved in the United States, for administration to sheep and currently marketed

Active Ingredient	Example Trade Name	Pharmaceutical Form	Type(s) of Sheep for Which Approved	Indications	Dose Rate and Route of Administration
Albendazole	Valbazen	Oral suspension	Nonpregnant	Control of internal parasites	7.5 mg/kg bw by mouth
Ceftiofur sodium	Naxcel	Injectable solution	Not specified	Respiratory disease	1.0–2.2 mg/kg bw im for 3 d
Chlortetracycline	Pfichlor, Chlorachel, Chlormax	Medicated premix	Breeding animals	Reduction of Campylobacter abortion incidence	80 mg/head/d in the feed
Chlortetracycline	Aureomycin, Pfichlor	Medicated premix	Growing animals	Increase weight gain and feed efficiency	20–50 g/t feed
Decoquinate	Deccox	Medicated premix	Young, nonlactating	Prevention of coccidiosis	0.5 mg/kg bw by mouth (13.6 g/t feed)
Ivermectin	Ivomec	Oral drench	Not specified	Control of internal parasites	0.2 mg/kg bw by mouth
Lasalocid	Bovatec	Medicated premix	Sheep in confinement	Prevention of coccidiosis	20–30 g/t of feed
Levamisole	Tramisole, Levasole	Oral suspension, tablet	Not specified	Control of nematode infections	8 mg/kg bw by mouth
Moxidectin	Cydectin	Oral drench	Not specified	Control of internal parasites	0.2 mg/kg bw by mouth
Neomycin	Neomix, Neosol, NeoMed	Soluble powder (for addition to drinking water or milk replacer)	Not specified	Treatment and control of gastrointestinal colibacillosis	22 mg/kg bw by mouth, divided doses daily for a maximum of 14 d

Neomycin type A medicated article for milk replacer or feed	Neomix 325 Medicated Premix	Medicated premix	Not specified	Treatment and control of gastrointestinal colibacillosis	22 mg/kg bw by mouth, for a maximum of 14 d
Neostigmine	Stiglyn	Injectable solution	Nonpregnant, nonlactating	Rumen atony, bowel evacuation, bladder evacuation	1–1.5 mg/45.36 kg (100 lb) bw sc
Oxytetracycline	Terramycin SP	Soluble powder (for addition to drinking water or milk replacer)	Not specified	Bacterial enteritis, bacterial respiratory infection	22 mg/kg bw daily in the drinking water or milk replacer
Oxytetracycline + polymyxin	Terramycin	Ophthalmic ointment	Not specified	Ocular infections	External application in the eye 2–4 times daily
Oxytetracycline	Terramycin-100 type A medicated article, TM-50 type A medicated article	Medicated premix	Not specified	Bacterial enteritis, bacterial respiratory infection	22 mg/kg bw daily (10–20 g/t of feed)
Penicillin G	Agricillin, Aqua-cillin	Injectable suspension	Not specified	Respiratory infection caused by Pasteurella multocida	6600 IU/kg bw im daily
Tilmicosin	Micotil	Injectable solution	Not specified	Respiratory infection associated with Mannheimia haemolytica	10 mg/kg bw sc
Vitamin E + sodium selenite	BO-SE	Injectable solution	Newborn, nonpregnant	Control of white muscle disease	2.5 mL/45.36 kg (100 lb) bw im or sc
Zeranol	Ralgro	Subcutaneous implant	Feedlot lambs	Increase weight gain and feed efficiency	One implant sc behind the ear

Abbreviations: bw, bodyweight; im, intramuscularly; sc, subcutaneously.
Data from Animal Drugs, FDA.

Table 3
Drugs approved in Canada for administration to sheep

Active Ingredient	Example Trade Name	Pharmaceutical Form	Indications	Dose Rate and Route of Administration
Acepromazine	Acepro-25, Atravet	Injectable solution	Sedation	0.05 mg–0.1 mg/kg bw im
Calcium borogluconate + electrolytes	CalMagPhos, Mag-Cal, Norcalciphos	Injectable solution	Electrolyte replacement	50–125 mL iv, sc
Ceftiofur sodium	Excenel sterile powder	Injectable solution	Respiratory infection associated with *Mannheimia haemolytica*	2 mg/kg bw once daily for 3 d im
Chlortetracycline	Aureomycin	Medicated premix	As an aid in reduction of losses caused by enterotoxaemia in feedlot lambs	22 mg/kg (0.0022 %) of complete feed by mouth
Dioctyl sodium sulfosuccinate	Anti-bloat, Bloat-Eze	Oral solution	Treatment of bloat	Range of 0.5–1 mL/kg bw by mouth
Equine chorionic gonadotrophin	Folligon, Novormon 5000	Injectable solution	Follicle stimulating	300–1000 IU im, iv, sc
Estradiol cypionate	—	Injectable solution	Anestrus	0.5–1 mg im
Ivermectin	Ivomec	Injectable solution, oral drench	—	200 µg/kg bw sc, by mouth
Lactated Ringer solution	Lact-R	Injectable solution	Dehydration and electrolyte disturbances	To effect iv
Lasalocid	Bovatec	Medicated premix	Prevention of coccidiosis	Mix 240 g (0.24 kg) of premix in 1 t (1000 kg) 100% dry matter basis of diet (including roughage) to provide 0.0036 % (36 ppm) of lasalocid sodium activity
Lidocaine or lidocaine + epinephrine	—	Injectable solution	Nerve block and anesthesia	Epidural, infiltration
Luteinizing hormone	Lutropin-V	Injectable solution	Breeding disorders	2 mL (2.5 mg) iv, sc
Mineral oil	—	Oral solution	Intestinal constipation	By mouth
Neomycin	Neomycin 325, Biosol	Oral solution	Bacterial enteritis	1 g powder/50 kg bw by mouth

Drug	Trade name	Form	Indication	Dosage
Neomycin + (methyl violet or gentian violet)	Keraplex, Co-op Pinkeye Spray	Spray for local application	Wound dressing, treatment of infectious keratoconjunctivitis	External application
Neomycin + sulfathiazole + sulfamethazine	Neorease, Scour Treat	Oral solution	Bacterial enteritis and pneumonia	10 mL/5 kg bw twice a day by mouth
Neomycin + methscopolamine	Scour solution	Oral solution	Bacterial enteritis	1 mL/5 kg bw in water or milk for 1–3 days
Neomycin + succinylsulfathiazole + atropine + hyoscyamine	Scour suspension	Oral solution	Bacterial enteritis	2 mL/kg bw divided twice a day by mouth
Oxytetracycline	Noromycin LP, Oxymycine LP	Injectable solution	Respiratory infection associated with *Mannheimia haemolytica*, mastitis, metritis, joint ill	3 mL/45 kg bw im, iv once a day for 3 d
Oxytetracycline	Terramycin-100 Premix	Medicated premix	(1) Bacterial enteritis and respiratory infection associated with *Mannheimia haemolytica* (2) As an aid in the reduction of losses caused by enterotoxemia in feedlot lambs	(1) 110 mg/kg complete feed (2) 22 mg/kg complete feed
Oxytocin	Oxy-20	Injectable solution	Treatment of obstetric disorders	30–50 IU
Penicillin G penicillin G + benzethine penicillin	Depocillin, Hi-pencin 300, Longisil	Injectable solution	Respiratory infection caused by *Pasteurella multocida*, metritis, wound infections	21,000 IU/kg bw (0.7 mL/10 kg) once a day im 0.5 mL/10 kg
Progesterone 5%	—	Injectable solution	Reproductive disorders	10–15 mg per animal daily, as needed im
Propylene glycol	Glycol-P	Oral solution	Prevention and treatment of pregnancy toxemia	Prevention: 50–100 mL daily; treatment: 75–125 mL daily for 10 d by mouth
Pyrilamine	—	—	Antihistamine	1 mL/45 kg bw
Sodium iodide	Sodide	Injectable solution	Expectorant	5–10 mL iv
Sulfamethazine	Sulfa 25	Soluble powder (for addition to drinking water or milk replacer)	Metritis, bacterial enteritis, mastitis, respiratory infections	225 mg/kg in water or milk replacer on day 1, 112.5 mg/kg on day 2–5

(continued on next page)

Table 3
(continued)

Active Ingredient	Example Trade Name	Pharmaceutical Form	Indications	Dose Rate and Route of Administration
Sulfamethazine	Sulfa 25	Bolus	Metritis, bacterial enteritis, mastitis, respiratory infections	1 bolus/80 kg bw by mouth on day 1, 1/2 bolus/80 kg bw on day 2–3
Sulfamerazine + sulfathiazole	Sulectim	Soluble powder (for addition to drinking water or milk replacer)	Bacterial enteritis, respiratory infections	454 g to 727 L (180 gallons) of drinking water for 5–10 days
Testosterone	Uni-test suspension	Injectable solution	Impotence, testicular deficiency	10–25 mg once a day im
Tetracycline	Onycin 250, Onycin 1000	Soluble powder (for addition to drinking water or milk replacer)	Bacterial enteritis, respiratory infection associated with *Mannheimia haemolytica*	Add in water 0.25 g of powder per 25 kg bw, every 12 h given as a drench for 4 or 5 d
Thiopental	Thiotal	Injectable solution	Anesthetic	iv
Tilmicosin	Micotil	Injectable solution	Respiratory infection associated with *Mannheimia haemolytica*	1 mL per 30 kg bw/1.5 mL per 45.36 kg (100 lb) bw sc
Vitamin A + vitamin D	Co-op A+D	Injectable solution	Control of respective deficiencies	im
Vitamin E + selenium	Dystosel, Selon-E	Injectable solution	Control of white muscle disease	Prevention: newborns 0.25 mL per animal; animals aged 2–8 wk 0.5 mL per animal; treatment: 0.5 mL per animal

Abbreviations: bw, bodyweight; im, intramuscularly; iv, intravenously; sc, subcutaneously.

Data from Health Canada Drug Product Database (drugs listed are not necessarily marketed; the list does not include all products approved for use in sheep in Canada).

Table 4
Drugs approved in the United States for administration to goats and currently marketed

Active Ingredient	Example Trade Name	Pharmaceutical Form	Type(s) of Animals for Which Approved	Indications	Dose Rate and Route of Administration
Albendazole	Valbazen	Oral suspension	Nonpregnant, nonlactating	Control of adult liver flukes	10 mg/kg bw by mouth
Ceftiofur sodium	Naxcel	Injectable solution	Not specified	Respiratory disease	1.0–2.2 mg/kg bw im for 3 d
Decoquinate	Deccox	Medicated premix	Young, nonlactating	Prevention of coccidiosis	0.5 mg/kg bw by mouth (13.6 g/t feed)
Fenbendazole	Safeguard, Panacur	Oral suspension	Nonlactating	Control of stomach worms	5 mg/kg bw by mouth
Morantel	Rumatel	Feed additive	Not specified	—	0.44 g/45.36 kg (100 lb) bw (0.44–4.4 g/0.45 kg [1 lb] of feed)
Neomycin	Neomix, Neosol, NeoMed	Soluble powder (for addition to drinking water or milk replacer)	Not specified	Treatment and control of gastrointestinal colibacillosis	22 mg/kg bw by mouth, divided doses daily for a maximum of 14 d
Neomycin type A medicated article for milk replacer or feed	Neomix 325 Medicated Premix	Medicated premix	Not specified	Treatment and control of gastrointestinal colibacillosis	22 mg/kg bw by mouth, for a maximum of 14 d

Abbreviations: bw, bodyweight; im, intramuscularly.
Data from Animal Drugs, FDA.

Table 5
Drugs approved in Canada for administration to goats

Active Ingredient	Example Trade Name	Pharmaceutical Form	Indications	Route of Administration
Acepromazine	Acepro-25, Atravet	Injectable solution	Sedation	im
Dioctyl sodium sulfosuccinate	Anti-bloat, Bloat-Eze	Oral solution	Treatment of bloat	By mouth
Mineral oil	—	Oral solution	Intestinal constipation	By mouth
Neomycin + sulfathiazole + sulfamethazine	Neorease, Scour Treat	Oral solution	Bacterial enteritis and pneumonia	By mouth
Progesterone 5%	—	Injectable solution	Reproductive disorders	im

Abbreviation: im, intramuscularly.
Data from Health Canada Drug Product Database (drugs listed are not necessarily marketed, the list does not include all products approved for use in sheep in Canada).

labeled for the condition being treated, which contains the needed ingredient, which is in the proper dosage form, and which is clinically effective, that labeled (ie, licensed) drug must be used. If those conditions are not all met, then extralabel use of a drug approved for a food animal may be considered. If there is no drug that is approved for a food animal that can be used in an extralabel manner to treat the condition, then a drug approved for humans or companion animals may be considered. If no drug approved for humans or companion animals can be used in an extralabel manner, then a compounded drug may be considered; however, this extralabel use must be compounded from approved drugs and must not be compounded from bulk or raw drug (also known as the active pharmaceutical ingredient [API]).

Other provisions of AMDUCA include the requirements for labeling of the drug (it must include the name and address of the veterinarian, the name and address of the dispensing pharmacy if applicable, the established name of the drug and, if there is more than one active ingredient, the established name of each ingredient, directions for use including identity of treated animals, dose, route, frequency, route and duration, cautionary statements, and the veterinarian's specified withdrawal time for any food that might be derived from treated animals) and the requirements for the veterinarian's keeping records for 2 years after prescribing (established name of drug and/or active ingredients, condition treated, species of animal treated, dosage prescribed, duration prescribed, number of animals treated, and specified withdrawal times).

Although technically illegal in the United States, the use of drugs in feed in an extralabel manner in minor species, such as sheep and goats, is the subject of some guidance from the FDA CVM.[4] Minor species are all species except horses, cattle, pigs, dogs, cats, chickens, and turkeys. The Compliance Policy Guide Section 615.115 states that the FDA does not ordinarily consider regulatory action against the veterinarian, producer, or feed mill provided the following are true.

1. The medicated feed is for use only in a minor species.
2. The medicated feed is approved (a) for use in a major species and the feed is formulated and labeled according to its approved labeling (ie, dosage, formulation,

nutrient content) or (b) for use in a food-producing minor species and the feed is approved in a major food-producing species.

3. The feed is limited to farmed or confined minor species.
4. The use of the medicated feed is only with the express prior written recommendation and oversight of a licensed veterinarian with a valid VCPR.
5. The extralabel use is limited to therapeutic use, when the health of the animal is threatened and suffering or death may result from the failure to treat.
6. There must be no labeled drug that could be used, or that drug must be clinically ineffective, and there must be no therapeutic dosage form drug that can be practically used under AMDUCA.

In addition, the veterinarian must establish an extended withdrawal time, must assure that the identity of treated animals is maintained, and must have written recommendations within 3 months before the use (with copies with the veterinarian and the producer). The producer must keep accurate feed records for at least 1 year from delivery of the feed, must maintain identity of treated animals, must assure withdrawal times are met, must use and dispose of any medicated feed in accordance with local, state, and federal regulations, and must follow safety provision of the approved product label.

In Canada, the regulations differ in that extralabel use of medicated feed may be prescribed by a veterinarian, as long as the drug is an approved drug product.[5] The medicated feed must be for a therapeutic purpose, rather than for a production purpose, such as growth promotion or feed efficiency. A valid VCPR must exist and all parties (client, prescribing veterinarian, and feed mill) must maintain a proper and valid veterinary prescription on file.

Illegal Extralabel Use of Drugs in the United States

Extralabel use of veterinary drugs is considered illegal under AMDUCA in the following cases.

1. Extralabel use of drugs in or on feed
2. Extralabel use from unapproved (nonlicensed) drugs or bulk drug (API)
3. Extralabel use outside a VCPR
4. Extralabel use of any of the drugs mentioned in **Box 1**
5. Any use that leads to a violative residue or higher than safe levels or tolerance.

Canadian regulations state that the following drugs may not be sold for administration to animals that produce food or are intended for consumption as food: chloramphenicol (or its salts or derivatives), 5-nitrofurans, clenbuterol (or its salts or derivatives), 5-nitroimidazoles, diethylstilbestrol, or other stilbene compounds.[6] Canadian policy regarding extralabel drug use in food animals states that veterinarians should preferentially not use the category 1 antimicrobials mentioned in **Table 6** extralabel, because of their importance in human health and the potential for selection for antimicrobial resistance in pathogens of human significance.

Withdrawal Time Estimation

If drugs are used in accordance with the label, the withdrawal times legally provided should be sufficient to prevent excess residues in meat or milk. In the United States, this withdrawal time is determined in the following way. During the approval process, the drug sponsor must present data to determine an NOEL (no observed effect level), which is the amount of drug expected to cause no harm if ingested by humans. Dividing this by a safety factor results in an acceptable daily intake (ADI)

> **Box 1**
> **Drugs prohibited for extralabel use in food-producing animals**
>
> Chloramphenicol
>
> Clenbuterol
>
> Diethylstilbestrol
>
> Dimetridazole
>
> Ipronidazole and other nitroimidazoles (such as metronidazole)
>
> Furazolidone, nitrofurazone, and other nitrofurans
>
> Sulfonamides in lactating dairy cattle (except approved uses of sulfadimethoxine, sulfabromomethazine, and sulfaethoxypyridazine)
>
> Fluoroquinolones
>
> Glycopeptides
>
> Phenylbutazone in female dairy cattle 20 months of age or older

of the drug. A safe concentration is then calculated by multiplying ADI by the average adult human weight and dividing by an estimate of amount of edible product consumed per day by the average adult (assumptions are that an adult consumes 300 g muscle, 100 g liver, 50 g kidney, 50 g fat, 1.5 L milk, and 100 g eggs). This safe concentration is the threshold that is then compared with the tissue concentrations of the drug in the animal products over time. Typically, the licensed dose of drug is administered in 20 target-species animals; then, 5 animals are killed at

Table 6
Category 1 antimicrobial drugs discouraged by Health Canada's policy for use in food-producing animals under extralabel provisions

Antimicrobial Drug Group	Example Drug
Carbapenems	Imipenem
Third- and fourth-generation cephalosporins	Cefotaxime
Fluoroquinolones	Enrofloxacin
Glycopeptides	Vancomycin
Glycylcyclines	Tigecycline
Ketolides	Telithromycin
Lipopeptides	Daptomycin
Monobactams	Aztreonam
Nitroimidazoles	Metronidazole
Oxazolidinones	Linezolid
Penicillin/β-lactamase inhibitor combinations	Ticarcillin-clavulanic acid
Polymyxins	Colistin
Streptogramins	Dalfopristin/quinupristin
Therapeutic agents for tuberculosis	Ethambutol, isoniazid, pyrazinamide, rifampin

Data from Anon. Health Canada categorization of antimicrobial drugs based on importance in human medicine. In: Health Canada, 2009.

each of 4 different time points after administration and the concentration of drug in various tissues is determined; control animals are also included in the study. The resulting time-concentration curve is used to statistically evaluate (using confidence intervals) the time point after drug administration at which the tissue concentration is predicted to be less than the safe concentration in 99% of the animals with 95% confidence.[7]

If drugs are used in an extralabel manner, withdrawal times on the label may be insufficient to prevent illegal residues for several reasons, including differences in formulations (eg, conventional vs long-acting, differing salts such as benzathine vs procaine), route of administration, metabolism, long half-lives resulting in accumulation of drug, increased dose, or differing administration frequency of the drug.[8] Therefore, it is particularly important to consider ways to accurately estimate the effects of extralabel use on withdrawal time estimates. One important resource in the United States for this information is the Food Animal Residue Avoidance Databank (FARAD), a national cooperative project sponsored by the US Department of Agriculture, with a primary mission to prevent or mitigate illegal residues of drugs, pesticides, and other chemicals in foods of animal origin. FARAD has personnel at the University of California-Davis, the University of Florida, and North Carolina State University, who can review their extensive database of residue information to provide estimates of withdrawal intervals to prevent illegal residues. Veterinarians can directly contact FARAD (see **Table 1**) with a withdrawal time question. FARAD also periodically publishes FARAD Digests in the *Journal of the American Veterinary Medical Association*. A compilation of published recommendations to date for withdrawal intervals for meat and milk for drugs and antidotes used in an extralabel manner (ie, drugs not currently approved for sheep or goats in the United States) are presented in **Table 7**.

In recent years, FARAD has branched out internationally with global or gFARAD. Cooperating gFARAD countries gain access to the FARAD database, as well as compiling drug information and tolerance (or maximum residue levels [MRLs]) data from their countries. For example, Canada has developed Canadian gFARAD, with a Web site and voicemail for customized withdrawal time estimates for extralabel uses of drugs and other chemicals (see **Table 1**).

If FARAD is not available or the veterinarian's location does not permit access to a gFARAD office, recommendations have been made on how practitioners can estimate a withdrawal time.[9] The apparent elimination half-life of the drug (the time for drug concentration to drop by 50%) and the tolerance (safe level, safe concentration, or MRL) are used to develop such an estimate. Given that after 10 elimination half-lives, more than 99.9% of the drug has been eliminated, multiplying the half-life by 10 and then rounding up to the nearest day provides an initial estimate of withdrawal interval. However, the serum elimination half-life may not be completely representative of the tissue elimination half-life in which residues are measured. Residues at harvest are determined from a target tissue, such as muscle or liver, not from plasma or serum; hence knowledge of the tissue elimination half-life is more useful. However, tissue elimination kinetics is often not publicly available, so veterinarians may have to use serum concentration data and assume homogeneous distribution of drug between tissues and serum. Although more than 99.9% of the drug may have been eliminated after 10 elimination half-lives, the less than 0.01% of the drug remaining may still be more than a safe concentration, tolerance, or MRL, and therefore may be illegal. If an estimate of the elimination half-life is available only in cattle, some comparative pharmacokinetic data suggest that sheep and goats eliminate drugs at a similar or faster rate than cattle, although this type of extrapolation should be performed with extreme caution, because individual drugs may have different pharmacokinetic

Table 7
Published recommendations from FARAD[a] for withdrawal times for drugs and antidotes used in sheep and goats

Drug	Year of Publication	Animal Species Referred To	Therapeutic Regime	Withdrawal Period	
				Meat	Milk
Acepromazine	1997[21]	Ruminants	<0.13 mg/kg bw iv OR <0.44 mg/kg bw im	7 d	48 h
Activated charcoal	2005[22]	Food animals	Not specified	Zero	Zero
Aspirin	1997[23]	Ruminants	All recommended doses	1 d	24 h
Atropine	2005[22]	Food animals	0.2 mg/kg bw iv or im; multiple administrations, as treatment of organophosphate toxicity	28 d	6 d
Butorphanol	1996[24]	Food animals	Not specified	48 h	[b]
Detomidine	1997[21,24]	Ruminants	<0.08 mg/kg bw iv or im	4 d	72 h
Dimercaprol	2005[22]	Food animals	—	5 d	5 d
EDTA	2005[22]	Food animals	Not specified	2 d	2 d
Epinephrine	2005[22]	Food animals	Not specified	Zero	Zero
Gentamicin	2005[25]	Sheep and goats	5 mg/kg bw im or sc	>18 mo	10 d; testing of milk is recommended
Guafenesin	1997[21]	Ruminants	<100 mg/kg bw iv	3 d	48 h
Ivermectin	2000[26]	Goats	0.4 mg/kg bw by mouth	14 d	9 d
Ivermectin	2000[26]	Goats	0.2 mg/kg bw sc	35 d	40 d
Ivermectin	2000[26]	Goats	0.5 mg/kg bw external use	[b]	7 d
Ketamine	1997[21]	Ruminants	<2 mg/kg bw iv or <10 mg/kg bw im	3 d	48 h
Ketoprofen	1997[23]	Sheep and goats	3.3 mg/kg bw iv or im, every 24 h for up to 3 d	7 d	24 h
Lidocaine + epinephrine	1997[21]	Ruminants	Infiltration; epidural	1 d	24 h
Methylene blue	2005[22]	Food animals	Not specified	14 d	4 d
Molybdate salts (ammonium molybdate, ammonium tetrathiomolybdate)	2005[22]	Food animals	Not specified	10 d	5 d

Drug	Year	Animal	Dose	Meat withdrawal	Milk withdrawal
Moxidectin	2000[26]	Goats	0.2 mg/kg bw by mouth	14 d	b
Moxidectin	2000[26]	Goats	0.5 mg/kg bw by mouth	23 d	b
Moxidectin	2000[26]	Goats	sc	b	b
Moxidectin	2000[26]	Goats	0.5 mg/kg bw external application	1 d	1 d
Oxytetracycline	1997[27]	Sheep and goats	6.6–11.0 mg/kg bw iv or im, once	Cattle withdrawal time is adequate	96 h and testing of milk
Oxytetracycline	1997[27]	Sheep and goats	>11.0 mg/kg bw iv or im, once 6.6–11.0 mg/kg bw iv or im, multiple doses	Cattle withdrawal time is adequate	144 h and testing of milk
Oxytetracycline (long-acting)	2003[28]	—	20 mg/kg bw im	28 d	96 h
Penicillamine	2005[22]	Food animals	Not specified	21 d	3 d
Pentobarbital	1996[24]	Food animals	Not specified	4 d	4 d
Phenylbutazone	2003[28]	—	Use discouraged	b	b
Pralidoxime (2-PAM)	2005[22]	Sheep	30 mg/kg bw every 8 h	28 d	6 d
Penicillin G (procaine)	2006	Sheep and goats	>6600 U/kg bw	Testing of urine is recommended	Testing of milk is recommended
Sodium nitrite	2005[22]	Food animals	Not specified, iv	24 h	48 h
Sodium thiosulfate	2005[22]	Food animals	Not specified, iv	24 h	b
Thiamylal	1997[21]	Ruminants	<5.5 mg/kg bw	1 d	24 h
Thiobarbital	1997[21]	Ruminants	<9.4 mg/kg bw	1 d	24 h
Vitamin K$_1$	2005[22]	Sheep and goats	0.5–2.5 mg/kg bw im, iv, or sc	Zero	Zero
Xylazine	1997[21]	Ruminants	0.016–0.1 mg/kg bw iv or 0.05–0.3 mg/kg bw im	5 d	72 h
Xylazine	1997[21]	Ruminants	0.3–2.0 mg/kg bw im	10 d	120 h
Yohimbine	1997[21]	Ruminants	<0.3 mg/kg bw iv	7 d	72 h

Abbreviations: bw, bodyweight; im, intramuscularly; iv, intravenously; sc, subcutaneously.

Veterinarians are advised to review current sources and contact FARAD to verify these recommendations, because new scientific evidence related to pharmacokinetics frequently affects the recommendations, and tolerances and residue levels may change over time.

[a] Veterinarians in Canada should consult the Canadian gFARAD because regulations and thus withdrawal times may be different.

[b] Relevant withdrawal periods not established.

properties in sheep or goats compared with those in cattle. Given the potential for error in making any of these estimates, veterinarians are cautioned to provide generous withdrawal time estimates or to make every effort to contact FARAD or other equally weighty sources to protect the food supply and to protect animal owners from the ramifications of illegal residues.

In the European Union, regulations stipulate that in cases of extralabel use of a drug, a withdrawal period of 28 days for meat or 7 days for milk should be prescribed and observed. This strategy raises the issue of withdrawal periods during extralabel use of drugs, which already have longer than the withdrawal periods mentioned earlier in other animal species. For example, moxidectin injectable solution has a licensed withdrawal period of 65 days for cattle meat and 82 days for sheep milk. Hence, it seems wrong to maintain a 28-day withdrawal period for meat of goats, if the drug would be administered under extralabel circumstances in that animal species. To avoid such circumstances, blanket statements, such as "Not to be used in animals producing milk for human consumption or for industrial purposes" or "Not to be used in animals younger than $\times\times$ months," have been devised and are enforced.

MONITORING OF DRUG USE
Residues in Foods

In the United States, the Food Safety and Inspection Service (FSIS) of the US Department of Agriculture is responsible for ensuring the safety of food products from animals. It publishes a yearly plan for which samples will be collected at harvest facilities in the next year, the so-called Blue Book[10] (see **Table 1**). It also publishes yearly reports on the previous year's sampling and findings, the Red Book[11] (see **Table 1**). The most recent report published is for the calendar year 2008, and data are reported on scheduled samples, as well as inspector-generated samples. Inspector-generated samples are those that were not regularly scheduled, but rather were collected by in-plant public health veterinarians because of the appearance of the animals ante or post mortem, suggesting medication use, previous history of the producer of animals with violative residues, or other suspicions raised during the on-site inspections. These samples may be tested via in-plant fast antimicrobial screen test (FAST) or kidney inhibition swab (KIS) test or they may be forwarded to the FSIS laboratory for testing. In-plant FAST-positive samples are also sent to the FSIS laboratory for testing for nonsteroidal antiinflammatory drugs.

In 2008, of 980 scheduled samples in goats, there was one sample with antibiotic violation (oxytetracycline); of 814 scheduled samples in lambs, there were 9 nonviolative positive samples (3 antimicrobials, one avermectin); of 472 scheduled samples in sheep, there were no violations.[11] Inspector-generated samples revealed the following: of 180 samples from goats there were no FAST-positive samples; of 370 samples from lambs there was one FAST-positive sample (sulfadimethoxine); and of 137 samples from sheep there were no FAST-positive samples.[11] Overall, these findings show a low level of violative residues in meat from sheep and goats in the United States.

Scheduled sampling for 2009 included the following: testing for antibiotic residues in 90 samples after random collection from goats, in 300 samples from lambs, and in 300 samples from sheep. The samples are tested for presence of antibiotics (including fluoroquinolones, which are currently illegal for use in sheep and goats in the United States) and avermectins. The confirmatory 7-plate bioassay tests for antibiotics include tetracyclines, aminoglycosides, macrolides, β-lactams, and fluoroquinolones. Samples from goats are also tested for β-agonists, such as clenbuterol.

Pharmacovigilance

Another important aspect of monitoring drug use, pharmacovigilance, involves the cataloging of adverse reactions to the drug product after approval, sometimes called phase IV or postmarketing surveillance. This area of data collection is undergoing considerable change, with the FDA CVM and the AVMA considering ways to appropriately and accurately gather data on adverse drug reactions. A major issue with adverse reactions is correct attribution of a reaction to the drug itself; another is who bears the burden of data collection and analysis. Drug sponsors are required to submit reports to the FDA CVM of any adverse reactions that are reported to the company. In addition, the FDA CVM has a form, Form FDA 1932a, "Veterinary Adverse Experience, Lack of Effectiveness or Product Defect Report", available online for submission directly to the FDA CVM (see **Table 1**), or the report can be submitted by telephone to 1-888-FDA-VETS. There are periodically published reports in the literature from various regulatory or epidemiologic experts, which examine adverse event data to attempt to attribute drugs to risks.[12–14] In Europe, pharmacovigilance procedures involve centralized (pan-European) and member-state (individual-country) responsibilities for reporting and follow-up of adverse reactions from veterinary drugs.[15]

OTHER REGULATIONS RELATED TO USE OF VETERINARY DRUGS IN SHEEP AND GOATS

Compounding

Compounding is not distinguished from manufacturing in the Federal Food Drug and Cosmetic Act; therefore, any manipulation of an approved drug not included in the license or use of an unapproved drug would be considered compounding and, technically, would be illegal for animal drugs. The FDA CVM has issued a Compliance Policy Guide for Compounding, which outlines the FDA's policy and regulatory priorities for compounded drugs.[16] The important parts of the Guide include the statement that compounding from bulk drugs (API) for food animals is considered a regulatory priority, as is compounding when not used for therapeutic purposes (AMDUCA authorizes compounding from approved drugs, but only when animal health is threatened).

Evidence of the regulatory priority of the use of bulk drugs for compounding for animals comes from the recent legal filing by the FDA CVM against Franck's Pharmacy in Florida, which was implicated in the death of polo ponies after they were administered a compounded vitamin product.[17] The issues with food animals of compounding from bulk drug include the potential for inclusion of toxic compounds resulting in unsafe food products, as well as the unpredictable bioavailability of compounded products, resulting in the potential for violative residues.[18]

Drug Use in Natural or Organic Farms

The regulations promulgated for the National Organic Program specifically state all synthetic substances that are permissible in animals being produced for certification as organic. At the time of writing (2010), these included aspirin, atropine, butorphanol, flunixin, furosemide, electrolytes, glucose, ivermectin, lidocaine, magnesium hydroxide, magnesium sulfate, mineral oil, oxytocin, poloxalene, and tolazoline, albeit, in most cases, with longer withdrawal times than those applied in conventional farms.[19,20] Veterinarians working with organic farmers must become familiar with the substances that are permissible in these operations, to assist producers in maintaining their organic status, as well as to assist them in understanding when it is appropriate to remove animals from the organic stream if they require nonlisted drugs (eg, antimicrobials). Animal welfare considerations and veterinary medical ethics do not provide for withholding of therapeutics just to maintain an animal in the organic arm of a farm.

Drug Use in Sheep or Goat Dairy Farms

Veterinarians working with sheep or goat dairy farms in the United States, which farm market products commercially, must be familiar with the Pasteurized Milk Ordinance. This ordinance relates to permissible drug uses, as well as drug storage and labeling on dairy farms (see **Table 1**).

SUMMARY

This article reviews laws and regulations related to drug use in sheep and goats, with special reference to legislation in the United States. The discussion includes the drug-licensing procedures (including issues related to minor species), legalities of extralabel drug use, withdrawal time estimation, and residues in sheep and goat tissues and products; it points out a few other important regulations related to organic production, dairy production, and compounding. Canadian and European regulations are also mentioned. Veterinarians working with sheep and goats must be familiar with regulations governing use of drugs in these species, to prevent legal action, fulfill their fiduciary responsibility to the producers, and help protect and provide for a wholesome and safe food supply.

REFERENCES

1. 21 U.S.C. 321. Definitions. In: Federal Food Drug and Cosmetic Act. 2009.
2. Anon. Guidance #61: Guidance for industry FDA approval of new animal drugs for minor uses and for minor species. Rockville (MD): Food and Drug Administration Center for Veterinary Medicine; 2008. p. 1–82.
3. Extralabel drug use in animals. Final rule, 21 CFR Part 530. Fed Regist 1996;61: 57731–46.
4. Anon. Compliance policy guide 615.115 Extra-label use of medicated feeds for minor species. Rockville (MD): Food and Drug Administration Center for Veterinary Medicine; 2001.
5. Anon. Policy on extra-label drug use (ELDU) in food producing animals. Ottawa, Ontario (Canada): Health Canada Veterinary Drug Directorate; 2010.
6. Anon. Food and Drug Regulations Part C Drugs C.01.610.1. Ottawa, Ontario (Canada): Canada Department of Justice; 2010. p. 771.
7. Anon. Guidance #3: Guidance for industry general principles for evaluating the safety of compounds used in food-producing animals. Rockville (MD): Food and Drug Administration Center for Veterinary Medicine; 2006. p. 1–42.
8. KuKanich B, Gehring R, Webb AI, et al. Effect of formulation and route of administration on tissue residues and withdrawal times. J Am Vet Med Assoc 2005;227: 1574–7.
9. Riviere JE, Webb AI, Craigmill AL. FARAD digest – primer on estimating withdrawal times after extralabel drug use. J Am Vet Med Assoc 1998;213:966–8.
10. Anon. Food Safety and Inspection Service 2009–National residue program scheduled sampling plans. Washington, DC: US Department of Agriculture; 2009. p. 1–178.
11. Anon. Food Safety and Inspection Service 2008–National residue program data. Washington, DC: US Department of Agriculture; 2009. p. 1–147.
12. Linnett PJ. APVMA veterinary pharmacovigilance program: suspected adverse experience reports for 2005. Aust Vet J 2006;84:418–20.

13. Muntener C, Bruckner L, Sturer A, et al. Vigilance for veterinary medicinal products: declarations of adverse reactions in the year 2008. Schweiz Arch Tierheilkd 2009;151:583–90.
14. Naidoo V, Sykes R. Overview of suspected adverse reactions to veterinary medicinal products reported in South Africa (March 2004–February 2006). J S Afr Vet Assoc 2006;77:164–7.
15. Woodward KN. Veterinary pharmacovigilance. Part 1. The legal basis in the European Union. J Vet Pharmacol Ther 2005;28:131–47.
16. Anon. Compliance policy guide 608.400–Compounding of drugs for use in animals. Rockville (MD): Food and Drug Administration Center for Veterinary Medicine; 2003.
17. Anon. FDA seeks injunction against Florida animal drug compounder. Rockville (MD): Food and Drug Administration; 2010. Available at: http://www.fda.gov/NewsEvents/Newsroom/PressAnnouncements/ucm208983.htm. Accessed November 28, 2010.
18. Riviere JE. Influence of compounding on bioavailability. J Am Vet Med Assoc 1994;205:226–31.
19. Anon. 7 CFR Sec. 205.603 Synthetic substances allowed for use in organic livestock production. Agricultural Marketing Service, US Department of Agriculture. College Park (MD): National Archives and Records Administration; 2009.
20. Anon. 7 CFR Sec. 205.60 Nonsynthetic substances prohibited for use in organic livestock production. Agricultural Marketing Service, US Department of Agriculture. College Park (MD): National Archives and Records Administration; 2009.
21. Craigmill AL, Rangel-Lugo M, Damian P, et al. Extralabel use of tranquilizers and general anesthetics. J Am Vet Med Assoc 1997;211:302–4.
22. Haskell SR, Payne M, Webb A, et al. Antidotes in food animal practice. J Am Vet Med Assoc 2005;226:884–7.
23. Damian P, Craigmill AL, Riviere JE. Extralabel use of nonsteroidal anti-inflammatory drugs. J Am Vet Med Assoc 1997;211:860–1.
24. Papich MG. Drug residue considerations for anesthetics and adjunctive drugs in food-producing animals. Vet Clin North Am Food Anim Pract 1996;12:693–706.
25. Gehring R, Haskell SR, Payne MA, et al. Aminoglycoside residues in food of animal origin. J Am Vet Med Assoc 2005;227:63–6.
26. Baynes RE, Payne M, Martin-Jimenez T, et al. Extralabel use of ivermectin and moxidectin in food animals. J Am Vet Med Assoc 2000;217:668–71.
27. Martin-Jimenez T, Craigmill AL, Riviere JE. Extralabel use of oxytetracycline. J Am Vet Med Assoc 1997;211:42–4.
28. Haskell SR, Gehring R, Payne MA, et al. Update on FARAD food animal drug withholding recommendations. J Am Vet Med Assoc 2003;223:1277–8.

Antimicrobial Resistance and Small Ruminant Veterinary Practice

Lisa C. Scott, MSc*, Paula I. Menzies, DVM, MPVM

KEYWORDS

• Antimicrobial resistance • Goat • Sheep • Small ruminant

ANTIMICROBIAL RESISTANCE

Antimicrobial resistance (AMR) is the ability of bacteria to resist the inhibitory effects of antimicrobial drugs.[1] Many bacteria are capable of developing resistance to antimicrobials, whether it is intrinsic or acquired resistance. In bacteria, resistance is carried on mobile genetic elements (plasmids). Therefore, one bacterium may develop multidrug resistance, cross-resistance (resistance to other antimicrobials in the same or related class), and/or coresistance (genes conferring resistance to related or unrelated classes of antimicrobials are linked, usually on the same transmissible element).[1]

At present, several countries monitor trends in antimicrobial use (AMU) and AMR in livestock. Surveillance programs from the United States, Canada, and Denmark report annually on the prevalence of AMR in bacteria isolated from food animals, foods, and humans.[2–4] Although these programs frequently monitor AMR in major livestock, such as cattle, swine, and poultry, they do not include small ruminants such as sheep and goats. Only one monitoring program continuously includes isolates collected from sheep.[5] Since 2000, the Norwegian monitoring program for AMR in the veterinary and food production sectors, NORM-VET, has monitored the prevalence of AMR in bacterial isolates from sheep; these include *Staphylococcus* spp (diagnostic samples), *Escherichia coli* (fecal and/or meat samples from slaughterhouses), *Enterococcus* spp (meat), and *Salmonella* spp (diagnostic or meat samples). Isolates of *Staphylococcus aureus* from goats (bulk milk samples and mastitis samples) were also included in selected years (1999, 2000, and 2003).[5]

In Sweden, *Salmonella* diagnoses in animals are notifiable to the government.[6] In 2005, the Swedish National Veterinary Institute, in collaboration with the Swedish

The authors have nothing to disclose.

Population Medicine Department, Ontario Veterinary College, University of Guelph, 2541 Stewart Building (#45), Guelph, ON N1G 2W1, Canada

* Corresponding author.

E-mail address: lscott@uoguelph.ca

Vet Clin Food Anim 27 (2011) 23–32

doi:10.1016/j.cvfa.2010.10.015

Animal Health Service, created a program called the Swedish Veterinary Antimicrobial Resistance Monitoring (SVARMpat). The purpose of this program was to increase surveillance of AMR in bacteria causing disease in various farm animals, including sheep. Annual reports include *Salmonella* isolates from sheep.[6]

IMPACT OF ANTIMICROBIAL RESISTANCE

An increasing prevalence of AMR, particularly to frequently used antimicrobials in livestock, could lead to reduced treatment options, forcing veterinarians to use more expensive drugs. In addition, infected animals may shed these bacteria, posing a threat to other farm animals, household pets, and humans, through direct contact or environmental contamination. Infected animals may also act as a reservoir for resistant bacteria, which then enter the food chain.

ANTIMICROBIAL RESISTANCE IN SHEEP AND GOATS

When testing for the presence of AMR, *E coli* are frequently used as an indicator because they are ubiquitous and provide insight into the prevalence of AMR that could spread to other animal or human pathogens. Additional zoonotic pathogens, such as *Salmonella* and *Campylobacter*, may be used, due to their effect on human health, while resistant staphylococci are often detected in sheep and goat clinical mastitis[7] and may represent a risk to human and animal health.

Published research on the prevalence of AMR in enteric bacteria isolated from sheep and goats is sparse. In addition, several studies focused on multiple animal and environmental sources and provided overall prevalence results,[8–12] further limiting our understanding on the prevalence of AMR in bacteria isolated from sheep and/or goats.

Some studies investigated the prevalence of AMR in bacterial isolates from meat and abattoir samples, as well as in bacteria from the rumen and respiratory tract of individual animals.[5,13–23] The following, however, presents findings on the prevalence of AMR at the farm level, where antimicrobial drug use by veterinarians may select for AMR in bacteria.

Table 1 summarizes previous findings on the prevalence of resistance and multidrug resistance in bacterial isolates from healthy sheep and goats, as well as from samples collected from animals with clinical or subclinical disorders in North America, Europe, and elsewhere. The prevalence of resistance varied between countries, sample sources, and bacteria, likely as a result of differences in location, management practices, study design, and/or a variety of host, agent, and environmental factors. Bacterial isolates from diagnostic samples displayed a higher prevalence of AMR than isolates of the same bacterial species isolated from healthy sheep samples. This is highlighted by 2 studies that examined the prevalence of fluoroquinolone resistance in *E coli* isolated from diarrhoeic lambs and healthy ruminants in the same geographic area in Spain.[26,29] The prevalence of resistance was much lower (<25%) in isolates from healthy sheep, which according to the investigators, may be a result of the increased likelihood of treating the diarrhoeic lambs with fluoroquinolones.[29]

A low prevalence of multidrug resistance was observed in a small number of studies, with the exception of 2 studies examining clinical isolates of *Campylobacter jejuni* (United States) and *Salmonella* Typhimurium DT104 (Europe).[24,27] The latter study only examined a few isolates, which may have influenced the observed prevalence. By contrast, no multidrug resistance patterns were found in a small number of *Salmonella* isolates recovered by SVARMpat[6] or in *E coli* isolates from healthy goats in Spain.[29] An additional study from the United States focused on multidrug resistance

Table 1
The prevalence of resistance and multidrug resistance in bacterial isolates from healthy sheep and goats, as well as from samples collected from animals with clinical or subclinical disorders in North America, Europe, and elsewhere

Location	Year of Study	Source of Bacteria	Bacteria	Number of Isolates	Proportion of Isolates Resistant to ≥1 Antimicrobial Drug	Proportion of Isolates Resistant to ≥2 Antimicrobial Drugs
Samples from Sheep						
USA[24]	2003–2007	Clinical samples	C jejuni	74	100%	100%
Canada[25]	2006–2007	Healthy animals	Campylobacter	162	46%	4%
Canada[25]	2006–2007	Healthy animals	E coli	849	13%	5%
Canada[25]	2006–2007	Healthy animals	Salmonella	4	0%	0%
Spain[26]	1993–1996	Clinical samples	E coli	57	26%	Not specified
Scotland[27]	1994–1995	Clinical samples	S Typhimurium DT104	7	100%	100%
Spain[28]	1996–1997	Clinical samples	S aureus	38	21%	21%
Sweden[6]	2006–2007	Clinical samples	S aureus	4	0%	0%
Spain[29]	1997–1998	Healthy animals	E coli	210	<1%	0%
United Kingdom[30]	1992–1995	Healthy animals	C jejuni	20	0%	0%
Iran[31]	Not provided	Healthy animals	E coli	155	8%	1%
Samples from Goats						
Spain[29]	1997–1998	Healthy animals	E coli	143	1%	0%
Italy[32]	2006	Clinical samples	S aureus	25	56%	4%
Italy[32]	2006	Clinical samples	Coagulase-negative staphylococci	75	41%	9%

in fecal *E coli* isolates from healthy sheep[9]; although the investigator stated that none of the isolates were resistant to 3 or more of the antimicrobials tested, the study is not included in **Table 1** because no quantitative data (eg, prevalence or individual AMR patterns) were provided.

Temporal trends in the prevalence of AMR in *Salmonella* spp was examined in 2 studies.[33,34] Both reported an increase in resistance of 54% and 12% to select antimicrobials in *S* Typhimurium (over 5 years) and in *S* Typhimurium DT104 (over 10 years), respectively. In both studies, AMR in *Salmonella* types other than *S* Typhimurium over the same time period was rare (prevalence: 0%–4%).

The Norwegian monitoring program has reported AMR in various bacteria isolated from sheep. *Salmonella* from diagnostic specimens were fully susceptible, while an overall low prevalence of resistance was observed in *S aureus* (<5%). *E coli* also displayed a low prevalence (<5%) of resistance to ampicillin, streptomycin, and sulfamethazine, which, according to the investigators, were being used therapeutically in sheep.[5]

Most goat studies reported increased prevalence of resistance in staphylococci isolated from subclinical and clinical cases of mastitis (Italy and Brazil).[32,35] A moderately high prevalence of resistance was observed in *S aureus* (56%) and coagulase-negative staphylococci (41%). A similar prevalence (40%) was reported by the Norwegian monitoring program in *S aureus* isolates examined from dairy goat herds.[5] However, the prevalence was much lower (8%) in *S aureus* isolated from goats with mastitis.

In summary, the overall prevalence of AMR in sheep varied widely and resistance was observed in different bacteria. Much less information is available for goats. Unfortunately, most sheep and goat studies are outdated, are focused on multiple animal species, or are varied in study design and location, making comparisons difficult. Resistance was observed to several antimicrobials important in human and animal medicine and, in some situations, even more so in clinical cases. Though multidrug resistance was reported, it was uncommon.

ANTIMICROBIAL DRUGS OF INTEREST

Antimicrobial drugs classified by the World Health Organization as critically important in human medicine[36] are also used in small ruminant medicine. Some of these are listed in **Table 2**. However, resistance is not limited to these antimicrobials, and cross-resistance and/or coresistance may occur.

Treatment practices in small ruminants vary depending on the country, due to differences in approved products, farming conditions, and diseases. In Canada and the United States, from a food production standpoint, sheep and goats are considered minor species. As a result, only a small number of antimicrobials are licensed for

Table 2
Antimicrobials considered by the World Health Organization as critically important in human medicine, which are also used in small ruminant health management

Antimicrobial Class	Antimicrobial Drug
Third-generation cephalosporins	Ceftriaxone
Macrolides	Erythromycin, telithromycin
Fluoroquinolones	Nalidixic acid, ciprofloxacin

Data from WHO Advisory Group on Integrated Surveillance of Antimicrobial Resistance (AGISAR). Critically important antimicrobials for human medicine. 3rd edition. World Health Organization 2010.

use on these animals. Although overall AMU is low,[37] there is a high reliance on extra-label drug use (ELDU). In Australia, sheep and goats are managed extensively on grassland, therefore few antimicrobials are used. Consequently, there are limited data on AMU in small ruminants in that country. The following paragraphs outline specific antimicrobials of concern in small ruminant medicine and the prevalence of AMR to those antimicrobial classes.

Sulfonamide and Trimethoprim-Sulfonamide Combinations

In Canada and the United States, some sulfonamides are licensed for use in sheep whereas sulfonamide combinations, including trimethoprim-sulfadoxine, are not.[38,39] These antimicrobials are the third most common antimicrobials used by producers in both Alberta and Ontario, Canada.[37,40] Sulfonamide or sulfonamide combinations are not licensed for use in either sheep or goats in all countries of Europe,[41] nor are they licensed for use in goats in Canada and the United States.[38,39]

Studies have detected sulfonamide resistance in bacteria from both sheep and goats. Isolates of E coli from healthy sheep have displayed a low prevalence of resistance to sulfisoxazole (3%, Ontario, Canada; 1 of 5 isolates, Spain), sulfamethoxazole (<2%, Norway) and trimethoprim-sulfamethoxazole (<1%, Canada).[5,25,41] A relatively higher prevalence of sulfonamide resistance was observed in C jejuni (27%) and C coli (39%) isolates from Brazil[12] and in S aureus isolates (24%) from bulk goat milk in Norway.[5] Although sulfonamide resistance generally appears to be infrequent, one Canadian study found that the use of sulfonamide and sulfonamide combinations was associated with increased odds of tetracycline resistance. However, the mechanism of this association is not completely understood.[25]

Tetracycline

Tetracycline is licensed for use in sheep and goats in Canada, the United States, and Europe.[38,39,41] According to sheep producers in Ontario, Canada, injectable tetracycline was the second most common class type of antimicrobial preparations used, while tetracycline administered in the feed and water was the sixth. After accounting for the number of sheep treated and the duration of treatment, tetracycline in the feed and water was used most frequently.[37]

Tetracycline resistance was observed in several different studies. In Scotland, up to 71% of Salmonella isolated from clinical cases were resistant to tetracycline. However, in Canada no tetracycline resistance was observed in 7 Salmonella isolates from healthy sheep.[25] Similarly, the prevalence of tetracycline resistance in E coli from healthy sheep ranged from very low in Greece and Iran (1%),[31,42] to moderate in Canada (12%)[25] and Spain (20%),[43] to high in the United States (33%)[44] and the United Kingdom (35%–49%).[45] On the other hand, the prevalence was much higher (76%) in E coli isolated from clinical cases in Spain.[46] Studies from Canada and Brazil isolated Campylobacter from healthy sheep and found that the prevalence of tetracycline resistance was higher in C coli (28%–79%) than in C jejuni (9%–31%). However, in the Canadian study, this may be a result of a much smaller sample size (19 isolates of C coli vs 142 C jejuni).[12,25] In the United States, 100% of C jejuni isolates associated with abortion cases across multiple states were resistant to oxytetracycline. This finding was important, as tetracycline was the only class of antimicrobials approved for the treatment of Campylobacter abortion in sheep in the United States.[24]

In E coli from healthy goats, the prevalence of tetracycline resistance has varied; 12% in the United States[44] and 86% in Europe.[42] According to the investigators who conducted the latter study, the E coli from goats displayed a significantly higher prevalence of AMR than those from cattle and sheep in the same study. The prevalence of tetracycline resistance also varied in subclinical and clinical isolates of S aureus (0%–16%) and coagulase-negative staphylococci (5%–12%) in Italy, Brazil, and Norway.[5,32,35]

It is evident that a moderate to high prevalence of tetracycline resistance has been observed in bacteria isolated from sheep and goats. Furthermore, one study demonstrated that the use of in-feed tetracycline in sheep is associated with increased odds of tetracycline resistance.[25] Minimizing the use of tetracycline, both as injectable solution and as in-feed additive, may reduce selection pressure for resistance and prolong their effectiveness.

Cephalosporins

Ceftriaxone, a third-generation cephalosporin, is considered a critically important antimicrobial in human medicine and is used to treat serious infections in humans (eg, acute bacterial meningitis and disease in children due to Salmonella).[36] From a public health standpoint, resistance to cephalosporins is a major concern, and reducing selection pressure by limiting cephalosporin use in animals may help slow the emergence of resistance to this class of antimicrobials in animal bacteria. In Canada and the United States, ceftiofur is the only cephalosporin licensed for use in sheep[38,39]; it is also licensed for use in goats in the United States. Although licensed for the treatment of respiratory disease, ceftiofur is one of the less commonly used antimicrobials in the Canadian sheep industry.[37] The US Food and Drug Administration is considering banning the extralabel use of cephalosporins, to preserve the drugs for use in humans.[46] At present, however, the call for the ban is suspended as the risks and benefits of using cephalosporins in animals are further assessed. Both the American Veterinary Medical Association and the American Sheep Industry Association have argued that banning the extralabel drug use of cephalosporins would "compromise the food safety system"[46] and would leave the sheep industry with few treatment options.[47] In most European countries, there are no cephalosporins licensed for use in small ruminants.[41]

Resistance to cephalosporins has previously been observed in bacteria from small ruminants. A very low prevalence of resistance to ceftriaxone and cefotaxime (<1%) was observed in E coli isolated from sheep in Spain.[48] No ceftriaxone resistance was observed in Salmonella or E coli isolated from Canadian sheep.[25] Resistance also remained very low (<1%) to other cephalosporins (cefoxitin and ceftiofur) in E coli and Salmonella isolated from healthy sheep in various countries.[5,25,29,48] However, a study from the United States found that 100% of C jejuni isolates from abortion cases were resistant to ceftiofur.[24]

Resistance to cephalothin in isolates of S aureus and coagulase-negative staphylococci from subclinical and clinical mastitis in goats ranged from 2% to 14% in Italy and Brazil, whereas no resistance was detected in S aureus isolated from clinical samples in Norway.[5,32,35] Resistance to other cephalosporins (ceftriaxone and cefoperazone) was not observed in any study.

Fluoroquinolones

Enrofloxacin is a synthetic fluoroquinolone, which is not licensed for use on sheep or goats in Canada or the United States, and ELDU is not allowed in either country.[38,49] Enrofloxacin is not licensed in European Union countries, but can be used in an extralabel manner to treat sheep and goats.[41] Ciprofloxacin is a fluoroquinolone classified as critically important in human medicine. A very low prevalence (<1%) of ciprofloxacin resistance has been observed in E coli from healthy sheep in Spain,[29,46,48] whereas no resistance has been detected in Salmonella or E coli isolated from healthy sheep in

Ontario, Canada.[25] The prevalence of resistance tends to be slightly more frequent to nalidixic acid, a first-generation quinolone and precursor of ciprofloxacin, also considered critically important in human medicine[36]; less than 1% nalidixic acid resistance in *E coli* from clinical cases has been observed in Spain,[27] while a range from less than 1% (Canada, Europe, Iran) to 27% (Europe) in *E coli* from healthy sheep has also been recorded.[25,29,31,42,46] A temporal decrease in nalidixic acid susceptibility (by 12%) has been observed in Great Britain.[33] A Canadian study found a low prevalence of multidrug resistance between ciprofloxacin and nalidixic acid (4%) in *C jejuni* from healthy Ontario sheep, despite no records of fluoroquinolone use in those flocks over the course of 1 year.[25] In *E coli* isolated from healthy goats in Spain, there was also a very low prevalence of resistance to nalidixic acid (<1%).[29] To date, evidence of ciprofloxacin and nalidixic acid resistance has been observed in sheep (particularly in Europe) and in one goat study. However, the prevalence is relatively low and may be a result of restricted fluoroquinolone use.

PRACTICES THAT INCREASE THE RISK OF ANTIMICROBIAL RESISTANCE

Very little research has been completed in sheep and none exists in goats that examine practices associated with increased risk of AMR. Antimicrobial use in livestock is known to select for AMR in bacteria[50]; through antimicrobial selection pressure, resistant strains possess survival and growth advantages over their susceptible competitors.[51,52] Two studies from Canada examined associations between AMU and AMR in *E coli* isolates from sheep.[21,25] One study found that injectable administration of penicillins, for prophylactic and/or group treatment reasons, clearly increased the odds of resistance to select antimicrobial drugs.[21] In the second study, injection of sulfonamides (including sulfonamide combinations) or administering tetracycline in the feed or water was associated with increased odds of tetracycline resistance. The second study did not find significant associations between AMU and tetracycline resistance in *Campylobacter* spp.[25] Despite the lack of research examining associations between AMU and AMR in sheep and goats, studies from sheep suggest certain AMU practices are associated with increased odds of resistance. A shifted focus to improve flock management and hygiene, in combination with limited use of all antimicrobials, could help slow the emergence of AMR.

SUMMARY

AMR is recognized as an emerging issue in the practice of veterinary medicine. Although little surveillance and research has been completed on the prevalence of AMR and associated risk factors in small ruminants, evidence of AMR is present in many countries. Furthermore, AMU practices in sheep have been shown to be associated with increased resistance, highlighting the issue of prudent use of these drugs.

REFERENCES

1. Guardabassi L, Courvalin P. Modes of antimicrobial action and mechanisms of bacterial resistance. In: Aarestrup FM, editor. Antimicrobial resistance in bacteria of animal origin. Washington, DC: ASM Press; 2006. p. 1–18.
2. FDA. National antimicrobial resistance monitoring system - Enteric Bacteria (NARMS): 2007 executive report. Rockville (MD): United States Department of Health and Human Services, Food and Drug Administration; 2007.
3. Government of Canada. Canadian integrated program for antimicrobial resistance surveillance (CIPARS) 2007 annual report. Guelph (ON): 2007.

4. Anon. Uses of antimicrobial agents and occurrence of antimicrobial resistance in bacteria from food animals, foods and humans in Denmark. Danish National Veterinary Institute, National Food Institute, Technical University of Denmark; 2009.

5. Anon. Norm norm-vet report. Tromø (Oslo): Norway National Veterinary Institute; 2009.

6. SVARM. Swedish veterinary antimicrobial resistance monitoring. Uppsala (Sweden): The National Veterinary Institute (SVA); 2010.

7. Fthenakis GC. Susceptibility to antibiotics of staphylococcal isolates from cases of ovine or bovine mastitis in Greece. Small Rumin Res 1998;28:9–13.

8. Pocurull DW, Gaines SA, Mercer HD. Survey of infectious multiple drug resistance among *Salmonella* isolated from animals in the United States. Appl Microbiol 1971;21:358–62.

9. Krumperman PH. Multiple antibiotic resistance indexing of *Escherichia coli* to identify high-risk sources of fecal contamination of foods. Appl Environ Microbiol 1983;46:165–70.

10. Sayah RS, Kaneene JB, Johnson Y, et al. Patterns of antimicrobial resistance observed in *Escherichia coli* isolates obtained from domestic- and wild-animal fecal samples, human septage, and surface water. Appl Environ Microbiol 2005;71:1394–404.

11. Heffernan HM. Antibiotic resistance among *Salmonella* from human and other sources in New Zealand. Epidemiol Infect 1991;106:17–23.

12. Aquino MHC, Filgueiras ALL, Ferreira MCS, et al. Antimicrobial resistance and plasmid profiles of *Campylobacter jejuni* and *Campylobacter coli* from human and animal sources. Lett Appl Microbiol 2002;34:149–53.

13. Bensink JC, Bothmann FP. Antibiotic-resistant *Escherichia coli* isolated from chilled meat at retail outlets. N Z Vet J 1991;39:126–8.

14. Little CL, Richardson JF, Owen RJ, et al. *Campylobacter* and *Salmonella* in raw red meats in the United Kingdom: prevalence, characterization and antimicrobial resistance pattern, 2003–2005. Food Microbiol 2008;25:538–43.

15. Molla W, Molla B, Alemayehu D, et al. Occurrence and antimicrobial resistance of *Salmonella* serovars in apparently healthy slaughtered sheep and goats of central Ethiopia. Trop Anim Health Prod 2006;38:455–62.

16. Enne VI, Cassar C, Sprigings K, et al. A high prevalence of antimicrobial resistant *Escherichia coli* isolated from pigs and a low prevalence of antimicrobial resistant *E. coli* from cattle and sheep in Great Britain at slaughter. FEMS Microbiol Lett 2008;278:193–9.

17. Gundogan N, Citak S, Yucel N, et al. A note on the incidence and antibiotic resistance of *Staphylococcus aureus* isolated from meat and chicken samples. Meat Sci 2005;69:807–10.

18. Shayegh J, Mikaili P, Sharaf JD, et al. Antimicrobial resistance evaluation of Iranian ovine and bovine *Pasteurella multocida*. J Anim Vet Adv 2009;8:1666–9.

19. Goodyear KL. Correspondence: veterinary surveillance for antimicrobial resistance. J Antimicrob Chemother 2002;50:611–8.

20. Berge AC, Sischo WM, Craigmill AL. Antimicrobial susceptibility patterns of respiratory tract pathogens from sheep and goats. J Am Vet Med Assoc 2006;229:1279–81.

21. Avery BP. Antimicrobial use in sheep and antimicrobial resistance among *Salmonella* spp. and *Escherichia coli* from cull ewes in Alberta. MSc thesis: University of Guelph; 2003.

22. Duffy G, Cloak OM, O'Sullivan MG, et al. The incidence and antibiotic resistance profiles of *Salmonella* spp. on Irish retail meat products. Food Microbiol 1999;16:623–31.

23. Flint HJ, Duncan SH, Stewart CS. Transmissible antibiotic resistance in strains of *Escherichia coli* isolated from the ovine rumen. Lett Appl Microbiol 1987;5: 47–9.

24. Sahin O, Plummer PJ, Jordan DM, et al. Emergence of tetracycline-resistant *Campylobacter jejuni* clone associated with outbreaks of ovine abortion in the United States. J Clin Microbiol 2008;46:1663–71.

25. Scott LC. Investigation of antimicrobial resistance in *Salmonella*, *Escherichia coli* and *Campylobacter* isolated from Ontario sheep flocks [MSc thesis]: University of Guelph; 2009.

26. Orden JA, Ruiz-Santa-Quiteria JA, García S, et al. Quinolone resistance in *Escherichia coli* strains isolated from diarrhoeic lambs in Spain. Vet Rec 2000; 147:576–8.

27. Low JC, Angus M, Hopkins G, et al. Antimicrobial resistance of *Salmonella enterica* Typhimurium DT104 isolates and investigation of strains with transferable apramycin resistance. Epidemiol Infect 1997;118:97–103.

28. Goni P, Vergara Y, Ruiz J, et al. Antibiotic resistance and epidemiological typing of *Staphylococcus aureus* strains from ovine and rabbit mastitis. Int J Antimicrob Agents 2004;23:268–72.

29. Orden JA, Ruiz-Santa-Quiteria JA, Cid D, et al. Quinolone resistance in potentially pathogenic and non-pathogenic *Escherichia coli* strains isolated from healthy ruminants. J Antimicrob Chemother 2001;48:421–4.

30. Piddock LJV, Ricci V, Stanley K, et al. Activity of antibiotics used in human medicine for *Campylobacter jejuni* isolated from farm animals and their environment in Lancashire, UK. J Antimicrob Chemother 2000;46:303–6.

31. Nazer AHK. Transmissible drug resistance in *Escherichia coli* isolated from healthy dogs, cattle, sheep and horses. Vet Rec 1978;103:587–9.

32. Virdis S, Scarano C, Cossu F, et al. Antibiotic resistance in *Staphylococcus aureus* and coagulase negative Staphylococci isolated from goats with subclinical mastitis. Vet Med Int 2010;517060:1–6.

33. Davies RH, Teale CJ, Wray C, et al. Nalidixic acid resistance in salmonellae isolated from turkeys and other livestock in Great Britain. Vet Rec 1999;144: 320–2.

34. Jones YE, Chappell S, McLaren IM, et al. Antimicrobial resistance in *Salmonella* isolated from animals and their environment in England and Wales from 1988 to 1999. Vet Rec 2002;150:649–54.

35. Da Silva ER, Siqueira AP, Martins JCD, et al. Identification and in vitro antimicrobial susceptibility of *Staphylococcus* species isolated from goat mastitis in the Northeast of Brazil. Small Rumin Res 2004;55:45–9.

36. WHO. WHO list of critically important antimicrobials (CIA). Report of the 1st meeting of the World Health Organization. 3rd edition. Copenhagen: Advisory Group on Integrated Surveillance of Antimicrobial Resistance (AGISAR); 2010.

37. Moon CS. Use of antimicrobial agents and other veterinary drugs on sheep farms in Ontario, Canada. MSc thesis: University of Guelph; 2009.

38. Anon. Compendium of veterinary products. Hensall (ON): Veterinary Purchasing Company; 2010.

39. Anon. Approved animal drug products. Rockville (MD): United States Food and Drug Administration, Department of Health and Human Services; 2010.

40. Avery BP, Rajić A, McFall M, et al. Antimicrobial use in the Alberta sheep industry. Can J Vet Res 2008;78:137–42.

41. Anon. Compendium of data sheets for animal medicines. Enfield (UK): United Kingdom National Office of Animal Health; 2010.

42. Vantarakis A, Venieri D, Komninou G, et al. Differentiation of faecal *Escherichia coli* from humans and animals by multiple antibiotic resistance analysis. Lett Appl Microbiol 2006;42:71–7.
43. Anon. FDA calls off ban on animal antibiotics. American Sheep Industry Association; 2010.
44. Bryan A, Shapir N, Sadowsky MJ. Frequency distribution of tetracycline resistance genes in genetically diverse, nonselected, and nonclinical *Escherichia coli* strains isolated from diverse human and animal sources. Appl Environ Microbiol 2004;70:2503–7.
45. Teale CJ, Martin PK. VLA antimicrobial sensitivity report. Norwich (UK): Veterinary Laboratory Agency, DEFRA; 2005.
46. Blanco J, Cid D, Blanco JE, et al. Serogroups, toxins and antibiotic resistance of *Escherichia coli* strains isolated from diarrhoeic lambs in Spain. Vet Microbiol 1996;49:209–17.
47. Cima G. JAVMA news, December 15, 2008: FDA revokes planned extralabel cephalosporin use ban. Schaumburg (IL): American Veterinary Medical Association; 2008.
48. Mora A, Blanco JE, Blanco M, et al. Antimicrobial resistance of Shiga toxin (verotoxin)-producing *Escherichia coli* O157:H7 and non-O157 strains isolated from humans, cattle, sheep and food in Spain. Res Microbiol 2005;156:793–806.
49. FDA. Reminder–extra-label use of fluoroquinolones prohibited. Rockville (MD): United States Food and Drug Administration, Department of Health and Human Services; 2009.
50. Schroeder CM, Zhao C, DebRoy C, et al. Antimicrobial resistance of *Escherichia coli* O157 isolated from humans, cattle, swine, and food. Appl Environ Microbiol 2002;68:576–81.
51. Wise R. The worldwide threat of antimicrobial resistance. Curr Sci 2008;95:181–7.
52. Barza M, Travers K. Excess infections due to antimicrobial resistance: the "attributable fraction. Clin Infect Dis 2002;34:S126–30.

Treatment of Emergency Conditions in Sheep and Goats

Elisa M. Ermilio, DVM[a], Mary C. Smith, DVM[b],*

KEYWORDS

- Emergency • Goat • Sheep • Small ruminant

The emergency treatment of small ruminant patients can be overwhelming for clinicians with limited experience with these species. This article outlines the diseases most frequently encountered in veterinary practice. Each section discusses clinical signs, causes, and treatment and/or procedures associated with small ruminant emergencies. Emphasis is placed on the treatment of critical patients, but practitioners should also be prepared to manage these conditions on a flock or herd level because most small ruminant emergencies stem from poor management.

ANEMIA

A common range of acceptable packed-cell volumes (PCV) for sheep is 27% to 45% and 22% to 39% for goats.[1–3] Small ruminant red blood cells (RBCs) are smaller than other species; therefore, hematocrit tubes should be centrifuged for a minimum of 10 minutes to ensure adequate packing of cells and accurate assessment of PCV.[1]

Diagnosis of anemia is primarily based on physical examination rather than on complete blood cell counts. Indicators of anemia in small ruminants include pale or icteric mucous membranes, tachycardia, tachypnea, and exercise intolerance, which are all evidence of insufficient oxygen transport to tissues. Other findings in animals with severe anemia may include melena, hematuria, and generalized weakness.[3,4] Restraint of an animal with severe anemia may lead to its demise, thus forced exercise or stressful handling should be avoided.

As in other animal species, anemia can be classified into 1 of the 3 groups: blood loss, RBC lysis, and decreased RBC production (**Table 1**). The most common cause of anemia in small ruminants is parasitism, especially infestation with *Haemonchus* spp causing severe decreases in both hematocrit values and total protein levels.[1,5]

The authors have nothing to disclose.
a Country Companions Veterinary Services, 9 Amity Road, Bethany, CT 06524, USA
b Department of Population Medicine and Diagnostic Sciences, College of Veterinary Medicine, Cornell University, 29 Tower Road, Ithaca, NY 14853, USA
* Corresponding author.
E-mail address: mcs8@cornell.edu

Table 1
Causes of anemia in small ruminants

Causes	Specific Causes	Accompanying Clinical Signs
Parasitism	*Haemonchus* spp, *Linognathus* spp, *Fasciola hepatica*	Often, reduced total blood protein levels
Trauma	Predation, aggressive animals in the flock or herd, postpartum period	Rough coat, pruritus, alopecia with external parasites
Surgical cause	Castration, dehorning, cesarean delivery	
Infectious cause	Blood parasites: *Anaplasma ovis*, *Eperythrozoon ovis*, *Babesia* spp Bacterial toxins: *Clostridium* spp, *Leptospira interrogans* serovars	Icteric mucous membranes with intravascular hemolysis Hemoglobinemia and hemoglobinuria
Nutritional problems	Administration of bovine colostrum (potentially), copper toxicity, nitrate or nitrite toxicity, consumption of poisonous plants (eg, kale, onions)	Potentially, fever and/or renal failure (hemoglobin is pyrogen and renotoxic substance)
Iatrogenic causes	Rapid IV administration of hypotonic fluids, water toxicity	
Chronic disorders	Any infectious disease, malnutrition, copper deficiency, cobalt deficiency	Nonregenerative anemia Often contributory to other types of anemia
Iron deficiency	Chronic parasitism, excess milk feeding with no mineral supplementation (newborns)	Primary bone marrow disease rare

In emergency management of severe anemia, the decision to transfuse should be based on prognosis of underlying condition, patient stability, availability of suitable donor, and economics of the flock or herd. There is no specific transfusion trigger, but the combination of clinical signs and disease chronicity may guide the veterinarian's choice. In long-standing conditions, the PCV may be extremely low (<10%) before signs are evident; these animals have had time to adapt and may not benefit from the stress of the procedure.[5] For acute severe blood loss, PCV is a poor indicator of need of transfusion because both the PCV and total protein level may take up to 12 hours to decrease after bleeding has started.[6] Otherwise healthy goats with substantial acute blood loss (up to 50% of RBC mass over 24 hours) have been found to be more appropriately treated with fluid replacement rather than blood products.[1,7] Clinical signs of shock, extreme weakness, anorexia, and/or respiratory distress all support a decision to transfuse.[5,6] Transfusions should be considered only temporary, with donor erythrocytes being cleared in an average of 8 days in goats[1]; however, normal bone marrow should begin a regenerative response within 5 days.[3]

Crossmatching small ruminant blood in anticipation of transfusion is of little use because of the minimal level of agglutinating antibody present in ruminant serum. Crossmatching can be performed if multiple transfusions are necessary.[1,2,6] In practice, selecting donors for single transfusions requires a stable animal with a normal PCV. A donor may give up to 20% of blood volume safely or about 10 to 15 mL/kg body weight (BW).[1,5,6] It has been suggested that the collected blood be mixed with 4% sodium citrate in a ratio of 4:1 to 10:1 for immediate use; the blood should be drawn aseptically and continuously swirled with anticoagulant during the procedure.[2,5,6] The preferred route of delivery of whole blood is through a blood filter set and sterile jugular catheter; a suitable rate of administration is 10 mL/kg/h for a recommended total of 10 to 20 mL/kg BW.[1,5] An increase in PCV by 3% can be expected from a transfused whole blood volume of 10 mL/kg BW.[5] Intraperitoneal infusion of whole blood is acceptable if jugular veins are not accessible; however, this route has slower absorption rates.[2,5]

Transfusion reactions are rare with reported rates of 2% to 3%.[1] Slow initial administration rates and monitoring of vital parameters during the transfusion are indicated. Signs of adverse reaction or anaphylaxis include pyrexia, trembling, urticaria, edema, tachycardia, and dyspnea; if none of these signs occurs within the first 15 to 30 minutes, the transfusion rate may be increased.[2,6,8] In case of a reaction, the transfusion should be stopped and antihistamines and/or epinephrine should be administered depending on the severity of the signs. Plasma transfusions may be administered with similar caution in anemic animals with concurrent hypoproteinemia; this condition is most commonly due to chronic parasitism or failure of passive transfer in neonates.[1]

POLIOENCEPHALOMALACIA

Polioencephalomalacia (PEM) is also known as cerebrocortical necrosis by the lesion it creates.[9] Stargazing, opisthotonos, circling, ataxia, and central blindness are common initial signs of PEM. Anorexia, depression, or diarrhea may be present just before or during initial presentation. Progression is often rapid and includes recumbency, dorsomedial strabismus, nystagmus, convulsions, and death in 1 to 3 days.[1,2]

The most common cause of PEM in ruminants is feeding on high-concentrate rations resulting in rumen acidosis and subsequent thiamine (vitamin B_1) deficiency. As the rumen pH decreases, it becomes a less favorable environment for thiamine-producing bacteria and more hospitable for thiaminase producers. Available thiamine concentration is drastically reduced, and impaired energy production and osmotic control result in neuronal swelling and death.[1,2] Any cause for alteration in rumen flora may precipitate PEM, such as sudden feed changes, moldy feed, or other disease states. Thiamine antagonists, such as the coccidiostat amprolium, can also induce PEM after an overdose.[2]

Sulfur toxicity is another reported cause of PEM, which is distinct from alterations in thiamine status. Sources of sulfur include forages, concentrates, molasses, water, and urinary acidifiers (ammonium sulfate).[2,9] Lead and salt toxicity may present similarly to both thiamine- and sulfur-related PEM because of the cerebral edema and histologic changes in the brain; however, these conditions are less common in small ruminants.[1,2]

Antemortem diagnostic testing is of little value in practice because of the rapid progression of the disease. The response to treatment is often the approach taken to clinical diagnosis. Rumen contents and feces (submitted frozen) can be tested for thiaminase activity if PEM is suspected. Tests for thiamine level and transketolase activity are not widely available; also, these test results are normal if PEM is caused by excess sulfur. Postmortem lesions include edema and softening of the cerebral cortex. Gyri appear flattened and in some cases may fluoresce under ultraviolet light.[1,2] Ration and water analysis are important in cases of sulfur excess.[9]

Thiamine supplementation at 10 mg/kg BW is the treatment of choice for PEM. Initial dosing is typically intravenous (IV) and is repeated every 6 hours (intramuscular [IM], subcutaneous [SC], or IV administration) for the first day. Dosing intervals may be tapered depending on the response to treatment; regaining appetite is a positive indicator.[2] Management of cerebral edema is accomplished with IV administration of mannitol at a dose rate of 1.5 g/kg BW or furosemide at 1 mg/kg BW.[1] Seizure control with diazepam, 0.5 to 1.5 mg/kg BW (IV), as needed and antiinflammatory doses of steroids may be indicated. Response to treatment should be swift, and euthanasia must be considered after 3 days of no clinical improvement. PEM caused by sulfur excess does not respond well to thiamine administration, and treatment is palliative and aimed at dietary changes on the flock or herd level.[2]

ENTEROTOXEMIA OR PULPY KIDNEY DISEASE

Proliferation of *Clostridium perfringens* type D and elaboration of toxins by the organism can cause enterotoxemia, also known as pulpy kidney disease, in all small ruminants older than 3 weeks, with young rapidly growing animals being at highest risk. The ε-toxin is the major virulence factor of this organism.[10] Clinical signs often occur after large carbohydrate or protein-dense meals, such as in feedlots or grazing lush pasture, or after a sudden feed change. Subsequent replication of type D bacteria and activation of ε-toxin by trypsin causes the disease.[2]

In peracute illness, both sheep and goats may simply be found dead. ε-Toxin causes a dramatic increase in vascular and intestinal permeability, thus allowing its own rapid systemic absorption.[11] Neurologic and pulmonary signs predominate in sheep: blindness, opisthotonos, convulsions, dyspnea (often with froth at the mouth), pulmonary edema, recumbency, and paddling before death are commonly observed.[12] Enterotoxemia in goats targets the gastrointestinal tract and may manifest as colic, distention, or diarrhea (fibrinohemorrhagic enterocolitis). Recumbency and convulsions are grave prognostic indicators. Glucosuria may be present in either species.[12,13]

Diagnosis of enterotoxemia requires compatible clinical history, identification of necropsy lesions, or recovery of the ε-toxin from gut contents or blood. *C perfringens* type D is commonly present in low numbers as normal flora in small ruminants, hence a positive culture of the organism is only suggestive of the disease. In goats, impression smears of the gut or feces may yield a largely monomorphic population of gram-positive rods, which supports enterotoxemia. Toxin-specific assays may be more definitive but require careful and timely collection of the sample because the toxins are extremely labile. Testing feces or gut contents for ε-toxin requires prompt freezing and shipment of samples.[1]

Even in cases of early and aggressive treatment of enterotoxemia, prognosis should be guarded. IV administration of antitoxin should be initiated if the disease is suspected.[1] Administration of fluids supplemented with bicarbonate and electrolytes, parenteral penicillin, and flunixin meglumine is indicated.[1,2] Vaccination is the cornerstone of preventing clostridial diseases. The combination vaccines (*C perfringens* type C, *C perfringens* type D, *Clostridium tetani*) convey reliable protection in sheep but may need to be administered more often in goats.[10] Vaccination of ewes and does 6 to 3 weeks before the expected start of the lambing season affords protection to newborn lambs or kids via the colostral antibodies.[14] In lambs or kids, vaccination may take place at the age of 4 and 8 weeks. Vaccination should also be performed in a whole group in the face of an outbreak.[1,10]

RUMINAL ACIDOSIS (GRAIN OVERLOAD)

Engorgement with carbohydrate-rich feeds leading to ruminal acidosis may follow a variety of management errors, including sudden access to feed and excessive meal size.[1,2] Rapidly fermented sugars and starches produce excess acid. This acid accumulates in the rumen and lowers pH therein, killing normal flora and drawing fluid into the rumen.[15] Clinical signs may include recumbency, colic, bloat, diarrhea, toxemia, and neurologic signs.[15,16] The rumen may feel sloshy because of the osmotic draw of water, which can be severe enough to produce hypovolemic shock.[15]

Diagnosis is based mainly on recent history of concentrate engorgement, which includes any cereal grain or carbohydrate-dense feed (bread, beet pulp, potatoes, fruits). Definitive diagnosis is made by rumen fluid analysis (via rumenocentesis), with pH less than 5.5 and shifts in normal flora to predominantly gram-positive rods.[2] The pH of urine and feces is also reduced; however, in severe cases, gut stasis precludes diarrhea.[15] Ancillary laboratory data are consistent with moderate to severe dehydration and metabolic acidosis.[2]

Treatment to correct acid-base and electrolyte abnormalities and restore a euvolemic state usually requires aggressive IV fluid therapy with supplemented bicarbonate. Multiplying the base deficit by (0.3 × BW in kg) provides milliequivalents of bicarbonate needed for replacement. If specific laboratory data are lacking, an approximate dose for a 50-kg goat would be 15 g of sodium bicarbonate.[1] Oral administration of fluids is contraindicated because of the limited absorption and further distension of the rumen.[2]

Small ruminants are often too small to reflux feed from an orogastric tube, but the tube may be helpful to remove and replace fluid with antacids (oral magnesium hydroxide or oxide at a dose rate of 1 g/kg BW).[1,2] Transfaunation can be done with rumen fluid obtained from any ruminant at slaughter or via an orogastric tube. After straining the fluid to remove fibrous contents, immediate administration is ideal; otherwise, the fluid should be covered with a layer of mineral oil to preserve anaerobic conditions.[2]

Severe cases warrant rumenotomy to manually remove feed and flush the rumen. Several techniques are described for this procedure, with emphasis on limiting the contamination of the peritoneal cavity.[17] Restricting the diet to grass hay and administering about 1 L of transfaunate are beneficial. Other treatments include thiamine supplementation 3 or 4 times a day to obviate PEM (described earlier), penicillin at 22,000 IU/kg BW (IM, twice a day), and flunixin meglumine at 1.1 to 2.2 mg/kg BW (IV).[2] Prevention with proper feed management is essential, with the addition of ionophores being helpful in reducing the lactate-producing bacteria in the rumen. In the United States, lasalocid and monensin are approved for use in nonlactating sheep and goats, respectively, in confinement feeding operations.[2] In Canada, only lasalocid is approved for use in sheep, whereas no product is licensed for use in goats.

HYPOCALCEMIA

Hypocalcemia occurs less frequently in small ruminants than in cattle. The condition occurs in late gestation and early lactation. It may also occur in association with forced exercise, pregnancy toxemia, or other mineral deficiencies. Initial clinical signs include ataxia, hyperactivity, muscle tremors (especially facial muscles), and anorexia; temperature may be within normal range or, possibly, only slightly reduced.[2] Progressively, the skin becomes cold and the pupils become dilated and show a sluggish light response; ultimately, in the case of no treatment, recumbency occurs. The heart beat is often muffled and rapid; bloating due to inability to eructate can occur before death. Diagnosis is often made on response to treatment, but blood calcium concentrations less than 7 mg/dL are definitive.[15]

Slow IV infusion of calcium should show immediate clinical response. A typical dose is 1 g calcium or approximately 50 to 75 mL of 23% calcium borogluconate solution per 45 kg BW.[2,15] Monitoring heart rate and rhythm during calcium administration is prudent, and treatment should be discontinued if arrhythmia occurs. A similar dosing can be given SC to provide a slower release of calcium.[2]

PREGNANCY TOXEMIA

Pregnancy toxemia in small ruminants occurs from a negative energy balance state in late gestation. Animals carrying twins or triplets require 180% or 240% more energy, respectively, than those with a single fetus. Obese ewes or does carrying multiple fetuses are at higher risk to develop the disease because of the limited space for adequate intake of feed.[18]

Early signs of the disorder include partial or complete anorexia with progression to recumbency, if left untreated. Neurologic signs, including bruxism, vigorous licking, stargazing, blindness, and tremors, may be seen preceding death.[15] Definitive diagnosis is made by detecting ketones in the urine or blood. With the use of recently available handheld meters, levels of β-hydroxybutyrate in blood can be determined; values greater than 1.5 mmol/L (about 15 mg/dL) are indicative of disease in sheep.[1,15,19] Glucose levels are variable throughout the course of the disease and are not helpful in diagnosis.

Treatment is aimed at restoring normal glucose metabolism and correcting dehydration. Deficits should be calculated by using the following formula: BW in kg × % dehydration = deficit in liters. For example, a 50 kg goat that is 10% dehydrated would have a 5 L deficit: $50 \times 0.1 = 5$.[18] Early in disease, oral replacement of glucose with 30 to 60 mL of propylene glycol twice a day may be sufficient, but severe cases require slow IV administration of 50% dextrose with a single dosing of 60 to 100 mL.[2] Valuable animals may justify the constant infusion of 5% to 8% dextrose solution in maintenance fluids until improvement is seen.[15] Hospitalized animals can be supported on partial parenteral nutrition consisting of dextrose and amino acids; total parenteral nutrition is contraindicated due to the lipid content.[18]

Owners must decide to prioritize the life of the pregnant female or that of the fetus, keeping in mind the high mortality rate of premature animals from metabolically unstable female patients. Reducing the glucose demand on the female animal by inducing lambing or kidding or casarean delivery could prevent relapse.[15] Administration of B vitamins, calcium, and highly palatable feed, coupled with free-choice access to water support the recovering ewe or doe.[2]

URINARY OBSTRUCTION

Urolithiasis and obstructive urinary tract disease are common problems in male small ruminants. Numerous resources are available for feed management strategies and surgical approaches to unblocking sheep and goats. This section focuses on medical treatment of the critical patient, with a brief review of surgical options.

Affected males may appear restless, dribble urine, or display tail twitching or signs of colic with obstruction. Crystals or blood may be seen on the hairs of the prepuce. Owners often mistake stranguria or dysuria for tenesmus. Goats often vocalize, as they strain, and some degree of rectal prolapse can occur.[20] Increased urethral pulsation may also be palpated per rectum.[2] Abdominal palpation or ultrasonography may reveal a large distended bladder or free fluid in the abdomen, which indicates bladder rupture. If urethral rupture occurs, urine accumulates in the SC tissues ventrally and around the prepuce ("water belly"). Anorexia, severe depression, and marked abdominal distension are signs of prolonged disease, with uremia and urinary tract rupture likely.[20]

Sedation with acepromazine (0.05–0.1 mg/kg BW, IV or IM) allows adequate muscle relaxation to place the animal on its rump and extrude the penis. Diazepam (0.1 mg/kg BW, IV and slowly) may be used for additional sedation; however, xylazine is contraindicated due to diuretic effects.[21] Cautious use of nonsteroidal antiinflammatory drugs is a crucial part of both pain control and reducing urethral swelling.

Once the penis is extruded, the urethral process should be carefully palpated for stones and may be incised if adhered to the prepuce or amputated with a scalpel or sharp scissors; this is a common place for obstruction.[20] The sigmoid flexure is another or additional site for blockage, requiring more intense management to correct.[21] Use of urethral catheterization is controversial. The presence of a urethral recess in the distal pelvic urethra precludes retrograde passage of a catheter in the bladder in most cases.[20,21] Some clinicians attempt gentle flushing with 2% lidocaine and saline solution (at a ratio of 1:3) to reduce spasms.[20] Another medical treatment option is the chemical dissolution of uroliths with the Walpole's solution (acetic acid and acetate). This procedure requires heavy sedation to place the animal in lateral recumbency and empty the bladder by using ultrasound-guided cystocentesis. The bladder is then filled with the Walpole solution and allowed to equilibrate. This step is continued until a target urine pH of 4 to 5 is reached. This procedure has been found to have a good (80%) success rate.[22]

Other diagnostic procedures include blood and urine examination, ultrasonographic examination, and abdominocentesis. Increased blood creatinine concentrations are expected, but serum urea nitrogen value is not consistently increased due to salivary excretion and recycling. Hyponatremia and hypochloremia are common, with other changes attributable to dehydration. If water belly or bladder rupture is suspected, it can be confirmed by aspiration of the edematous tissues around the prepuce or by abdominocentesis. The fluid obtained should have a creatinine concentration that is 1.5 to 2.0 times that of the peripheral blood and may smell like urine when heated.[20] Fluid therapy should begin immediately, especially if surgery is anticipated, to correct electrolyte imbalances and reduce anesthetic risks associated with hyperkalemia-induced arrhythmias. After unblocking, diuresis is important for reducing azotemia and flushing the urinary tract.[21] Stone analysis guides diet changes to prevent stone reformation and reblocking.[20]

If medical management is unsuccessful, as is often the case, several surgical approaches can be performed. Perineal urethrostomy and penile amputation should be considered salvage procedures for slaughter animals. Urethrostomy and urethrotomy have been shown to have poor long-term prognosis, due to stricture formation, but if a stone is readily palpated, a simple urethrotomy may easily unblock the animal. Tube cystostomy is considered the most successful surgical approach in terms of short- and long-term resolution (76%–90% and 86%, respectively). Although preserving breeding ability, tube cystostomy has the major drawback of expense and prolonged hospital stays. Percutaneous tube placement can unblock the animal for less expense but is more likely to have complications requiring a second procedure.[21] Bladder marsupialization is used after failure of tube cystostomy or if breeding is not required.[20] This procedure eliminates urinary continence and is associated with urine scalding, which is problematic for the pet animal and owner. Laser lithotripsy is currently under investigation but may become a viable option for valuable rams or bucks.[21]

ACUTE MASTITIS

Staphylococcus aureus and *Mannheimia haemolytica* are the causal agents of the most severe and life-threatening cases of mastitis in small ruminants; the latter organism is implicated less often in goats than sheep and is transmitted to the teat of the dam by the sucking young animals.[2,23] Development of peracute mastitis, because of the production of necrotizing virulence factors by the invading bacteria, occurs quickly and produces fever, anorexia, and lameness due to severe udder pain.[1] Typically, only one gland is affected. The affected gland becomes erythematous and hot but turns cold and cyanotic with disease progression; this explains the term "bluebag" used by farmers. Mammary secretion is watery and serous, with blood-tinted or brown discoloration or fibrin clots.

In acute mastitis, mortality can reach 80% if left untreated; alternatively, toxin-induced thrombosis of the vessels in the affected gland may lead to sloughing of mammary tissue over several days if the dam survives.[2] The decision to treat should be undertaken with consideration of production status, economics of the flock or herd, and welfare of the animal, especially because the disease is a serious welfare concern. Even mild cases of mastitis can render the gland less productive due to the development of intramammary fibrosis and can lead to malnutrition and losses in young stock. Because ewes or does can be chronic carriers, culling of chronically infected animals is prudent[24] to reduce infection risks for healthy animals in the farm.

If treatment is elected, systemic and intramammary antibiotics (eg, oxytetracycline or β-lactams) are common empirically used drugs. Parenteral administration of tilmicosin can be used in sheep but should be avoided in goats due to occasional adverse reactions. However, penetration of the gland is variable and antibiotics may have little effect on the outcome. Management of an animal with peracute mastitis should include fluid therapy and administration of flunixin meglumine (1–2 mg/kg BW, IV or IM).[2,25] Further medical options include the use of diuretics and regular removal of the mammary secretion aided with oxytocin administration. Partial mastectomy, although expensive, can be life saving in severe cases of peracute mastitis, especially in animals of high genetic potential. The operation should be performed under general anesthesia. During surgery, it is prudent to have stored blood or a blood-donor animal accessible because hemorrhage can be dramatic.[1,2]

BLOAT

Frothy and free gas bloat occur in both sheep and goats and can be life-threatening emergencies.[1] Feedlot rations (high in concentrates), large quantities of lush pasture or alfalfa feeding, and transitioning to new rations are significant risk factors for developing frothy bloat. As gas production from fermentation combines with excessive rumen mucus, stable foam is created, which covers the cardia and prevents eructation. Free gas bloat, secondary to obstruction of the esophagus from intraluminal foreign body or poorly chewed feed, is less common. Extraluminal compression of the esophagus or vagus nerve due to thoracic lymph node enlargement or abscess formation in the abdomen or thorax can also cause free gas bloat.[26]

Bloat is easily recognizable as a progressive distension of the left paralumbar fossa; it may also present early with anxiety or signs of colic. Respiratory distress develops as the rumen continues to press on the diaphragm. Excessive salivation is noted if feed obstructs the esophagus, and the course may be prolonged if small amounts of gas can intermittently escape. Free gas bloat can frequently be completely relieved with the passage of a stomach tube; however, in the presence of froth, gas does not flow and the distension does not resolve. Froth may be present on the tube after removing it, thus confirming the diagnosis. Various surfactant solutions can be delivered via the stomach tube to break down froth, including poloxalene (44–100 mg/kg BW) or dioctyl sodium sulfosuccinate (30 mL); cooking oil (about 100 mL) may be used if other products are unavailable.[1,2]

Rumen trocharization should be reserved for severe cases, in which there is not enough time to pass a tube. This procedure carries the risk of peritonitis, so animals treated in this manner should be placed on a course of broad-spectrum antibiotics.[1] If trocharization and infusion of surfactants do not relieve clinical signs, an emergency rumenotomy is warranted.[2]

RESPIRATORY DISTRESS

Dyspneic patients require prompt treatment. A quick assessment of respiratory pattern and effort before handling or restraining the animal can be beneficial because the stress of the examination may be fatal. Inspiratory difficulty, exemplified by stertor, stridor, or flared nostrils, indicates large or upper airway disease. In contrast, open-mouthed breathing and exaggerated abdominal push are associated with expiratory and lower airway disease. The normal resting respiratory rate for small ruminants is 10 to 30 breaths per minute (lambs/kids, 20–40 breaths per minute), but ambient temperature, extrapulmonary disease, pain, or the mere presence of the veterinarian decreases the objectivity of this range.[1]

On closer examination (wearing gloves), the first step to any distressed patient is ensuring a patent airway. Obstructions of the upper airways caused by regional lymphadenopathy or abscess formation (eg, caseous lymphadenitis), neoplasia, or foreign body may require emergency tracheostomy. If available, sedatives or induction drugs (short-acting barbiturates, ketamine, xylazine, propofol, anesthetic gas) facilitate intubation and oxygen delivery. The relative size of the trachea is small, with the average dairy goat requiring an endotracheal tube that is only 11 to 12 mm in diameter and 35 cm long.[1] In-hospital oxygen delivery using intranasal catheters (5F–10F red rubber catheter placed with local lidocaine and sutured or glued to the nares) or flow-by delivery with a mask is always beneficial.[27]

Diseases of the lower airway and lung parenchyma are best defined by careful auscultation and imaging modalities. The absence of lung sounds may be due to obesity, effusion, pneumothorax, thoracic masses (such as thymoma), or, rarely, diaphragmatic hernia. Careful cranial auscultation in the axilla is essential to diagnose the most common form cranioventral pneumonia.[1,28]

Ultrasonography is helpful to diagnose pleural effusion, adhesions, atelectasis, consolidation, and abscesses that reach the pleural surface.[2,29] Sector scanners are preferred over linear array transducers due to small intercostal spaces.[1] Ultrasonography is also a useful tool for needle placement for thoracocentesis in cases of pleural effusion. The site should be clipped, prepared, and blocked, with an 18-gauge needle or catheter inserted off the cranial border of the rib, to avoid nerves and vasculature. If ultrasonography is not available, needle placement in the seventh intercostal space at the level of the costochondral junction works well.[2] Pneumothorax is also relieved by thoracocentesis; usually, as much air or fluid as possible should be removed during the procedure. The exception is in cases of acute hemothorax, in which the patient may benefit from absorption of blood; therefore, only enough air or fluid should be withdrawn to relieve respiratory distress.[30] The use of radiography in distressed patients is often impractical but may help to confirm a diagnosis or give clients a more accurate prognosis. Techniques and equipment used for small animals are suitable for small ruminants but sedation may be required.[1,2]

Many respiratory emergencies are caused by diseases originating outside the respiratory tract. Certain poisonous plants cause changes to hemoglobin and oxygen dissociation, resulting in hypoxia. For example, cyanide poisoning or nitrite or nitrate poisoning results in fully saturated hemoglobin and methemoglobinemia, respectively, but these forms are unable to efficiently exchange gases in tissues.[2] Other hypoxic conditions may stem from severe anemia or bloat. Xylazine can cause severe respiratory depression, hypoxemia, and pulmonary edema. In sheep, even at therapeutic doses, the drug can occasionally damage the capillary endothelium and incite intra-alveolar hemorrhage and edema. These changes dissipate with time, but affected animals may become acutely cyanotic or die during the sedation period. It is recommended to never exceed a dose rate of 0.15 mg/kg BW of xylazine given IV for any small ruminant, to use a tuberculin syringe to draw up dosages accurately, and to have specific reversal agents readily available for administration.[1]

Other monitoring and diagnostic procedures after acute stabilization of a respiratory emergency include following trends in blood gas parameters and oxygen saturation. Screening for severe hypoxemia with portable pulse oximeters is more practical but less sensitive.[27] Venous blood gas samples are of benefit for assessing ventilation and acid-base status.[1]

DYSTOCIA AND OBSTETRIC EMERGENCIES

Although fetal postural abnormalities are the most common cause of dystocia,[2] the manipulations and detailed approaches to use are outside the scope of this article. Determining if there is a deviation from normal parturition is a critical first step in obstetric evaluations. A common rule of thumb for overzealous farmers and clinicians to follow is the 30-minute rule: (1) wait to examine the dam until 30 minutes after the chorioallantois has ruptured or after contractions begin, (2) if presentation is normal wait an additional 30 minutes before manipulating a fetus, and (3) finally, wait an additional 30 minutes after a normal delivery to examine for multiples.[2,31] An exception, however, would be meconium staining indicating fetal distress and the need for timely intervention.[1] Regardless of the cause, vaginal examinations should be performed with thorough cleaning, gloved hands (for operator's and animal's safety), gentle manipulation, and copious amounts of lubrication.

Delays in progression of labor may be due to several causes. Ringwomb, or incomplete dilation of the cervix, is more common in sheep and may be heritable in some instances. Correction with gentle manual stretching can be attempted, being mindful of the risk of tearing; however, a cesarean delivery is usually required.[2] Uterine inertia may explain slow progression and can be resolved with SC or IV administration of calcium or a caesarean delivery (especially, if other disorders are concurrent); IV administration of calcium should be avoided in case of toxicity.[1] A vaginal prolapse can predispose to inadequate cervical dilation and thus dystocia. Although the prolapse is often easily replaced in the first place, these animals should be individually monitored before lambing or kidding is imminent; thereafter, they should be removed from the flock or herd.[31] Uterine torsion, hydrops, and prepubic tendon rupture are all sporadic conditions that delay parturition and require veterinary attention; these conditions are approached as in cattle.

Manual correction of a dystocia is made easier with epidural analgesia. The skin above the first and second caudal vertebrae is clipped and prepared, and an 18- to 21-gauge, 2.5- to 4-cm-long needle is inserted into the epidural space with an angle that is perpendicular to the slope of the tail head; a dose of 1 mL/45 kg BW of 2% lidocaine solution provides relief for about 1 hour.[2] A 2 mL dose of combined 2% lidocaine and xylazine (0.07 mg/kg BW) limits straining and provides longer pain relief.[31] Moreover, it is best to avoid IV administration of xylazine because of the hypotensive and hypoxic effects for the dam and neonates.[31,32] In cases with a possibility for cesarean delivery, ultimately, a high (lumbosacral) epidural for more complete spinal analgesia might be useful.[33] The palpable depression between the sixth lumbar and first sacral vertebras is prepared and the skin blocked before administration. Paralysis of the rear legs can persist for several hours, and nerve damage and mothering ability must be considered, especially for larger recumbent patients.[32]

Indications for a fetotomy in small ruminants include an emphysematous fetus, inability to untangle dead multiples, or a friable uterus. Disarticulation of a head at the atlantooccipital joint is often sufficient to resolve the dystocia, when front limbs are retained.[2] SC fetotomy can easily remove a front limb of a dead fetus to create more room; a circumferential skin incision is made proximal to the carpus to remove the limb.[31] Administration of a nonsteroidal antiinflammatory drug and an antibiotic before surgery is usually indicated because often the fetus has been dead for some time.[2] As described, epidural anesthesia reduces straining and provides additional pain relief during the procedure. Epinephrine (1 mL of 1:1000 solution IM) may also be used to relax the uterus and provide more room for manual corrections.[31]

Fetal monsters, uterine tears, ringwomb, pregnancy toxemia, and the presence of a live fetus during dystocia are indications for selecting a cesarean delivery over fetotomy. The procedure is largely the same as in cattle, with a left-flank approach most common, using local blocks with a 2% lidocaine solution for analgesia.[33] High epidurals, paravertebral blocks, and gas anesthesia are also acceptable methods of achieving surgical anesthesia.[31,33] Blindfolding the animal and/or administration of diazepam (0.2–0.4 mg/kg BW, IV) can help in restraint. The uterus can be closed in 1 or 2 layers, with an inverting pattern, using absorbable suture; postsurgical parenteral administration of antibiotics is usually necessary.[31] Subsequent fertility in small ruminants undergoing a cesarean delivery to correct a dystocia does not seem to be affected.[34]

Postpartum conditions that present as emergencies include uterine prolapse and septicemia or toxemia from retained fetal membranes. Any condition that weakens the dam or prolongs delivery may increase the risk of a uterine prolapse, usually occurring within 12 to 18 hours post partum.[2] The prognosis is generally excellent if the uterus is cleaned thoroughly and replaced promptly, with little risk of recurrence in subsequent parturitions. Replacement is aided by a caudal epidural and elevation of the hindquarters.[31] Administration of tetanus toxoid prophylactically and oxytocin is justified, but systemic antibiotics and suturing the vulva may not be necessary in all cases. Diffuse necrosis or injury to the uterus (especially if prolapsed for >36 hours) may require removal.[1] Retained fetal membranes in a systemically ill animal are addressed with antibiotics, such as oxytetracycline, and antiinflammatory drugs. Manual removal of retained fetal membranes should not be performed in small ruminants.[2]

In newborn lambs or kids, mortality is often associated with hypothermia and/or hypoglycemia. Reservoirs of brown fat around the heart and kidneys can only sustain normal temperatures for about 5 hours in neonates and when combined with an inattentive mother or a delay in nursing, these factors can be rapidly fatal.[31] Malnutrition may be more common in animals born in large litters, as well as in newborns from ewes or does in which induction of parturition took place because it may take several days for these animals to reach full milk production.[35] Excellent instructions for warming neonates and managing hypoglycemia are available from the Ontario Ministry of Agriculture, Food and Rural Affairs.[36] In case of apnea, neonates may be manually stimulated with vigorous rubbing and suction of fluid from the nares. If a heartbeat is palpable, doxapram hydrochrloride (1.0–1.5 mg/kg BW, IV or sublingually) can be used as a respiratory stimulant.[1] Routine care of the umbilicus and proper colostrum management cannot be overemphasized in preventing critical conditions in newborn lambs or kids.

SUMMARY

This article addresses some of the more common small ruminant emergencies that veterinary practitioners may encounter. In many cases, knowledge of comparative medicine may help the clinician properly approach the emergency, although small ruminants often have specific disease issues, which require specialized knowledge.

REFERENCES

1. Smith MC, Sherman DM. Goat medicine. 2nd edition. Ames (IA): Wiley-Blackwell; 2009. p. 871.
2. Pugh DG. Sheep and goat medicine. Philadelphia: Saunders; 2002. p. 468.
3. Smith BP. Large animal internal medicine. 4th edition. St Louis (MO): Mosby Elsevier; 2009. p. 821.
4. Polizopoulou ZS. Haematological tests in sheep health management. Small Rumin Res 2010;92:88–91.
5. Navarre CB. Anemia in goats other than haemonchosis. In: Proceedings of the North American Veterinary Conference. Orlando (FL); 2007. p. 261. Available at: http://www.ivis.org/proceedings/navc/2007/LA/100.asp?LA=1. Accessed November 28, 2010.
6. Divers TJ. Blood component transfusions. Vet Clin North Am Food Anim Pract 2005;21:615–22.
7. Awad M, Ahmed I, Gohar H, et al. Comparative studies on fluid resuscitation in goat under surgical hypovolemic shock. In: Proceedings of the 25th World Buiatrics Congress. Budapest (Hungary); 2008. p. 114–5. Available at: http://www.ivis.org/proceedings/wbc/wbc2008/part4.pdf. Accessed November 28, 2010.
8. Feldman BF, Sink CA. Clinical considerations in transfusion practice. In: Feldman BF, Sink CA, editors. Practical transfusion medicine. Ithaca (NY): International Veterinary Information Service (www.ivis.org); 2008.
9. Gould DH. Polioencephalomalacia. J Anim Sci 1998;76:309–14.
10. Van Metre DC. Clostridial infections of the ruminant GI tract. In: Proceedings of the North American Veterinary Conference. Orlando (FL); 2006. p. 52–5. Available at: http://www.ivis.org/proceedings/navc/2006/LA/020.asp?LA=1. Accessed November 28, 2010.
11. Finnie JW. Pathogenesis of brain damage produced in sheep by Clostridium perfringens type D epsilon toxin: a review. Aust Vet J 2003;81:219–21.
12. Uzal FA, Songer JG. Diagnosis of Clostridium perfringens intestinal infections in sheep and goats. J Vet Diagn Invest 2008;20:253–65.
13. Scholes SFE, Welchman B, Hutchinson JP, et al. Clostridium perfringens type D enterotoxemia in neonatal lambs. Vet Rec 2007;160:811–2.
14. Socié-Jacob M, Bolkaerts B, Wiggers L, et al. Effect of vaccination against enterotoxaemia of pregnant ewes on antitoxin alpha and epsilon antibodies in colostrum, milk, and lambs after colostrum intake. In: Proceedings of the 25th World Buiatrics Congress. Budapest (Hungary); 2008. p. 111. Available at: http://www.ivis.org/proceedings/wbc/wbc2008/part4.pdf. Accessed November 28, 2010.
15. Van Saun RJ. Nutritional diseases of small ruminants: diagnosis, treatment, and prevention. In: Extension publications. University Park (PA): Penn State College of Agriculture and Sciences. Available at: http://vbs.psu.edu/extension/resources/pdf/small-ruminant/Sm%20Rum%20nutr%20disease.pdf. Accessed November 28, 2010.
16. Van Saun RJ. Rumen disease for the non-ruminant practitioner. In: Proceedings of the North American Veterinary Conference. Orlando (FL); 2007. p. 1754–7. Available at: http://www.ivis.org/proceedings/navc/2007/SAE/630.asp?LA=1. Accessed November 28, 2010.
17. Niehaus AJ. Rumenotomy. Vet Clin North Am Food Anim Pract 2008;24:341–7.
18. Navarre CB. Fluid therapy for pregnancy toxemia. In: Proceedings of the North American Veterinary Conference. Orlando (FL); 2007. p. 262–3. Available at: http://www.ivis.org/proceedings/navc/2007/LA/101.asp?LA=1. Accessed November 28, 2010.

19. Braun JP, Trumel C, Bézille P. Clinical biochemistry in sheep: a selected review. Small Rumin Res 2010;92:10–8.
20. Navarre CB. Urolithiasis in goats. In: Proceedings of the North American Veterinary Conference. Orlando (FL); 2007. p. 255–7. Available at: http://www.ivis.org/proceedings/navc/2007/LA/098.asp?LA=1. Accessed November 28, 2010.
21. Ewoldt JM, Jones ML, Miesner MD. Surgery of obstructive urolithiasis in ruminants. Vet Clin North Am Food Anim Pract 2008;24:455–65.
22. Janke JJ, Osterstock JB, Washburn KE, et al. Use of Walpole's solution for treatment of goats with urolithiasis: 25 cases (2001–2006). J Am Vet Med Assoc 2009;234:249–52.
23. Mavrogianni VS, Cripps PJ, Papaioannou N, et al. Teat disorders predispose ewes to clinical mastitis after challenge with *Mannheimia haemolytica*. Vet Res 2006;37:89–105.
24. Mørk T, Waage S, Tollersrud T, et al. Clinical mastitis in ewes; bacteriology, epidemiology and clinical features. Acta Vet Scand 2007;49:23.
25. Fthenakis GC. Field evaluation of flunixin meglumine in the supportive treatment of ovine mastitis. J Vet Pharmacol Ther 2000;23:405–7.
26. Cheng KJ, McAllister TA, Popp JD. A review of bloat in feedlot cattle. J Anim Sci 1998;76:299–308.
27. Macintire DK. Stabilization of respiratory emergencies. In: Proceedings of the North American Veterinary Conference. Orlando (FL); 2006. p. 256–8. Available at: http://www.ivis.org/proceedings/NAVC/2006/SAE/088.asp?LA=1. Accessed November 28, 2010.
28. Scott PR. Lung auscultation recordings from normal sheep and from sheep with well-defined respiratory tract pathology. Small Rumin Res 2010;92:104–7.
29. Scott PR, Sargison ND. Ultrasonography as an adjunct to clinical examination in sheep. Small Rumin Res 2010;92:108–19.
30. Hawkins EC. Rescuing patients in respiratory distress. In: Proceedings of the North American Veterinary Conference. Orlando (FL); 2006. p. 1297–9. Available at: http://www.ivis.org/proceedings/navc/2006/SAE/461.asp?LA=1. Accessed November 28, 2010.
31. Smith MC. Dystocia management and neonatal care. In: Proceedings of the North American Veterinary Conference. Orlando (FL); 2008. p. 312–4. Available at: http://www.ivis.org/docarchive/proceedings/navc/2008/la/108.pdf. Accessed November 28, 2010.
32. George LW. Pain control in food animals. In: Steffey EP, editor. Recent advances in anesthetic management of large domestic animals. Ithaca (NY): International Veterinary Information Service (www.ivis.org); 2003.
33. Scott PR. The management and welfare of some common ovine obstetrical problems in the United Kingdom. Vet J 2005;170:33–40.
34. Brounts SH, Hawkins JF, Baird AN, et al. Outcome and subsequent fertility of sheep and goats undergoing cesarean section because of dystocia: 110 cases (1981–2001). J Am Vet Med Assoc 2004;224:275–81.
35. Rowe JD. Sharing obstetrical tips with clients. In: Proceedings of the North American Veterinary Conference. Orlando (FL); 2006. p. 285–6. Available at: http://www.ivis.org/proceedings/navc/2006/LA/112.asp?LA=1. Accessed November 28, 2010.
36. Ontario Ministry of Agriculture Food & Rural Affairs Website. Hypothermia in newborn lambs. Factsheet 431/23. Available at: www.omafra.gov.on.ca. Accessed November 28, 2010.

Anesthesia and Analgesia in Sheep and Goats

Apostolos D. Galatos, DVM, PhD

KEYWORDS

• Anesthesia • Analgesia • Goat • Pain • Sheep • Welfare

Physical or chemical restraint, with or without local anesthesia, has been extensively used to perform diagnostic or minor surgical procedures in small ruminants. However, anesthetic and analgesic techniques are required when specific diagnostic procedures and painful surgery are to be performed. Apart from improving animal welfare standards, anesthesia and analgesia are essential to make the procedures easier and improve both animal and personnel safety.

Economic considerations and the limited number of anesthetics and analgesics licensed for use in small ruminants may dictate the use of a technique. Inhalational anesthesia is seldom feasible and economically justified, except when the economic value of the animal is high. Injectable anesthesia is easy and relatively safe to perform and its advantages overcompensate for the extra cost because the quality of pain management is improved, thus avoiding its deleterious effects.

Doses of drugs used for sedation, analgesia, and anesthesia vary greatly depending on the anesthetic protocol, the physical condition of the animal, the route of administration, and the particular indication. Lower doses should be administered when combinations of drugs are used or high-risk animals are involved. A detailed list of all the possible doses and combinations of drugs is beyond the scope of this article. The reader is referred to specific texts, in which information for dose adjustment can be found.[1–5] After administration of the drugs, adequate withdrawal times should be allowed. Most of these drugs have short half-lives, leaving no residues after a few days.[1]

PHYSIOLOGIC CONSIDERATIONS

Secretion of large volumes of saliva continues during anesthesia in small ruminants and may contribute to airway obstruction or aspiration. Anticholinergics, instead of markedly decreasing salivation, lead to increased viscosity of the saliva, thus making the obstruction of the airway possible.

The author has nothing to disclose.
Department of Surgery, Faculty of Veterinary Medicine, University of Thessaly, Trikalon 224, GR-43100 Karditsa, Greece
E-mail address: agalatos@vet.uth.gr

Vet Clin Food Anim 27 (2011) 47–59
doi:10.1016/j.cvfa.2010.10.007
0749-0720/11/$ – see front matter © 2011 Elsevier Inc. All rights reserved.

vetfood.theclinics.com

Regurgitation and the ensuing aspiration of ruminal contents, which may lead to either asphyxiation or pneumonia, are common during deep surgical anesthesia or when intubation of the trachea is attempted in a lightly anesthetized animal, especially when the animal is in lateral or dorsal recumbency.[2] Because the rumen cannot be emptied completely, withholding food and water does not preclude regurgitation and aspiration, but the maintenance of the animal in sternal recumbency minimizes the risk. The best way to avoid the aspiration of ruminal contents and saliva and protect the airway from obstruction is to intubate the trachea with a cuffed endotracheal tube. If this technique is not feasible, the head may be positioned in such a way that the larynx is elevated relatively to the thoracic inlet and mouth, so ruminal contents and saliva drain out of the mouth.

When small ruminants are positioned in lateral or dorsal recumbency, the rumen and other abdominal viscera or the gravid uterus interfere with ventilation, resulting in hypoxemia and hypercapnia,[2] whereas the abnormal positioning leads to pulmonary ventilation-perfusion mismatch.[1] Furthermore, lateral or dorsal recumbency, heavy sedation, and anesthesia impair eructation; gas produced through continuous fermentation of ingesta accumulates in the rumen and leads to tympany, which further aggravates the respiratory distress.[1,2] The abdominal viscera, particularly when the animal is in dorsal recumbency, also compress the major abdominal vessels and impede venous blood return, thus decreasing cardiac output, blood pressure, and tissue perfusion.[1,2] Although hypoxemia and hypercapnia can be avoided, if oxygen is administered and intermittent positive pressure ventilation performed, this is not always feasible, especially in the field. Therefore, dorsal recumbency should be avoided or kept to a minimum. Withholding food for 12 to 18 hours and water for 8 to 12 hours in adult animals ameliorates the detrimental effects on cardiorespiratory function because it decreases the severity of tympany,[3] although the volume of ruminal contents is not greatly affected.[2] In emergencies, the passage of a stomach tube or percutaneous insertion of a needle into the rumen can remove the accumulated gas.

PREANESTHETIC PREPARATION

Besides withholding food and water, thorough physical examination, appropriate laboratory tests (complete blood test and serum biochemistry profile or, at least, packed cell volume and plasma total protein), and accurate assessment of body weight (BW) are essential before anesthesia. Venous catheterization permits the rapid and safe administration of anesthetics and fluids and may prove valuable during emergencies. In small adult ruminants, a 14 to 16 gauge, 18 to 20 gauge, or 20 to 22 gauge catheter is appropriate for the jugular, cephalic, or auricular vein, respectively.[3] Prior application of a local anesthetic facilitates venipuncture.[3]

SEDATION AND PREMEDICATION

It has long been claimed that premedication is rarely necessary[3–5] and often undesirable in small ruminants because it may increase the incidence of regurgitation and prolong recovery.[3] However, premedication makes the handling and induction of anesthesia of intractable animals safer, greatly reduces the requirements for anesthetics and thus the incidence and the intensity of any adverse effects, provides preemptive analgesia, and smoothes recovery.[2,3] In most cases, the advantages of premedication seem to far outweigh its disadvantages. The drugs used for sedation can also be used in smaller doses for premedication.

Acepromazine and other phenothiazines are not frequently used in small ruminants.[3] They do not have an analgesic effect and their sedative effect is limited[1,2,5]; however, they seem to reduce the dose required of both injectable induction agents and inhalant anesthetics.[6] The effects of phenothiazines on heart rate, respiratory function, arterial blood gases, and uterine blood flow are minimal, but hypotension and hypothermia are likely to occur, especially in hypovolemic or debilitated animals or if large doses are administered.[1,2,4] Furthermore, the risk of regurgitation is increased, and prolapse and trauma of the penis may occur.[1,3] Induction and recovery are smooth, but recovery may be delayed.[1]

Xylazine is the most commonly used α_2-adrenoceptor agonist; romifidine, detomidine, medetomidine, and dexmedetomidine are used to a lesser extent.[3,7] They are all potent sedatives with analgesic and muscle relaxant effects.[1,7] Sedation depends on the dose and animal temperament.[3] Goats seem to be more sensitive than sheep to xylazine, and variations in the analgesic effect of xylazine between different breeds of sheep have also been reported.[3,4] α_2-Adrenoceptor agonists may cause respiratory depression,[7,8] hypercapnia,[3] and significant hypoxemia,[7,8] which may outlast the duration of sedation.[9] Occasionally, clinical signs of pulmonary edema and fatalities have been reported in sheep.[3,5,7,9] Different possible mechanisms that lead to hypoxemia and pulmonary edema have been proposed.[7] Adverse effects can be reversed if α_2-adrenoceptor antagonists are administered less than 10 minutes after their onset.[7] α_2-Adrenoceptor agonists also cause profound bradycardia, especially after intravenous (IV) administration,[7,8] and a biphasic response characterized by initial hypertension and subsequent hypotension.[8,9] This complication is uncommon after xylazine administration, and only hypotension is usually evident.[2,7] Increased urine production associated with hyperglycemia and hypoinsulinemia may also occur.[2,8] α_2-Adrenoceptor agonists should be used with extreme caution or better avoided in animals with preexisting cardiopulmonary disease, hypovolemia or debilitation, or urinary tract obstruction. They should also be used with caution or even avoided during the last third of pregnancy because xylazine has an oxytocin-like effect on the uterus of pregnant ruminants,[2,10] potentially leading to abortion; however, detomidine seems to be safer.[2,11]

α_2-Adrenoceptor antagonists, such as atipamezole, yohimbine, or tolazoline, can reverse the adverse effects of agonists and shorten recovery time, but analgesia is also reversed.[3,5,8] Administration of half the dose by slow IV injection and the other half by intramuscular injection may prevent excitement.[8]

Benzodiazepines have anxiolytic, mild sedative, muscle relaxant, and anticonvulsant, but not analgesic, effects.[2,3,5] The cardiovascular and respiratory effects of benzodiazepines are minimal and transient[2]; therefore, they are safe to use in animals with preexisting cardiopulmonary disease or cardiovascular compromise. However, decreases in minute ventilation and a transient hypoxemia may occur.[2] Diazepam and midazolam are the most commonly used benzodiazepines. Because diazepam is a tissue irritant and its absorption and the degree of sedation are unpredictable after intramuscular administration,[2,5] slow IV administration is preferred to avoid transient excitement.[12] Midazolam is water-soluble and, therefore, preferable for both intramuscular and IV injection and is nonirritant, with a shorter action and greater potency than diazepam.[2] Diazepam and midazolam are usually used in conjunction with ketamine to improve muscle relaxation or with opioids. If necessary, flumazenil may be used to reverse their effects.

Premedication with anticholinergics is generally considered unnecessary and is not routinely recommended for small ruminants.[2–5] Large repeated doses, which produce tachycardia and mydriasis, are required to prevent salivation completely,[3–5,13] whereas smaller doses make saliva more viscous and liable to obstruct the airway.[1–3,5] Further-more, anticholinergics may adversely affect gastrointestinal motility[2] and promote accumulation of gas in the rumen, increasing the incidence of tympany.[4] IV administra-tion of anticholergenics is preferred if intraoperative bradycardia develops.[4,5] However, it might be a wise precaution to administer them preoperatively to prevent the occur-rence of bradycardia during ophthalmic surgery or manipulation of the viscera.[13] Glycopyrrolate may be a better choice in many cases because it has a longer duration of action than atropine and does not readily cross the placenta.[4]

ANALGESIA

Analgesia is an integral part of anesthesia; however, most of the sedatives and anes-thetics have mild, if any, analgesic effects. Therefore, it is mandatory to use specific analgesic agents. However, the use of analgesic agents is not common in small rumi-nant practice.

Sheep seem to be stoical, often showing only subtle signs of pain; however, this does not mean that they do not experience pain. Conversely, goats are evidently sensitive to pain and not tolerant of painful procedures. Sudden deaths have occurred after surgery and have been attributed to catecholamine-induced ventricular fibrilla-tion resulting from inadequate analgesia.[12] Irrespective of how animals express pain, most of its biologic consequences are similar across all mammalian species,[14] even if the argument that pain perception may be suppressed in neonatal animals[15] proves to be correct. Unrelieved pain has detrimental effects, causing severe stress and behavioral changes as well as cardiopulmonary, neuroendocrine, metabolic, immunologic, and thermoregulatory disorders.[14] Postoperative pain, resulting from tissue injury, may lead to peripheral and central sensitization and disinhibition.[14] As a result, analgesics are less effective when administered after the painful stimulus has been established. It is highly beneficial to institute both preemptive analgesia, that is, analgesia established before pain initiates, and multimodal analgesia, that is, inhibition of all the mechanisms that are responsible for pain production.[14] Therefore, analgesia should begin in the preoperative period and continue throughout surgery and at least until the third postoperative day by using various techniques and classes of analgesic agents that act on various parts of the pain pathways. The notion that analgesics should be administered only when the animal is in obvious pain is erroneous. Assessment of pain in small ruminants is not always easy; bleating may be increased in goats, but tachypnea, inappetence, grinding of teeth, immobility, or abnormal gait may be the only signs observed, especially in sheep.[5]

Opioids are effective analgesics, especially for visceral pain, but analgesia has a short duration in sheep. Morphine, pethidine, butorphanol, buprenorphine, fentanyl, hydromorphone, and oxymorphone can be used.[3,4] Although their use can be associ-ated with adverse behavioral effects from central nervous system stimulation, which mask their sedative effects, such effects are not common when they are administered in conjunction with a sedative or in animals in pain.[2] Respiratory depression is not a problem when high doses are avoided. When fentanyl patches (50–100 μg/hour) are used, analgesia may last up to 3 days, but the animals should be observed for excessive sedation or signs of excitement.[16,17] Epidural injection of morphine at a dose rate of 0.1 mg/kg BW provides analgesia for procedures on the perineum, hindlimbs, and abdomen, lasting for 6 to 12 hours.[2,3,5]

Nonsteroidal antiinflammatory drugs (NSAIDs) are not as potent analgesics as opioids but they are longer-acting and therefore useful, especially when used in conjunction with other analgesics,[18] to provide both preemptive and prolonged postoperative analgesia in small ruminants.[14] Apart from their peripheral antiinflammatory effects, NSAIDs also have centrally mediated analgesic effects. However, they may cause abomasal ulceration and, therefore, should be used cautiously for no longer than 3 days; dose rate should not exceed recommendations.[2] Flunixin meglumine provides excellent visceral analgesia lasting 6 to 12 hours but has less potent effects for many musculoskeletal injuries.[14] Phenylbutazone seems to provide excellent musculoskeletal pain relief but offers little benefit for the treatment of visceral pain.[14] Carprofen, ketoprofen, and meloxicam may also be used.

α_2-Adrenoceptor agonists provide short-term visceral analgesia that does not outlast sedation and their adverse effects limit their use in small ruminants.[3,4] Their epidural administration provides analgesia for procedures on the perineum, hindlimbs, and abdomen, but systemic absorption occurs, resulting in sedation and cardiorespiratory effects.[3,4]

The analgesic effects of ketamine have been recognized. An IV loading dose of 1.5 mg/kg BW may be used followed by infusion at 15 µg/kg/min.[19] In goats, epidural administration at a dose rate of 2.5 mg/kg BW, with or without xylazine, provides analgesia lasting only 15 to 30 minutes.[20]

Lidocaine, although a local anesthetic, has systemic analgesic effects.[2] In goats, an IV loading dose of 2.5 mg/kg BW followed by infusion at 0.1 mg/kg/min, with or without ketamine, reduced isoflurane requirements.[19] Infusion of lidocaine and ketamine had similar results in sheep undergoing orthopedic surgery.[21]

LOCAL AND REGIONAL ANESTHESIA AND ANALGESIA

Local and regional anesthetic and analgesic techniques are popular and useful in small ruminant practice. Their extensive discussion and description is beyond the scope of this article, and the reader is referred to other texts.[5,11,12,22–26] Local and regional anesthesia have long been considered as alternatives to general anesthesia,[2] their advantages being the low cost, the need for minimal equipment,[25] the minimal cardiovascular and respiratory depression and, at least in the standing animal, the low risk of regurgitation and aspiration.[5,25] However, it is often preferable to be applied in conjunction with general anesthesia. Furthermore, as soon as the action of the local anesthetic ends, pain recurs at the postoperative period and should be alleviated by the administration of the same or other analgesics.

The simplest technique is to infiltrate the surgical site with a local anesthetic. However, local anesthetics are less effective in inflamed tissue because its relatively low pH prevents the disassociation of their active basic form.[14,23] Furthermore, local infiltration may result in the administration of large doses and, although effective when used in superficial layers, it may be ineffective during abdominal surgery, in which anesthesia of the whole body wall, including the peritoneum, is required.[2] In such cases, inverted "L" block or, preferably, paravertebral nerve block or cranial epidural block should be used.[2,11]

Paravertebral block of the dorsal and ventral branches of the thirteenth thoracic nerve and the first, second, or third lumbar nerves can be quickly performed, and although technically more demanding, the procedure uses a small anesthetic dose and offers better anesthetic and surgical conditions. To block the dorsal and ventral branches of the thirteenth thoracic nerve, a needle is inserted vertically, at a point 2.5 to 3 cm from the midline, until it strikes the anterior edge of the transverse process of the first lumbar vertebra. Then it is "walked off" the edge and advanced deeper until it penetrates the intertransverse ligament. As the needle is withdrawn, the local anesthetic is injected both below and above the ligament. To block each one of the first, second, or third lumbar nerves, the needle strikes the posterior edge of the transverse process of the first, second, or third lumbar vertebrae, respectively, before it is "walked off" the edge and advanced deeper.

For cranial epidural block, the animal is restrained in sternal recumbency with the spine flexed, and the lumbosacral space is identified by locating a depression, which is in the midline between the last lumbar vertebra and the first sacral vertebra and approximately 3 cm caudal to the line joining the anterior borders of the ilium. The needle is inserted at a 90° angle and advanced until the ligamentum flavum (interarcuate ligament) is penetrated, which is recognised as a loss of resistance. Depending on the dose of the anesthetic, the cranial epidural block may anesthetize the whole body behind the diaphragm; however, the animal is unable to stand. Of major concern is the hypotension that may develop because of the blockade of the sympathetic tone, which causes vasodilation, when large doses are used.[2] Moreover, the doses should be decreased to two-thirds of that recommended during late pregnancy or in obese animals because epidural space volume is reduced as a result of vessel engorgement or fat deposition, respectively.[23] For perineal surgery, cranial or caudal epidural block can be used. For caudal epidural block, either the sacrococcygeal or the first intercoccygeal space is selected, located by palpation during slight vertical movement of the tail. The needle is introduced usually at a 10° to 20° angle and advanced to the epidural space. Caudal epidural block permits the animal to remain standing but is not indicated for anesthesia of the udder or male genitalia.[2] For udder anesthesia, cranial epidural block is preferred, but paravertebral and perineal nerve block can also be used, whereas ring block, inverted "V" block, teat cistern infusion, and IV regional anesthesia can be used for teat surgery.[25] Pudendal or dorsal penile nerve blocks can be used for surgery of the penis, whereas intratesticular injection or, preferably, injection into each spermatic cord at the scrotal neck is used for castration or vasectomy.

For lower limb surgery of 60 to 90 minutes duration, it is preferable to perform IV regional anesthesia, without adrenaline, but in conjunction with sedation.[2,25] Exsanguination of the limb by using an Esmarch bandage offers better anesthesia and reduced bleeding.[2,22] Various techniques have been described for dehorning and disbudding.[24–26] However, general anesthesia may be preferred in very young animals to avoid toxicity[2,5] and in adults with large horns to provide better anesthetic and surgical conditions.[2,25,26]

Lidocaine 2% is the most commonly used local anesthetic and provides anesthesia for 45 to 90 minutes.[26] Depending on the technique, anesthesia is evident within 5 to 20 minutes.[24] Mepivacaine 2% has more rapid onset and may produce anesthesia for 1.5 to 3 hours, whereas bupivacaine 0.5% has slow onset but provides anesthesia for 4 to 8 hours.[2,26] Lidocaine patches have been used in ruminants, with variable results.[14,25] Recently, a spray-on product formulation containing lidocaine and bupivacaine has been tried and its postoperative application to mulesing, castration, and tail-docking wounds showed seemingly good results.[27] These results probably could be further augmented if the product is used in conjunction with other analgesic techniques providing both preemptive and postoperative analgesia.[18]

Large or repeated doses of local anesthetics may induce systemic toxicity, especially in young animals or animals of low BW.[2,5,26] Clinical signs usually include opisthotonos and convulsions, but hypotension, apnea, and death may also occur.[2,5,26] Toxicity results from high plasma concentrations of the local anesthetic, which depends on the dose, degree of absorption, site of injection, concurrent administration of adrenaline, health status of the animal, and individual variations.[2] It is generally accepted that the total doses of lidocaine or mepivacaine should not exceed 6 to 10 mg/kg BW and that of bupivacaine should not exceed 3 to 4 mg/kg BW.[2,5,26] Diluted solutions (ie, with 1% or 0.5% concentration) should be used especially in young animals to prevent toxicity.[12,26] If convulsions occur, they can be controlled with an IV dose of 0.1 mg/kg BW of diazepam or 5 mg/kg BW of thiopental.[26]

The addition of adrenaline (5–20 μg/mL, ie, 1:200,000–1:50,000) decreases the potential for toxicity and prolongs local anesthesia. However, vasoconstriction causes local ischemia, often leading to tissue necrosis and, when injected near or in the surgical site, wound dehiscence.[22] Therefore, adrenaline should not be used near wounds or at the ring blocks of the teat, tail, or toes.

INJECTABLE ANESTHESIA

Injectable anesthetics can be used for both induction and maintenance of short-term anesthesia. Induction of anesthesia with IV administration of injectable anesthetics is preferable to induction with intramuscular administration or inhalational anaesthetics because it reduces the incidence of regurgitation and aspiration of ruminal contents.

Ketamine is commonly used in small ruminants for induction and maintenance of anesthesia. It is a dissociative anesthetic with analgesic effects, which provides mild cardiovascular stimulation and largely maintains the swallowing and cough reflexes[2,3,5]; however, aspiration can still occur,[13] and endotracheal intubation can be performed.[3,5,28] Apnea is not uncommon, especially after rapid IV injection,[13] and significant salivation can be seen.[28] The eyes remain open. Immediately after IV administration of ketamine (10 mg/kg BW), propofol (3 mg/kg BW), or thiopental (8 mg/kg BW) in goats to induce anesthesia that was maintained with halothane for 30 minutes, heart rate, blood pressure, respiratory rate, and arterial blood gases were quite similar with all 3 induction agents; however, intubating conditions were less satisfactory, and recovery times were longer when ketamine was administered.[28] When used alone, ketamine provides poor muscle relaxation, and the peripheral reflexes are maintained.[2] Therefore, it is strongly recommended to administer ketamine in conjunction with an α_2-adrenoceptor agonist or a benzodiazepine to improve muscle relaxation and sedation and facilitate induction and endotracheal intubation.[2] Tiletamine, another dissociative anesthetic used in conjunction with zolazepam, provides rapid and smooth induction, good anesthesia, and smooth recovery.[29,30]

Combinations of ketamine and α_2-adrenoceptor agonists, benzodiazepines, or acepromazine have been used to induce anesthesia in small ruminants.[1-5,11,12] If maintenance with an inhalant anesthetic is not feasible, anesthesia may be prolonged by incremental doses, and analgesics should be administered. The choice of a specific drug cocktail depends on the degree of analgesia, the duration of anesthesia required, as well as the animal's physical status. The combination of ketamine and benzodiazepines is preferable for debilitated animals because cardiorespiratory depression is minimal.[2] The combination of ketamine and α_2-adrenoceptor agonists enhances the degree of analgesia and prolongs anesthesia, but respiratory depression may be severe and the recovery delayed when large doses are used.[2,5] Administration of oxygen may be needed to avoid hypoxemia.[2,13]

After IV injection of 2.5% thiopental at a dose rate of 7 to 20 mg/kg BW, induction is smooth and rapid; anesthesia lasts for 5 to 10 minutes[5] and is suitable for endotracheal intubation.[28] However, apnea, usually lasting for 1 to 2 minutes, is common,[13,26] especially after rapid administration of large doses.[2] To avoid apnea, an initial dose of 5 to 7 mg/kg BW can be administered, followed by incremental doses every 20 to 30 seconds.[5] Doses of 5 to 10 mg/kg BW are adequate for induction when premedication has been used.[2] Thiopental causes respiratory and some cardiovascular depression,[4,26] has no analgesic effect and, when it is used in nonpremedicated small ruminants, muscle relaxation and the quality of recovery are relatively poor.[2,3] Because of the accumulation of thiopental, its use for the maintenance of anesthesia for more than 15 minutes is not recommended[1,3,4] because recovery would be delayed.[3,26] In goats, recovery times after an induction dose of thiopental were at least double compared with those after induction with propofol.[28] However, thiopental can be included in drug cocktails to maintain anesthesia for as long as 1 hour[26] in healthy small ruminants. Perivascular leakage must be avoided because its solutions are irritating.[2]

Compared with thiopental, propofol has the advantage of being noncumulative; recovery is rapid[28,31] and smooth, even after constant-rate infusion.[2,5,31–33] Propofol seems almost ideal for the maintenance of injectable anesthesia.[2] After IV injection at a dose of 3 to 7 mg/kg BW,[3,5,28] induction is smooth and rapid, although myoclonic activity of the face or limbs may occur[34]; anesthesia lasts for 5 to 10 minutes[26] and is suitable for endotracheal intubation.[5,28,34] Anesthesia can be maintained with a constant infusion of 0.3 to 0.6 mg/kg/min.[3,5,31–33] Propofol has no analgesic effect and its cardiopulmonary effects are similar to those of thiopental.[2,4] Apnea is common[5,33] and has been suggested to be attributed to the rapid rate of administration[34]; therefore, slow administration may prevent apnea.[2] However, because apnea may also occur when administration is slow,[33] it has been argued that its incidence might be also influenced by the induction dose.[28] Hypoventilation, hypoxemia, and hypercapnia occur when anesthesia is maintained with propofol,[2,31,32] and supplementary oxygen and ventilation should be provided, preferably after endotracheal intubation.[2,5,31] In goats, induction with a combination of detomidine, butorphanol, and propofol and maintenance with propofol provided anesthesia for castration and ovariectomy.[31] A combination of ketamine and propofol for induction and maintenance of anesthesia in sheep has also been tried.[33] Unused propofol should be discarded because of the risk of contamination.

Guaifenesin is not an anesthetic but a muscle relaxant that acts centrally, with no effect on diaphragmatic function, and mild, if any, analgesic and sedative effects.[1,3] Cardiovascular and respiratory depression is minimal.[1] It should be used in 5% solutions to avoid potential hemolysis and, in case of perivascular administration, tissue necrosis.[3] It is not often used alone in small ruminants,[5] but it can be used in combination with thiopental or ketamine[11,26] to induce and maintain short-term anesthesia. It can also be used as a constant-rate infusion, being part of a solution of xylazine (50 mg), ketamine (500 mg), and guaifenesin (500 mL of a 5% solution),[1,26,35] often referred to as triple drip. Anesthesia is induced in 5 to 10 minutes by the rapid administration of 0.5 to 2 mL/kg BW of the above-mentioned mixture and maintained by infusion at 2 to 2.6 mL/kg/hour.[1,11,35] A constant level of anesthesia is produced, and recovery is smooth but not rapid[35]; however, administration of oxygen, preferably after endotracheal intubation, is strongly recommended to avoid severe and potentially fatal hypoxemia, especially in debilitated animals or during prolonged anesthesia (ie, >0.5–1 hour).[1,5,35]

ENDOTRACHEAL INTUBATION

It is widely accepted that endotracheal intubation is necessary not only during inhalational anesthesia but also during injectable anesthesia maintained for longer than 5 to 10 minutes, especially if dorsal recumbency is to be adopted, to prevent the aspiration of ruminal contents or saliva and permit unimpeded administration of oxygen and assisted or controlled ventilation if apnea occurs.[1,2] Intubation should be done quickly, with the animal adequately anesthetized and preferably held in sternal recumbency, to reduce the risk of aspiration, with the head and neck fully extended. If regurgitation occurs during intubation, the animal should be positioned in lateral recumbency, the head lowered to allow drainage of fluids and any material scooped out of the mouth. Tubes of 5 to 14 mm internal diameter should be used in small ruminants; tubes required for goats are 1 to 2 sizes smaller than those required for sheep of the same BW.[1,2,13] Various techniques for endotracheal intubation have been described.[1,5,13] Orotracheal intubation is preferable to nasotracheal intubation.[2] It is easier to intubate the trachea under direct vision with the aid of a long-bladed (ie, 25–35 cm) laryngoscope. Using a guide tube or placing the animal into dorsal recumbency facilitates intubation.[5,13] In the absence of a laryngoscope, blind intubation can be performed rapidly, although it takes some practice, with the animal held in sternal or lateral recumbency, by gripping the larynx externally by one hand while the endotracheal tube is inserted into it by the other.[13] Once inserted, the cuff is inflated and the tube is left in place until coughing and swallowing reflexes are regained during recovery.

INHALATIONAL ANESTHESIA

Although the use of inhalational anesthesia is seldom feasible and economically justified in small ruminants, compared with injectable anesthesia, it is by far the safest and most satisfactory, especially for debilitated, pregnant, very young or aged animals or prolonged (ie, >1 hour) and complicated surgical procedures.[1,4,11,13,26] Easy control of the anesthetic depth and rapid recovery are among its major advantages. Inhalational anesthetics can be used for facemask induction in small ruminants weighing less than 50 to 100 kg,[3] and especially in young or debilitated animals.[13,26] However, although recovery is rapid, this technique is generally not recommended, especially in large, healthy, adult animals[26] because anesthetic consumption and environmental pollution are excessive, induction is delayed, the risk of regurgitation and aspiration is increased, and endotracheal intubation may not be easily feasible.[2] It is preferable to use inhalational anesthetics only for maintenance of anesthesia induced with an injectable anesthetic. Halothane can be used, but isoflurane and sevoflurane are superior because they do not sensitize the myocardium to catecholamine-induced arrhythmias, are only partially eliminated through metabolism,[2,4] and are expected to provide somewhat faster induction [2] and recovery.[36] However, they all cause dose-dependent cardiovascular and respiratory depression, which may be severe.[2,5] Nitrous oxide is not recommended because it increases the risk of ruminal tympany.[11] Small animal anesthetic circuits can be used to deliver inhalational anesthetics in small ruminants. Vaporizer should be set at 3% to 5%, 2% to 5%, or 4% to 6% when halothane, isoflurane, or sevoflurane, respectively, is used for induction; during maintenance, the vaporizer setting should be adjusted to 1% to 2%, 1.5% to 3%, or 2.5% to 4% when halothane, isoflurane, or sevoflurane, respectively, is used.[3,5] Oxygen flow rate should be 2 to 4 L/min during induction and reduced to 0.5 to 1 L/min during maintenance.[5]

INTRAOPERATIVE MONITORING AND SUPPORTIVE THERAPY

Small ruminants should be monitored continuously throughout anesthesia[26] to establish appropriate anesthetic depth and avoid complications. Monitoring equipment permits electrocardiography, assessment of arterial hemoglobin O_2 saturation and end-tidal CO_2 and inhalant anesthetic concentration, measurement of blood pressure, and analysis of the arterial blood gases, thus allowing for an accurate assessment of anesthetic depth and cardiovascular, respiratory, and central nervous system depression. If the monitoring equipment is not available, the assessment of the anesthetic depth in small ruminants is difficult; if in doubt, the anesthetic depth should be reduced until signs of light anesthesia are obvious. Rotation of the eye is not a useful indicator of anesthetic depth in small ruminants.[3] The corneal reflex should be maintained during anesthesia. Mydriasis may indicate both light and deep anesthesia; however, mydriasis, in conjunction with absence of the palpebral reflex and continuous passive flow of ruminal fluid from the mouth signify deep anesthesia. Movement of the limbs or head or chewing on painful stimulation and peristaltic activity of the esophagus perceptible under the skin and accompanied by swallowing motions indicate inadequate anesthesia. Heart rate should be within normal values, that is, 80 to 150 beats/min[26]; however, the heart rate varies with age and decreases when anesthesia is deep.[3] Decreased pulse pressure, palpated at the common digital, caudal auricular, radial, and saphenous arteries, indicates increased anesthetic depth but not mean arterial or perfusion pressure,[3] and the method is greatly subjective. Mucus membranes should be pink, and the capillary refill time should be 1 to 2 seconds, giving an indication of adequate tissue perfusion.[3] Respiratory rate should be between 20 and 40 breaths/min[26]; if a rebreathing bag is used, the tidal volume can be estimated. Response to pain can be used to estimate the anesthetic depth[3]; however, intraoperative analgesia is mandatory.

Lactated Ringer solution or other balanced electrolyte solutions should be infused at a rate of 5 to 10 mL/kg/hour IV, especially during prolonged anesthesia, to correct any preexisting dehydration, replace intraoperative losses, increase cardiac output, avoid hypotension, and ensure tissue perfusion.[3,11] In emergencies, more rapid administration may be necessary. Small ruminants younger than 3 months should also receive 5% dextrose solution at 2 to 5 mL/kg/hour to prevent hypoglycemia. When significant blood loss occurs, that is, more than 20 mL/kg BW, colloids (10–20 mL/kg BW) or hemoglobin (20 mL/kg BW) are preferable.[37] Blood transfusion may be necessary when the hematocrit is less than 20% to 25%.[1] If metabolic acidemia develops, sodium bicarbonate should be administered.

Young small ruminants may become hypothermic during anesthesia, and measures to avoid hypothermia may be essential[26]; however, hypothermia is rarely a problem in adult animals.[3] Hypoventilation and apnea are not uncommon in anesthetized small ruminants, thus, supplementary oxygen and assisted or controlled ventilation should be provided, especially during prolonged anesthesia.[2,3] Hypotension, that is, mean arterial blood pressure less than 65 to 70 mm Hg,[5,11] may be treated by rapid fluid administration and reduction of the anesthetic depth.[5] Additional treatment includes IV administration of dobutamine (0.5–5 µg/kg/min, administered to effect), dopamine (2–10 µg/kg/min, administered to effect), or adrenaline (0.02–0.06 mg/kg BW).[2,3,5,26]

RECOVERY FROM ANESTHESIA

Recovery from anesthesia is usually uneventful.[2,3,5] However, the potential for complications exists; therefore, small ruminants should remain under supervision in a quiet, comfortable, dry, and warm place. The duration of recovery depends on the type and amount of drugs used. To avoid ruminal tympany and regurgitation, small ruminants should be placed in sternal recumbency, with the endotracheal tube left in place and its cuff inflated, until swallowing and coughing reflexes are evident. If regurgitation had occurred during anesthesia, the oral cavity and pharynx should be lavaged and drained[1-3] and the endotracheal tube removed, with its cuff inflated in an attempt to remove any material that may have relocated to the trachea.

SUMMARY

Anesthesia and analgesia are essential in the management of sheep and goats. Local anesthesia should be considered as a part of the entire anesthetic protocol and not as an alternative to general anesthesia. Injectable anesthetics can be used for the induction and maintenance of short-term anesthesia. However, inhalational anesthesia should be considered for high-risk animals or prolonged and complicated surgical procedures. The detrimental effects of pain must be avoided by establishing preemptive and multimodal analgesia.

REFERENCES

1. Thurmon JC, Benson GJ. Anesthesia in ruminants and swine. In: Howard JL, editor. Current veterinary therapy 3: food animal practice. Philadelphia: WB Saunders; 1993. p. 58–76.
2. Valverde A, Doherty TJ. Anesthesia and analgesia in ruminants. In: Fish R, Danneman PJ, Brown M, et al, editors. Anesthesia and analgesia in laboratory animals. 2nd edition. London: Academic Press; 2008. p. 385–411.
3. Riebold TW. Ruminants. In: Tranquilli WJ, Thurmon JC, Grimm KA, editors. Lumb & Jones' veterinary anesthesia and analgesia. 4th edition. Ames (IA): Blackwell; 2007. p. 731–46.
4. Carroll GL, Hartsfield SM. General anaesthetic techniques in ruminants. Vet Clin North Am Food Anim Pract 1996;12:627–61.
5. Hall LW, Clarke KW, Trim CM. Anaesthesia of sheep, goats and other herbivores. In: Veterinary anaesthesia. 10th edition. London: WB Saunders; 2001. p. 341–66.
6. Doherty TJ, Rohrbach BW, Geiser DR. Effect of acepromazine and butorphanol on isoflurane minimum alveolar concentration in goats. J Vet Pharmacol Ther 2002;25:65–7.
7. Kästner SBR. A2-agonists in sheep: a review. Vet Anaesth Analg 2006;33:79–96.
8. Carroll GL, Hartsfield SM, Champney TH, et al. Effect of medetomidine and its antagonism with atipamezole on stress-related hormones, metabolites, physiologic responses, sedation, and mechanical threshold in goats. Vet Anaesth Analg 2005;32:147–57.
9. Celly CS, McDonell WN, Young SS, et al. The comparative hypoxaemic effect of four α_2 adrenoceptor agonists (xylazine, romifidine, detomidine and medetomidine) in sheep. J Vet Pharmacol Ther 1997;20:464–71.
10. Sakamoto H, Misumi K, Nakama M, et al. The effects of xylazine on intrauterine pressure, uterine blood flow, maternal and fetal cardiovascular and pulmonary function in pregnant goats. J Vet Med Sci 1996;58:211–7.
11. Ivany JM, Muir WW. Farm animal anesthesia. In: Fubini SL, Ducharme NG, editors. Farm animal surgery. St Louis (MO): WB Saunders; 2004. p. 97–112.
12. Gray PR, McDonell WN. Anaesthesia in goats and sheep. Part I. Local analgesia. Compend Contin Educ Pract Vet 1986;8(Suppl):S33–9.
13. Gray PR, McDonell WN. Anaesthesia in goats and sheep. Part II. General anesthesia. Compend Contin Educ Pract Vet 1986;8(Suppl):S127–35.
14. Anderson DE, Muir WW. Pain management in ruminants. Vet Clin North Am Food Anim Pract 2005;21:19–31.
15. Johnson CB, Sylvester SP, Stafford KJ, et al. Effects of age on the electroencephalographic response to castration in lambs anaesthetized with halothane in oxygen from birth to 6 weeks old. Vet Anaesth Analg 2009;36:273–9.
16. Ahern BJ, Soma LR, Boston RC, et al. Comparison of the analgesic properties of transdermaly administered fentanyl and intramuscularly administered buprenorphine

during and following experimental orthopedic surgery in sheep. Am J Vet Res 2009; 70:418–22.

17. Carroll GL, Hooper RN, Boothe DM, et al. Pharmacokinetics of fentanyl after intravenous and transdermal administration in goats. Am J Vet Res 1999;60: 986–91.

18. Paull DR, Colditz IG, Lee C, et al. Effectiveness of non-steroidal anti-inflammatory drugs and epidural anaesthesia in reducing the pain and stress responses to a surgical husbandry procedure (mulesing) in sheep. Aust J Exp Agric 2008; 48:1034–9.

19. Doherty T, Redua MA, Queiroz-Castro P, et al. Effect of intravenous lidocaine and ketamine on the minimum alveolar concentration of isoflurane in goats. Vet Anaesth Analg 2007;34:125–31.

20. Aithal HP, Pratap AK, Singh GR. Clinical effects of epidurally administered ketamine and xylazine in goats. Small Rumin Res 1997;24:55–64.

21. Raske TG, Pelkey S, Wagner AE, et al. Effect of intravenous ketamine and lidocaine on isoflurane requirement in sheep undergoing orthopedic surgery. Lab Anim 2010;39:76–9.

22. Brock KA, Heard DJ. Field anesthesia techniques in small ruminants. Part I. Local analgesia. Compend Contin Educ Pract Vet 1985;7(Suppl):S417–25.

23. Benson GJ, Thurmon JC. Regional analgesia. In: Howard JL, editor. Current veterinary therapy 3: food animal practice. Philadelphia: WB Saunders; 1993. p. 77–88.

24. Skarda RT. Local and regional anesthesia in ruminants and swine. Vet Clin North Am Food Anim Pract 1996;12:579–626.

25. Skarda RT, Tranquilli WJ. Local and regional anesthetic and analgesic techniques: ruminants and swine. In: Tranquilli WJ, Thurmon JC, Grimm KA, editors. Lumb & Jones' veterinary anesthesia and analgesia. 4th edition. Ames (IA): Blackwell; 2007. p. 643–81.

26. Lin HC, Pugh DG. Anesthetic management. In: Pugh DG, editor. Sheep and goat medicine. Philadelphia: WB Saunders; 2002. p. 405–19.

27. Lomax S, Sheil M, Windsor PA. Use of local anaesthesia for pain management during husbandry procedures in Australian sheep flocks. Small Rumin Res 2009;86:56–8.

28. Prassinos NN, Galatos AD, Raptopoulos D. A comparison of propofol, thiopental or ketamine as induction agents in goats. Vet Anaesth Analg 2005;32:289–96.

29. Taylor JH, Botha CJ, Swan GE, et al. Tiletamine hydrochloride in combination with zolazepam hydrochloride as an anaesthetic agent in sheep. J S Afr Vet Assoc 1992;63:63–5.

30. Carroll GL, Hartsfield SM, Hambleton R. Anesthetic effects of tiletamine-zolazepam, alone or in combination with butorphanol, in goats. J Am Vet Med Assoc 1997;211:593–7.

31. Carroll GL, Hooper RN, Slater MR, et al. Detomidine-butorphanol-propofol for carotid artery translocation and castration or ovariectomy in goats. Vet Surg 1998;27:75–82.

32. Lin HC, Purohit RC, Powe TA. Anesthesia in sheep with propofol or with xylazine-ketamine followed by halothane. Vet Surg 1997;26:247–52.

33. Correia D, Nolan AM, Reid J. Pharmacokinetics of propofol infusions, either alone or with ketamine, in sheep premedicated with acepromazine and papaveretum. Res Vet Sci 1996;60:213–7.

34. Pablo LS, Bailey JE, Ko JCH. Median effective dose of propofol required for induction of anesthesia in goats. J Am Vet Med Assoc 1997;211:86–8.

35. Lin HC, Tyler JW, Welles EG, et al. Effects of anesthesia induced and maintained by continuous intravenous administration of guaifenesin, ketamine, and xylazine in spontaneously breathing sheep. Am J Vet Res 1993;54:1913–6.
36. Hikasa Y, Hokushin S, Takase K, et al. Cardiopulmonary, hematological, serum biochemical and behavioral effects of sevoflurane compared with isoflurane or halothane in spontaneously ventilating goats. Small Rumin Res 2002;43:167–78.
37. Posner LP, Moon PF, Bliss SP, et al. Colloid osmotic pressure after hemorrhage and replenishment with Oxyglobin Solution, hetastarch, or whole blood in pregnant sheep. Vet Anaesth Analg 2003;30:30–6.

Control of *Brucella ovis* Infection in Sheep

Anne L. Ridler, BVSc, PhD[a],*, David M. West, BVSc, PhD[b]

KEYWORDS

- *Brucella ovis* • Disease control • Epididymitis
- Reproduction • Sheep

The approach to control of *Brucella ovis* depends on flock and farm characteristics, disease prevalence, and the economics of control. In flocks where eradication and prevention of reintroduction is feasible, control is based on test and slaughter. Use of antimicrobials can be considered in some circumstances. In flocks where eradication and prevention of reinfection is not feasible, efforts should be directed at minimizing the economic effects. This is usually achieved by vaccination or less effectively by removal of grossly diseased animals.

TRANSMISSION AND EFFECTS

B ovis has a predilection for the genital tract of sheep and, primarily, causes epididymitis and reduced fertility in rams. Infection may be introduced into a flock after the purchase of infected rams or via straying rams. Because it causes few obvious clinical signs, it can go undetected for some time. Transmission occurs between rams in direct contact or between rams mating the same ewe during the same breeding season.[1,2] Once infected, the majority of rams continue to shed *B ovis* in semen for at least 2 to 4 years,[2–5] but ewes seem only transiently infected. Apart from acting as a source of infection from ram to ram during mating, ewes are generally considered not important in the epidemiology of the disease, although *B ovis* is known to be a rare cause of abortion marked by severe placentitis.

The economic consequences of *B ovis* infection vary depending on disease prevalence and mating ratios. Infected rams are often subfertile or infertile, so infection may result in reduced conception rates or a protracted lambing period.[6,7] In countries

The authors have nothing to disclose.

[a] Department of Veterinary Clinical Sciences, The Royal Veterinary College, Hawkshead Lane, North Mymms, Hertfordshire AL9 7TA, UK
[b] Institute of Veterinary, Animal and Biomedical Sciences, Massey University, Private Bag 11-222, Palmerston North 4442, New Zealand
* Corresponding author.
E-mail address: aridler@rvc.ac.uk

where disease-free status within flocks is possible, control of *B ovis* is of particular economic importance for pedigree flocks to prevent sale of diseased rams.

ERADICATION
Overview

B ovis has been successfully eradicated from flocks, and from entire countries, using a test-and-slaughter approach.[8,9] Only rams are included in the testing program. Testing is based on scrotal palpation—with particular attention to the shape, size, and consistency of the epididymides[10]; serologic examination; and bacteriologic examination of semen samples,[11] where appropriate. The process may become prolonged and expensive when flock prevalence is high or if the disease has been present in the flock for some time. Hence, consideration of prevalence of the disease, chronicity of infection, value of the rams, and expenses of testing should be made before embarking on such a program. In some cases, culling the entire ram flock may be the most economical approach.[12]

Testing Methods

On a flock basis, detection of lesions of epididymitis by scrotal palpation may indicate that infection by *B ovis* is present. In some countries, scrotal palpation, with subsequent serologic testing of any rams with epididymitis and a proportion of others, is used as a rapid and inexpensive flock screening test.[13] This cannot be used for diagnosis in individual rams, however, because only approximately 35% of infected rams develop detectable lesions.[14]

Serologic testing is generally utilized for individual-animal and flock diagnosis. The most commonly used serologic tests are a complement fixation test (CFT), enzyme-linked immunosorbent assay (ELISA), and gel diffusion test (GDT). Depending on where and how testing is performed, the cutoff values used, and the chronicity of infection, the approximate respective sensitivity and specificity of these tests have been reported as follows: CFT, 96% and 99%; ELISA, 97% and 99%; and GDT, 92% and 100%.[15,16] A few serum samples are anticomplementary in the CFT. Due to the test sensitivities being less than 100%, a minimum of 2 tests at appropriate intervals is required. In infected flocks, retesting should be performed at 4- to 8-week intervals; experimental studies where rams were infected by inoculating semen onto mucus membranes resulted in seroconversion after 2 to 5 weeks and shedding of the organism in semen after 4 to 9 weeks.[17–19] A shorter testing interval is preferred to identify new infections as rapidly as possible and to prevent further transmission. If the interval is too short, then not all infected rams would have seroconverted.

Some rams exposed to *B ovis* do not develop a persistent infection and do not shed the organism in the semen but may be still be seropositive.[18] For the purposes of test-and-slaughter programs, it is generally assumed that all seropositive rams are potentially contagious and should be culled.

Test-and-slaughter programs can be compromised by rams that give false-negative serologic reactions, so in infected flocks the option of using 2 or more serologic tests should be considered for the second and subsequent testing periods. In some cases, semen collection and bacterial culture can be valuable when used at the second or subsequent testing periods to screen seronegative rams.[20] Shedding of *B ovis* in semen can be intermittent[5,14]; hence, a single negative sample does not guarantee that an animal is negative. *B ovis* requires selective media for reliable isolation[21]; it is a slow-growing organism that is easily overgrown; therefore, samples should be collected as aseptically as possible and sent to a laboratory with expertise in *B ovis* isolation. Slaughter followed by culture and histopathology of the epididymides and accessory sex glands can be considered in extreme cases where it is fundamental to establish whether or not a ram is infected.[20]

Other Considerations

Ideally, eradication programs should be undertaken outside the breeding season and it is essential that all susceptible males are included. There has been debate about whether or not young rams are susceptible; however, infection has been documented in 4- to 6-month-old rams.[22–24] It is reasonable to assume that ram lambs at approximately or beyond the age of puberty, which have been in direct contact with infected rams, potentially are infected.

Transmission of *B ovis* between rams occurs only when in direct contact, so groups of infected and noninfected rams can be kept on the same property provided they are strictly separated at all times. Splitting a ram flock into multiple small groups can help limit transmission during a test-and-slaughter program. Similarly, some farmers choose to manage the disease by keeping the infected rams separate from newly purchased, noninfected rams. Over time, the infected rams are culled and the ram flock becomes disease-free.[12] In this situation, it is essential that each group of rams are mated to separate groups of ewes.

Once a flock is free of infection, it can remain disease-free by purchasing only noninfected rams and ensuring straying of rams does not occur. Male deer can develop *B ovis* infection and transmission can occur from rams to deer.[25] Although there is currently no evidence that transmission can occur from deer to rams, it is wise to keep rams and male deer separate from one another.

ANTIBIOTIC ADMINISTRATION

Administration of antibiotics has been successfully used to treat infected rams. Experimental treatment for 7 to 21 days with long-acting oxytetracycline or chlortetracycline alone or in combination with dihydrostreptomycin resulted in cessation of shedding of *B ovis* and improvement of sperm motility in 80% to 100% of rams.[26–28] After treatment, it is prudent to keep rams isolated, collect at least 2 semen samples for bacterial culture to ensure cessation of shedding, and undertake post-treatment semen evaluation. The cost of treatment and follow-up testing is likely to mean that antibiotic therapy is only warranted in the case of valuable rams. Successfully treated rams remain seropositive for some time after resolution of infection, which needs to be considered if a test-and-slaughter program is implemented.

VACCINATION

Vaccination is considered the most viable method of control in countries or areas with a high incidence of infection.[29] In the past, a vaccine containing live *B abortus* strain 19 and killed *B ovis* organisms was used[30] as was also a vaccine containing killed *B ovis* organisms in adjuvant.[31] Both vaccines had the disadvantage of low efficacy and development of *B ovis* antibodies, which interfered with subsequent testing programs.[32] In addition, the former vaccine resulted in colonization of *B abortus* strain 19 and shedding in semen and occasionally development of epiphysitis and lameness.

B melitensis Rev1 vaccine, a modified live vaccine developed for the control of *B melitensis* infection, is now considered the best available vaccine against infection by *B ovis*.[29] The vaccine is administered via a subcutaneous injection or intraconjunctival inoculation. Experimentally, 56% to 100% of vaccinated rams that were challenged with *B ovis* after vaccination did not develop infection; potential genital lesions were less severe than in nonvaccinated animals.[33,34] It is not clear whether or not revaccination improves the immunity achieved with a single dose.[29] For practical purposes, Rev1 vaccination will result in a decrease in the incidence and economic consequences of B ovis but will not eradicate the disease from the flock. The disadvantages of using this vaccine include the development of both B melitensis and B ovis antibodies, which can interfere with serologic diagnosis,[33,34] and the increased risk of human disease by accidental self-inoculation.[35] Moreover, this vaccine is prohibited for use in countries considered free from B melitensis. Innovative vaccine approaches are currently being investigated,[35] which raises the possibility of more effective vaccines in the future.

REMOVAL OF GROSSLY DISEASED RAMS

In flocks where eradication of B ovis is not feasible, annual scrotal palpation and removal of rams with epididymitis can be practiced in an effort to reduce possible effects on flock reproductive performance. The cost of constantly replacing diseased rams, however, makes this an expensive option, and more rational control methods are recommended.

ACCREDITATION PROGRAMS

Some countries, for example, New Zealand and Australia, have established voluntary accreditation programs, allowing individual flocks to achieve accredited disease-free status. In some places (eg, Colorado), it is required that ELISA-positive rams be either castrated or slaughtered to control this disease. Additionally, all rams sold for breeding purposes and all rams entering Colorado must first have a negative test. Colorado also defines a certified-free flock status. Other US states have similar programs. This is of particular benefit to pedigree breeders and is likely reasonably effective at reducing spread of disease in countries where most rams sold to commercial farms are from pedigree flocks. Generally, these programs are based on an initial screen, where the whole ram flock is serologically tested twice; if all rams test negative, they achieve accredited-free status. Annual retests are based on scrotal palpation of all rams and serologic testing of any with lesions and a proportion of the remainder.[12]

SUMMARY

Approach to control of B ovis would vary in different countries and areas depending on farm and flock characteristics and economic factors. Eradication by a test-and-slaughter approach is the most desirable option in areas where it is logistically and financially feasible. Vaccination is used in areas with a high incidence of infection where eradication is difficult. Voluntary accreditation programs have been established in some countries and are of particular benefit to pedigree ram breeders.

REFERENCES

1. Buddle MB. Observations on the transmission of Brucella infection in sheep. N Z Vet J 1955;3:10–9.
2. Hartley WJ, Jebson JL, McFarlane D. Some observations on natural transmission of ovine brucellosis. N Z Vet J 1955;3:5–10.
3. Buddle MB. Studies on Brucella ovis (N.Sp.), a cause of genital disease of sheep in New Zealand and Australia. J Hyg 1956;54:351–64.

4. Worthington RW, Stevenson BJ, de Lisle GW. Serology and semen culture for the diagnosis of *Brucella ovis* infection in chronically infected rams. N Z Vet J 1985; 33:84–6.
5. Ridler AL, West DM, Stafford KJ, et al. Persistence, serodiagnosis and effects on semen characteristics of artificial *Brucella ovis* infection in red deer stags. N Z Vet J 2006;54:85–90.
6. McGowan B, Devine DR. Epididymitis of rams. The effect of naturally occurring disease upon fertility. Cornell Vet 1960;50:102–6.
7. Swift BL, Weyerts PR. Ram epididymitis. A study on infertility. Cornell Vet 1970;60: 204–12.
8. Ryan FB. Eradication of ovine brucellosis. Aust Vet J 1964;40:162–5.
9. Reichel MP, Baber DJ, Armitage PW, et al. Eradication of *Brucella ovis* from the Falkland Islands 1977–1993. Vet Rec 1994;134:595–7.
10. Gouletsou PG, Fthenakis GC. Clinical evaluation of reproductive ability of rams. Small Rumin Res 2010;92:45–51.
11. Tsakmakidis IA. Ram semen evaluation. Development and efficiency of modern techniques. Small Rumin Res 2010;92:126–30.
12. West DM, Bruere AN, Ridler AL. In: The sheep: health, disease and production. Palmerston North (New Zealand): VetLearn Foundation; 2009.
13. Reichel MP, West DM. *Brucella ovis* accreditation in New Zealand. Surveillance 1997;24:19–20.
14. Hughes KL, Claxton PD. *Brucella ovis* infection 1. An evaluation of microbiological, serological and clinical methods of diagnosis in the ram. Aust Vet J 1968;44:41–7.
15. Worthington RW, Weddell W, Penrose ME. A comparison of three serological tests for the diagnosis of *B. ovis* infection in rams. N Z Vet J 1984;32:58–60.
16. Reichel MP, Ross G, Drake J, et al. Performance of an enzyme-linked immunosorbent assay for the diagnosis of *Brucella ovis* infection in rams. N Z Vet J 1999;47: 71–4.
17. Laws L, Simmons GC, Ludford CG. Experimental *Brucella ovis* infection in rams. Aust Vet J 1972;48:313–7.
18. Plant JW, Eamens GJ, Seaman JT. Serological, bacteriological and pathological changes in rams following different routes of exposure to *Brucella ovis*. Aust Vet J 1986;63:409–11.
19. Webb RF, Quinn CA, Cockram FA, et al. Evaluation of procedures for the diagnosis of *Brucella ovis* infection in rams. Aust Vet J 1980;56:172–5.
20. West DM, Bruce RA. Observations on the eradication of *Brucella ovis* infection from a ram flock. N Z Vet J 1991;39:29–31.
21. Brown GM, Ranger CR, Kelley DJ. Selective media for the isolation of *Brucella ovis*. Cornell Vet 1971;61:265–80.
22. Clapp KH. Epidemiology of ovine brucellosis in South Australia. Aust Vet J 1962; 38:482–6.
23. Burgess GW, McDonald JW, Norris MJ. Epidemiological studies on ovine brucellosis in selected ram flocks. Aust Vet J 1982;59:45–7.
24. Bulgin MS. *Brucella ovis* epizootic in virgin ram lambs. J Am Vet Med Assoc 1990; 196:1120–2.
25. Ridler AL, West DM, Stafford KJ, et al. Transmission of *Brucella ovis* from rams to red deer stags. N Z Vet J 2000;48:57–9.
26. Kuppuswamy PB. Chemotherapy of brucellosis in rams. N Z Vet J 1954;2:110–8.
27. Marin CM, Jimenez de Bagues MP, Barberan M, et al. Efficacy of long-acting oxytetracycline alone or in combination with streptomycin for treatment of *Brucella ovis* infection of rams. Am J Vet Res 1989;50:560–3.

28. Dargatz DA, Smith JA, Knight AP, et al. Antimicrobial therapy for rams with *Brucella ovis* infection of the urogenital tract. J Am Vet Med Assoc 1990;196: 605–10.
29. Blasco JM. *Brucella ovis*. In: Neilson K, Duncan JR, editors. Animal brucellosis. Boca Raton (FL): CRC Press; 1990. p. 351–70.
30. Buddle MB. Production of immunity against ovine brucellosis. N Z Vet J 1954;2: 99–109.
31. Buddle MB. Production of immunity in rams against *Brucella ovis* infection. N Z Vet J 1962;10:111–5.
32. McDiarmid JJ. Observations on *Brucella ovis* CFT results. N Z Vet J 1978;26: 286–7.
33. Blasco JM, Marin CM, Barberan M, et al. Immunization with *Brucella melitensis* Rev 1 against *Brucella ovis* infection of rams. Vet Microbiol 1987;14:381–92.
34. Marin CM, Barberan M, Jimenez de Bagues MP, et al. Comparison of subcutaneous and conjunctival routes of Rev 1 vaccination for the prophylaxis of *Brucella ovis* infection in rams. Res Vet Sci 1990;48:209–15.
35. Estein SM, Fiorentino MA, Paolicchi FA, et al. The polymeric antigen BLSOmp31 confers protection against *Brucella ovis* infection in rams. Vaccine 2009;27: 6704–11.

Pharmaceutical Control of Reproduction in Sheep and Goats

José A. Abecia, DVM, PhD[a],*, Fernando Forcada, DVM, PhD[a],
Antonio González-Bulnes, DVM, PhD[b]

KEYWORDS

- Estrous control • Goat • Melatonin • Progestagen
- Prostaglandin • Reproductive management • Sheep

Sheep and goats are seasonally polyestrous, that is, they present a seasonal pattern of reproduction, to ensure that lambs and kids are born at the optimal time of the year (temperature and pasture availability), usually in the spring. The breeding season of these species are a succession of estrous cycles, 16 to 18 (average: 17) days (sheep) or 18 to 24 (average: 21) days (goats) in length. The cycle, which usually begins in late summer or early autumn in response to shortening day-length and ends in the late winter or early spring, is termed the ovulatory period. The variation is breed- and age-dependent. The anovulatory period covers the late spring to mid-summer, with the transition period mid-summer to the onset of the ovulatory period. This seasonal breeding pattern results in a clear period of lambing/kidding and, if animals are milked, a seasonal pattern of milk production.

Following the laws of supply and demand, this situation causes a seasonal pattern of meat and milk prices with prices lowest when the supply of meat/milk is the highest (late spring to early fall) and vice versa to take advantage of higher prices in winter and early spring, induction of "out-of-season" estrous cycles may be practiced, which will enable spring breeding and therefore fall lambing/kidding, resulting in winter production of milk and production of lambs and kids for the winter markets (eg, Christmas). Several methods to control the reproduction of small ruminants have been developed in the last few decades and are employed worldwide. Some of these involve either an environmental manipulation (light control)[1] or exposure to a male during the transition period (ram or buck effect).[2] Some others are based on administration of exogenous

The authors have nothing to disclose.
[a] Dept de Producción, Animal y Ciencia de los Alimentos, Facultad de Veterinaria, Universidad de Zaragoza, Miguel Servet 177, 50013 Zaragoza, Spain
[b] Dept de Reproducción, INIA, Ctra de la Coruña, km 5,9, 28040 Madrid, Spain
* Corresponding author.
E-mail address: alf@unizar.es

hormones that modify the physiologic chain of events involved in the sexual cycle (pharmacologic methods), which are able to modify the luteal phase of the cycle (progesterone/progestagen and prostaglandins) or the annual pattern of reproduction (melatonin).

Use of exogenous hormones for controlling reproduction has enabled other benefits. For many years artificial insemination (AI) of sheep and does was impractical, mainly due to the difficulty of detecting estrus in these animal species; use of progestagens to induce estrus has allowed the increased use of AI since the 1970s.[3] Multiple ovulation and embryo transfer (MOET) programs are also possible with the use of estrous synchronization and AI. Synchronization of estrous allows control and shortening of lambing and kidding, with synchronization of weaning and uniform batching of animals to slaughter; it also allows more efficient use of labor and animal facilities. Finally, hormonal treatments have also been used to induce estrus in peripubertal ewe-lambs and doelings, to bring forward their first mating. The aim of this review is to describe the pharmacologic methods to control reproduction of sheep and goats available, namely administration of progesterone/progestagens, prostaglandins, and melatonin. Because these methods are based on administration of hormones or analogues that participate in the natural endocrinology of these species, it is necessary to provide a brief overview of the physiology of reproduction. The authors have chosen sheep as representative of the small ruminant species.

Modifications to the activity of the hypothalamic-pituitary axis through changes in pulsatile gonadotropin-releasing hormone (GnRH) and luteinizing hormone (LH) control the seasonal changes; such modifications reflect differences in sensitivity to the negative feedback of circulating estradiol.[4] The increasing day-length during spring might be responsible for the onset of the breeding season at the end of the summer, whereas the long, but decreasing day-lengths from the summer solstice to the autumnal equinox seem to ensure the normal duration of the subsequent reproductive season. The pineal gland is directly involved in the ewe's perception of photoperiod. The retina receives photoperiodic information, which follows a multistep neural pathway to the pineal gland, where it modulates the rhythm of melatonin secretion.[5] Because melatonin is only released at night, the duration of secretion lengthens as days shorten. This change in the duration of melatonin secretion is processed neurally and regulates the secretion of GnRH; this is the hormonal basis of the treatment with exogenous melatonin.

Other methods that use progesterone, its analogues, and/or prostaglandins, are based on their effects on the luteal phase of the cycle. The estrous cycle is divided into 2 phases: follicular and luteal. After ovulation, the follicle is transformed into a corpus luteum (CL) that produces progesterone, which in turn is responsible for controlling LH secretion from the pituitary. This article describes how administration of progesterone or its analogues is able to modify the cycle, mimicking the activity of the CL. In the absence of fertilization, the uterus releases prostaglandins to lyse the CL to start a new cycle; this is the mechanism used by exogenous prostaglandins administered to control CL life.

It is a prerequisite that in all cases of pharmaceutical control of reproduction, male animals to be used (rams or bucks) must be of confirmed fertility. Appropriate clinical evaluation of male animals[6] or examination of semen samples[7] should be performed before attempting the pharmaceutical treatment.

PROGESTERONE AND ANALOGUES (PROGESTAGENS)

The first methods attempting to control the sexual cycle of sheep were published in the late 1940s.[8,9] Treatment consisted of 14 daily subcutaneous injections of 10 mg of progesterone, in 2 mL of corn oil; treatment reduced the range within which the animals were bred to 8 days. In some subsequent investigations pregnant mare serum (PMSG) and human chorionic gonadotropins (hCG) were given in addition to progesterone treatment.[10] Because progesterone not only suppresses pituitary gonadotropin release but also affects the female genital tract, the low fertility often encountered by these pioneering works was related to a persisting effect of progesterone on the uterine and tubal environment. Thus, a progestational agent whose activity ceases relatively abruptly after the end of treatment should give better results. This hypothesis was proposed by Southcott and colleagues,[11] who successfully used in sheep an analogue of progesterone, 6-methyl-17-acetoxyprogesterone, to induce synchronization of estrus. In addition, the intravaginal route of administration of progesterone or analogues was found to facilitate the abrupt removal of those hormones. Two methods are commercially used for this administration: polyurethane sponges impregnated with progestagen; and the controlled internal drug release (CIDR) dispenser (an inert silicone elastomer) usually impregnated with natural progesterone.

Since the early 1960s, intravaginally inserted pessaries impregnated with progestagen treatments have been applied to synchronize sheep estrous cycles and have been found to be equally effective in estrous synchronization in goats.[12,13] The most commonly used commercial forms of progestagens are fluorogestone acetate (FGA) (at 20–40 mg/sponge) and medroxiprogesterone acetate (MPA) (at 60 mg/sponge). Both progestagens seem to be effective inhibitors of the estrous cycle. FGA and MPA are not available in all countries (eg, United States and Canada) but are widely available in other sheep-rearing countries (eg, Australia, United Kingdom, Europe). The CIDR was designed in New Zealand in the late 1980s[14] and contains 0.30 g progesterone. Recently, the US Food and Drug Administration and the Canadian Veterinary Drug Directorate have approved the CIDR (progesterone solid matrix) for inducing estrus in ewes during seasonal anoestrus.

Melengestrol acetate (MGA), another synthetic progestagen used in the feed for suppressing estrus in feedlot heifers, has also been used to induce estrus in sheep and goats. There are several protocols suggested, but all include feeding MGA either in a total mixed ration or as a supplement fed every 8 to 12 hours, usually for a period of 8 to 14 days. The daily dose used is most often 0.25 mg/head/d, and most protocols have it administered twice per day at a dose of 0.125 mg.[15,16]

At the time of removal of progesterone or progestagen, animals are treated with equine chorionic gonadotropin (eCG, formerly pregnant mare serum gonadotropin or PMSG), a placental glycoprotein hormone prepared from the serum of pregnant mares. eCG has simultaneous FSH- and LH-like activities. For progestagen treatment to be effective it is necessary to have sufficient gonadotropin available to initiate the preovulatory events, increasing endogenous gonadotrophins with exogenous FSH[17] provided from the administration of eCG. This method can be applied throughout the year, as it induces estrous activity (during the anovulatory season when its use is obligatory) and also aids in synchronizing the estrous cycle (during the ovulatory season when its use is optional). However, its use during the ovulatory season leads to increased ovulation rates, that is, increased numbers of lambs born, and should be given cautiously. eCG products are currently not available in the United States, and veterinarians have used a product (PG600), which contains 400 IU of eCG and 200 IU of hCG per 5-mL dose, in combination with MGA pretreatments. However, it has been concluded that eCG is a better choice than PG600 as the gonadotropin to use at the time of progestagen withdrawal to prepare ewes for AI during a predetermined time frame.[18]

Proposed Protocols

In sheep, progestagen-impregnated intravaginal sponges or CIDRs are inserted intravaginally for 12 to 14 days. Ewes will be in estrus for mating or AI approximately 48 hours after device removal. The treatment includes eCG coincidentally with sponge removal; dose of eCG varies from 250 to 500 IU, depending on age (250–300 IU in ewe lambs, 350–500 IU in adult ewes), season (400–500 IU during anestrus, 300–350 IU during the breeding season), and breed (lower dose for prolific breeds). For mating of animals, a ram to ewe ratio of 1:10 is recommended in season but should be lower at 1:5–7 out of season. Insemination can be performed from 47 (intrauterine) to 55 (cervical) hours after removal of the device.

In goats, progestagen-impregnated sponges are inserted intravaginally for 16 to 18 days; CIDR devices are left in place for 18 to 21 days. Most does will be in estrus approximately 48 hours after device removal. The treatment includes eCG 2 days before sponge removal; dose of eCG varies from 500 to 800 IU, depending on the same factors described above. Insemination using a laparoscopic or cervical technique should be performed within 48 hours after device removal.

Sheep and goats in the ovulatory season will return to estrus 16 to 18 (sheep) or 20 to 22 (goats) days after removal of the devices if pregnancy does not occur. If outside the breeding season, the induced estrus is followed by only one other, 16 to 18 (sheep) or 20 to 22 (goats) days after removal of the devices; thereafter, no further cycles take place until the breeding season.

PROSTAGLANDINS AND ANALOGUES

Intravaginal devices with progesterone or progestagens are the most commonly used tools for estrous synchronization, but are not without their drawbacks. Their main advantages are availability in the market and simplicity of application. However, their use in season may lead to lower conception rates than nonhormonal natural services, about 80%,[19,20] due to alterations in patterns of LH release,[21] in quality of ovulations,[22] and/or in sperm transport and survival in the female reproductive tract.[23] Moreover, use of progestagens is under review in some countries,[24] due to issues related with public health (output of chemical residues in food, which has led to them being banned in the United States and has caused the enforcement of the regulation in maximum residue limits in the European Union) and animal welfare (causes of potential problems, such as vaginitis and/or sponge retention). Thus, pharmaceutical companies and researchers worldwide are developing possible alternatives, based on reducing the length or the dose of treatments by using more effective releasing systems, where the effect on the ovary is similar to classic protocols.[25]

An alternative during the ovulatory season is based on the elimination of the CL to induce a follicular phase with ovulation. The luteolytic factor in ruminants is the prostaglandin $F_{2\alpha}$ ($PGF_{2\alpha}$)[26]; hence, administration of exogenous $PGF_{2\alpha}$ or its analogues can be used to induce a controlled luteolysis. The most universal prostaglandin analogues used for veterinary purposes are cloprostenol and luprostiol, which are less expensive than the original molecule. A commonly used protocol in sheep and goats is 125 μg of cloprostenol or 7.5 mg luprostiol. $PGF_{2\alpha}$ treatments have the advantages of being effective after being applied by intramuscular injection,[27] of improving animal welfare, and to be quickly and almost totally (99%), metabolized,[28] decreasing residues. These facts favor the use of $PGF_{2\alpha}$ or its analogues as an alternative method for estrous synchronization. However, to be effective, $PGF_{2\alpha}$ has to be applied in the presence of a CL. Thus, animals outside the ovulatory season will not respond to the treatment. $PGF_{2\alpha}$ should only be used during ovulatory season in breeds from temperate areas[27]; however, in tropical breeds, with a continuous breeding season and no seasonal anoestrus, $PGF_{2\alpha}$ can be applied throughout the entire year.[29,30]

Thus, for estrous synchronization in a group of females, it is necessary to use 2 injections of $PGF_{2\alpha}$ or analogues, 9 to 10 days apart, which assures that almost all the animals will be in mid-luteal phase at the second dose and that all will respond with estrous behavior and ovulation. This protocol is effective in synchronizing estrus, but fertility of the ewes at first service has been reported to be reduced when compared with progestagen treatments and natural services,[31,32] reaching only about 70% pregnancy rate. A possible explanation for this drop in fertility may be that, by using a 9- to 10-day interval, the presence of a CL is assured, but it may induce a disruption of ovulatory follicular dynamics, disturbing functionality and final maturation of the preovulatory follicles and normal luteogenesis, and/or a variability in the timing of ovulation after $PGF_{2\alpha}$-induced luteolysis.[33,34]

Follicular function may be compromised during the mid-luteal phase of the estrous cycle, because higher progesterone concentrations induce lower amounts of LH in blood; LH is crucial for the final growth and maturation of preovulatory follicles.[35,36] Thus, the most desirable moment for $PGF_{2\alpha}$ treatments would be during either early or late luteal phase of the estrous cycle. Data from different research groups indicate a greater number of females showing estrous signs, an earlier appearance of such behavior, and a greater number of females ovulating after being treated early in the luteal phase.[29,37,38] These facts may be related to the presence during the early luteal phase of large-growing follicles from the first wave of development.[39,40] Conversely, follicular waves during mid-luteal stages may be poorly synchronized owing to a high variability between individuals, with a mixture of animals having growing, static, or regressing follicles.[33,41]

The CL in the small ruminant is responsive to $PGF_{2\alpha}$ from day 3 of the estrous cycle.[42,43] The luteolytic efficiency, percentage and timing of appearance of estrus, preovulatory release of LH and ovulation, and functionality of subsequent CLs are similar whether treating at day 3 or 5 of the cycle. So to avoid the risk of treating animals at day 1 or 2 of the cycle, which will not respond to $PGF_{2\alpha}$,[42] it is better to administer the treatment at day 5. In addition, treating in the early luteal phase favors maturation of follicles and synchronization of the preovulatory LH peak and ovulation, because restoration of required LH pulsatility would be earlier in the presence of younger CLs secreting less progesterone.[37] This protocol is suitable for timed AI.[44,45]

The timing of the preovulatory LH surge and ovulation may be narrowed by applying the "male effect" coincidentally with the second $PGF_{2\alpha}$ injection. The male effect is commonly used for inducing an LH surge, estrus, and ovulation during the transition season; however, it also induces increases in LH secretion during the ovulatory season, in cycling,[46] progestagen-treated,[47] and prostaglandin-treated sheep.[48] Moreover, the combination of $PGF_{2\alpha}$ during the early luteal phase with the male effect may be an adequate alternative for synchronizing estrus prior to artificial AI in the absence of previous estrus detection; fertility rates inseminating between 48 and 55 hours after prostaglandin injection vary between 44% and 62.5%.[48]

Proposed Protocol

Treatment consists of 2 doses of $PGF_{2\alpha}$ or analogues, by administering them 10 days apart, and exposure to the male effect coincidentally with the second dose (using vasectomized males if AI is to be employed). Dose is product dependent. A male to female ratio of 1:10 is recommended. Ewes will be in estrus for mating or AI approximately 48 hours after the second $PGF_{2\alpha}$ dose; insemination can be performed between 48 and 55 hours after the second injection.

COMBINATION OF PROGESTAGENS AND PROSTAGLANDINS

A possibility for reducing the exposure of animals to intravaginal devices and progestagen treatments is, of course, shortening the treatment period. In order for exposure to progesterone or progestagens to be effective, it should be longer than the luteal phase (ie, longer than the time of permanence of a CL in an ovary). Thus during the ovulatory season, to reduce the time of exposure it is necessary to eliminate the CL, usually by administration of exogenous $PGF_{2\alpha}$ or its analogue; this was first described in goats.[49] A sponge or CIDR is maintained intravaginally for 11 days instead of 18 days, while a single dose of $PGF_{2\alpha}$ is applied at day 9, that is, 2 days before sponge removal. eCG is administered coincidentally with the $PGF_{2\alpha}$, which allows a longer time of activity and a better recruitment and maturation of follicles and oocytes. Thus, fertility after insemination with frozen-thawed spermatozoa is improved when compared with classic protocols (61% vs 57%). At present, the time of permanence of intravaginal devices can be further decreased, to 5 to 7 days, both in sheep and goats; the effect on the ovary is similar to classic protocols and the fertility may be improved.[25,45,50,51]

Proposed Protocol

Treatment consists of insertion intravaginally of a sponge or CIDR for 11 days. On day 9 of the insertion, a single dose of $PGF_{2\alpha}$ is given and, if during the anovulatory season, a dose of eCG is also administered. At day 11, the sponge is removed and the males are introduced 24 hours later. This protocol can be revised to insertion for 9 days and injection of $PGF_{2\alpha}$ at day 7.

MELATONIN

The discovery of melatonin by Lerner and colleagues[52] opened up a new area of research in the field of seasonality of reproduction. In fact, most of the research related to melatonin and the pineal gland in the first 30 years after the discovery of the hormone related to properties of that hormone to regulate reproduction in photoperiod-dependent breeding animals. Photoperiodic information is received at the level of the retina and transmitted, via a multistep neural pathway, to the pineal gland, where the message modulates the rhythm of melatonin secretion.[53]

Most of the species tend to have births at the end of winter and spring, the most favorable period for the progeny to survive. Plasma melatonin concentrations are high during the night and baseline during the day, while the changing duration of the nocturnal melatonin secretion is a passive signal that provides information to the hypothalamus-pituitary-gonadal axis concerning the time of the year. Due to their gestation length, both sheep and goats are short-day breeders; their reproductive activity takes place during fall and winter (ie, as length of daylight decreases). Therefore, in these animal species melatonin can be considered as "progonadotropic." Photoperiodic treatments or different ways to administer melatonin to advance or induce a season of reproduction have been investigated during the last 30 years. Although the actions of melatonin occur at multiple levels and melatonin receptors have been identified in different organs and sites of the body, the main effect to modify the photoperiodic perception by the animal is exerted at the hypothalamic-pituitary level. In sheep, a significant increase of LH-releasing hormone (LHRH) secretion after 40 days and high LHRH and LH pulsatility after 74 days of melatonin treatment has been reported in anestrous ewes.[54] In fact, melatonin stimulates GnRH and LH secretion during the anestrus by reducing tyrosine hydroxylase activity in the median eminence.[55]

Melatonin Implants

Melatonin implants for subcutaneous application have been commercially available since the 1990s in several European countries (United Kingdom, France, Spain, Greece, Italy, Portugal, Turkey), as well as on other continents (eg, Algeria in Africa, Australia in Oceania) but are not available in North America. These implants have been widely used to advance the breeding season of anestrous ewes and goats. Melatonin implants induce high plasma concentrations of melatonin for 24 h every day, without suppressing the endogenous secretion of the pineal hormone during the night. Thereby, implants cause a short day-like response by lengthening the duration of the melatonin signal.[56] The implants contain 18 mg of melatonin and are designed to maintain high plasma melatonin concentrations for at least 60 days, although most of them continue to release the hormone for longer than 100 days.[57] The implant release maintains daytime plasma concentrations of melatonin above 100 pg/mL, in both ewes[58] and does.[59]

Proposed Protocol

The protocol for melatonin application is simple and less demanding than the traditional treatment of induction-synchronization of estrus using progestagens. Initially, each ram in a flock is subcutaneously injected with 3 melatonin implants, deposited at the base of the ear. Subsequently, the rams are taken away from the ewes in the flock. Seven days later, ewes in the flock are also injected, each with a single melatonin implant at the base of the ear. Rams are introduced to ewes 40 days after melatonin implantation in the females. It is important to observe this period, to give time to the ewes to respond to the new photoperiodic signal induced by the treatment.[54,60]

The time of treatment is important to guarantee a good efficacy. Melatonin implants inserted around the summer solstice have been widely used as a means of advancing the breeding season in ewes in areas with latitude more northern than N 45° or more southern than S 45°.[61,62] However, the breeding season starts earlier in animals in latitudes more southern than N 40° or more northern than S 40°[63]; in these areas, melatonin implants can be used at around the time of the spring equinox.[64] Of course, the need to use melatonin in latitudes between N 20° and S 20° is limited, as ewes in those areas have a throughout-the-year breeding pattern.

Melatonin in goats is necessary to induce cyclicity during anoestrus in a breeding system in which the bucks remain with the does[65] and to optimize the ovulatory activity induced by the male effect in temperate latitudes. In those areas, it is recommended that administration of melatonin to does is performed around the time of the spring equinox.[66,67] A maximum response can be obtained when melatonin administration follows up a photoperiodic treatment of long days for 2 to 3 months, starting around the winter solstice.[64,66] On commercial farms, long days in open barns are simulated with 2 artificial light periods per 24 hours, according to the flash method[68]: from 06:00 to 09:00 and from 22:00 to 24:00. In fact, melatonin treatment can be replaced by natural photoperiod when the long-day treatment is finished before the end of March, and a good response has been reported either after natural mating in response to male effect,[69] or after AI in seasonal goats treated with artificial photoperiod and progestagens and induced to ovulate by the male effect.[70] However, application of melatonin implants in goats is still not fully established.

A vast amount of knowledge on the practical use of melatonin to improve reproduction in sheep is now available. Melatonin implants can be used to advance the onset of the breeding season and/or to increase productivity after mating. Both fertility and

Table 1
Summary of the features of the main pharmacologic treatments available to control reproduction in small ruminants

Hormone	Pharmaceutical Form	Route of Administration	Dose	Season for Use	Time for Introduction of Male Animals into the Females	Optimum Male:Female Ratio	Comments
Progesterone	CIDR	Intravaginal × 12–14 d	20–40 mg FGA	All year	36–48 h after removal of devices	1:5	Can be used in combination with eCG
Progestagen	Sponge	Intravaginal × 12–14 d	20–40 mg FGA, 60 mg MPA	All year	36–48 h after removal of sponges	1:5	Can be used in combination with eCG
	Melengestrol acetate	In feed × 8–14 days	2.5 mg MGA split in 2 feedings	All year	26–48 h after removal of feed	1:5	eCG injected 8 h after last feeding
eCG	Injectable solution	Intramuscular	250–500 IU	All year			Must be used after administration of progesterone or progestagens
Prostaglandin or synthetic analogues	Injectable solution	Intramuscular/ Subcutaneous	125 μg cloprostenol, 7.5 mg luprostiol	Breeding period	48 h after administration	1:10	Two injections with a 10-d interval
Melatonin	Implant	Subcutaneous	Rams: 3×18 mg; Ewes: 18 mg	Outside of breeding season	40 d after administration to ewes	1:20	Males separated from females for 45 d before introduction

litter size of treated ewes are improved; the number of lambs produced can be increased by 15% to 30%. The mechanisms by which melatonin improves reproductive performance are not fully understood, as the pineal hormone can act at different body sites. Effects at hypothalamus-pituitary level have been previously mentioned, and an effect at ovary level seems to be consistent, either by reducing atresia during late folliculogenesis to increase ovulation rate[71] or as a luteotropic agent[72] to improve fecundity rate and therefore litter size. A significant interaction, melatonin × level of nutrition, on ovulation rate has been reported by several investigators[58,73]; the effects of exogenous melatonin in enhancing the ovulation rate are more pronounced in ewes on a low plane of feed intake as compared with ewes on high-plane intake. Concerning the potential response to the male effect, melatonin seems to increase the number of cyclic ewes before the introduction of rams. Moreover, administration of melatonin leads to an increased proportion of ewes exhibiting full-length cycles in response to the contact with the rams,[74] probably as a consequence of its luteotropic effect. Therefore, the lambing period tends to be more compact in melatonin-treated ewes when the male effect is used.

Administration of melatonin during anestrus seems to improve the quality of gametes. It has been reported that melatonin implants in rams can improve fertility rate, either by increasing sperm progressive motility from days 45 to 90 after implantation[75] or by preventing capacitation and apoptosis of spermatozoa.[76] Oocyte quality, evaluated by in vitro developmental kinetics and blastocyst output, has also been found to be increased after melatonin administration in ewes[77] and does.[78]

SUMMARY

The possibilities to control reproduction in small ruminants using pharmacologic substances are well described and contrasted, and are useful tools that help to increase farm profitability. The various methods that can be used are summarized in **Table 1**. Moreover, a new approach claims the use of "biostimulation" in place of exogenous hormones and drugs to control and improve the productivity of sheep and goats.[24] This may be a long-term phenomenon, so it makes sense for animal producers in all countries to begin to move toward clean, green, and ethical practices.

Small ruminant species are short-day breeders, which is a crucial factor affecting the offer of lambs and kids throughout the year. An appropriate management of reproduction allows ewes and does to breed in the spring to increase the supply of product to the marketplace on a year-round basis. Pharmaceutical control of reproduction is possible, usually through administration of hormones or analogues related to the natural estrous cycle, such as progesterone, prostaglandins, and/or melatonin.

REFERENCES

1. Vesely JA. Induction of lambing every 8 months in 2 breeds of sheep by light control with or without hormonal treatment. Anim Prod 1975;21:165–74.
2. Schinckel PG. The effect of the presence of the ram on the ovarian activity of the ewe. Aust J Agric Res 1954;5:465–9.
3. Robinson TJ, Moore NW, Lindsay DR, et al. Fertility following synchronization of oestrus in sheep with intravaginal sponges. 1. Effects of vaginal douche, supplementary steroids, time of insemination, and numbers and dilution of spermatozoa. Aust J Agric Res 1970;21:767–81.
4. Karsch FJ, Dahl GE, Evans NP, et al. Seasonal changes in gonadotropin-releasing hormone secretion in the ewe. Alteration in response to the negative feedback action of estradiol. Biol Reprod 1993;49:1377–83.

5. Karsch FJ, Bittman EL, Foster DL, et al. Neuroendocrine basis of seasonal reproduction. Recent Prog Horm Res 1984;40:185–232.
6. Gouletsou PG, Fthenakis GC. Clinical evaluation of reproductive ability of rams. Small Rumin Res 2010;92:45–51.
7. Tsakmakidis IA. Ram semen evaluation: development and efficiency of modern techniques. Small Rumin Res 2010;92:126–30.
8. Dutt RH, Casida LE. Alteration of the estrual cycle in sheep by use of progesterone and its effects upon subsequent ovulation and fertility. Endocrinology 1948;43:208–17.
9. O'Mary CC, Pope AL, Casida LE. Effect on their subsequent lambing records of the estrual periods in a group of ewes and the use of progesterone in the synchronization. J Anim Sci 1950;9:499–503.
10. Braden WH, Lamond R, Radford M. Control of the time of ovulation in sheep. J Agric Res 1960;11:389–401.
11. Southcott WH, Braden AWH, Moule GR. Synchronization of oestrus in sheep by orally active progesterone derivative. Aust J Agric Res 1962;139:901–6.
12. Robinson TJ. Use of progestagen-impregnated sponges inserted intravaginally or subcutaneously for control of oestrous cycle in sheep. Nature 1965;206:39–41.
13. Ritar AJ, Maxwell WMC, Salamon S. Ovulation and LH-secretion in the goat after intravaginal progestagen sponge PMSG treatment. J Reprod Fertil 1984;72: 59–63.
14. Welch RAS, Andrewes WD, Barnes DR, et al. CIDR dispensers for oestrus and ovulation control in sheep. In: Proceedings of the 10th International Congress on Animal Reproduction & Artificial Insemination, vol. 3. Urbana (IL); 1984. p. 354–5.
15. Gordon IR. Controlled reproduction in sheep and goats. Oxford (UK): CAB International; 1996. p. 480.
16. Daniel JA, Sterle SW, McFadin-Buff EL, et al. Breeding ewes out-of-season using melengestrol acetate, one injection of progesterone, or a controlled internal drug releasing device. Theriogenology 2001;56:105–10.
17. Powell MR, Kaps M, Lamberson WR, et al. Use of melengestrol acetate-based treatments to induce and synchronize estrus in seasonally anestrous ewes. J Anim Sci 1996;74:2292–302.
18. Cline MA, Ralston JN, Seals RC, et al. Intervals from norgestomet withdrawal and injection of equine chorionic gonadotropin or P.G. 600 to estrus and ovulation in ewes. J Anim Sci 2001;79:589–94.
19. Langford GA, Marcus GJ, Batra TR. Seasonal effects of PMSG and number of inseminations on fertility of progestagen treated sheep. J Anim Sci 1983;57:307–12.
20. Simonetti L, Blanco MR, Gardon JC. Estrus synchronization in ewes treated with sponges impregnated with different doses of medroxyprogesterone acetate. Small Rumin Res 2000;38:243–7.
21. Scaramuzzi RJ, Downing JA, Campbell BK, et al. Control of fertility and fecundity of sheep by means of hormonal manipulation—review. Aust J Biol Sci 1988;41: 37–45.
22. Killian DB, Kiesling DO, Warren JE Jr. Lifespan of corpora lutea induced in estrous-synchronized cycling and anestrous ewes. J Anim Sci 1985;61:210–5.
23. Hawk HW, Conley HH. Sperm transport in ewes administered synthetic progestagen. J Anim Sci 1971;33:255–6.
24. Martin GB, Milton JT, Davidson RH, et al. Natural methods for increasing reproductive efficiency in small ruminants. Anim Reprod Sci 2004;82–83:231–45.
25. Letelier CA, Contreras-Solis I, García-Fernández RA, et al. Ovarian follicular dynamics and plasma steroid concentrations are not significantly different in

ewes given intravaginal sponges containing either 20 or 40 mg of fluorogestone acetate. Theriogenology 2009;71:676–82.

26. McCracken JA, Carlson JC, Glew ME, et al. Prostaglandin F 2 identified as a luteolytic hormone in sheep. Nature New Biol 1972;238:129–34.

27. Douglas RH, Ginther OJ. Luteolysis following a single injection of PGF2α in sheep. J Anim Sci 1973;37:990–3.

28. Light JE, Silvia WJ, Reid RC. Luteolytic effect of prostaglandin F2 alpha and two metabolites in ewes. J Anim Sci 1994;72:2718–21.

29. Acritopoulou S, Haresign W. Response of ewes to a single injection of an analogue of PGF-2 alpha given at different stages of the oestrous cycle. J Reprod Fertil 1980;58:219–21.

30. Godfrey RW, Gray ML, Collins JR. A comparison of two methods of oestrous synchronisation of hair sheep in the tropics. Anim Reprod Sci 1997;47:99–106.

31. Godfrey RW, Collins JR, Hensley EL, et al. Estrus synchronization and artificial insemination of hair sheep in the tropics. Theriogenology 1999;51:985–97.

32. Boland MP, Gordon IR, Kelleher DL. The effect of treatment by prostaglandin analogue (ICI-80996) or progestagen (SC-9880) on ovulation and fertilization in cyclic ewes. J Agric Sci 1978;91:727–30.

33. Barrett DMW, Bartlewski PM, Cook SJ, et al. Ultrasound and endocrine evaluation of the ovarian response to PGF2a given at different stages of the luteal phase in ewes. Theriogenology 2002;58:1409–24.

34. Gonzalez-Bulnes A, Veiga-Lopez A, Garcia P, et al. Effects of progestagens and prostaglandin analogues on ovarian function and embryo viability in sheep. Theriogenology 2005;63:2523–34.

35. Campbell BK, Scaramuzzi RJ, Webb R. Control of antral follicle development and selection in sheep and cattle. J Reprod Fertil Suppl 1995;49:335–50.

36. Gonzalez-Bulnes A, Souza CJ, Campbell BK, et al. Systemic and intraovarian effects of dominant follicles on ovine follicular growth. Anim Reprod Sci 2004; 84:107–19.

37. Deaver DR, Stilley NJ, Dailey RA, et al. Concentrations of ovarian and pituitary hormones following prostaglandin F2a-induced luteal regression in ewes varies with day of the estrous cycle at treatment. J Anim Sci 1986;62:422–7.

38. Houghton JAS, Liberati N, Schrick FN, et al. Day of estrous cycle affects follicular dynamics after induced luteolysis in ewes. J Anim Sci 1995;73:2094–101.

39. Ginther OJ, Kot K, Wiltbank MC. Association between emergence of follicular waves and fluctuations in FSH concentrations during the estrous cycle in ewes. Theriogenology 1995;43:689–703.

40. Bartlewsky PM, Beard AP, Cook SJ, et al. Ovarian antral follicular dynamics and their relationships with endocrine variables throughout the oestrous cycle in breeds of sheep differing in prolificacy. J Reprod Fertil 1999;115:111–24.

41. Viñoles C, Rubianes E. Origin of the preovulatory follicle after induced luteolysis during the early luteal phase in ewes. Can J Anim Sci 1998;78:429–31.

42. Rubianes E, Menchaca A, Carbajal B. Response of the 1-5 dayaged ovine corpus luteum to prostaglandin F2alpha. Anim Reprod Sci 2003;78:47–55.

43. Hacket AJ, Robertson HA. Effect of dose and time injection of prostaglandin PGF2α in cycling ewes. Theriogenology 1980;13:347–51.

44. Menchaca A, Miller V, Gil J, et al. Prostaglandin F2alpha treatment associated with timed artificial insemination in ewes. Reprod Domest Anim 2004;39:352–5.

45. Menchaca A, Miller V, Salveraglio V, et al. Endocrine, luteal and follicular responses after the use of the short-term protocol to synchronize ovulation in goats. Anim Reprod Sci 2007;102:76–87.

46. Hawken PA, Beard AP, Esmaili T, et al. The introduction of rams induces an increase in pulsatile LH secretion in cyclic ewes during the breeding season. Theriogenology 2007;68:56–66.

47. Evans ACO, Duffy P, Crosby TF, et al. Effect of ram exposure at the end of progestagen treatment on estrus synchronization and fertility during the breeding season in ewes. Anim Reprod Sci 2004;84:349–58.

48. Contreras-Solis I, Vasquez B, Diaz T, et al. Efficiency of estrous synchronization in tropical sheep by combining short-interval cloprostenol-based protocols and "male effect". Theriogenology 2009;71:1018–25.

49. Corteel JM, Leboeuf B, Baril G. Artificial breeding of adult goats and kids induced with hormones to ovulate outside the breeding season. Small Rumin Res 1988;1:19–35.

50. Menchaca A, Rubianes E. New treatments associated with timed artificial insemination in small ruminants. Reprod Fertil Dev 2004;16:403–13.

51. Menchaca A, Rubianes E. Pregnancy rate obtained with short-term protocol for timed artificial insemination in goats. Reprod Domest Anim 2007;42:590–3.

52. Lerner AB, Case JD, Takahashi Y, et al. Isolation of melatonin, the pineal gland factor that lightens melanocytes. J Am Chem Soc 1958;80:2587.

53. Bittman EL, Karsch FJ, Hopkins JW. Role of pineal gland in ovine photoperiodism: regulation of seasonal breeding and negative feedback effects of estradiol upon luteinizing hormone secretion. Endocrinology 1983;113:329–36.

54. Viguié C, Caraty A, Locatelli A, et al. Regulation of LHRH secretion by melatonin in the ewe. I. Simultaneous delayed increase in LHRH and LH pulsatile secretion. Biol Reprod 1995;52:1114–20.

55. Viguié C, Thibault J, Thiéry JC, et al. Characterization of the short day-induced decrease in median eminence tyrosine hydroxylase activity in the ewe: temporal relationship with the changes in LH and prolactin secretion and short day-like effect of melatonin. Endocrinology 1997;138:499–506.

56. Malpaux B, Viguié C, Skinner DC, et al. Control of the circannual rhythm of reproduction by melatonin in the ewe. Brain Res Bull 1997;44:431–8.

57. Forcada F, Abecia JA, Zúñiga O, et al. Variation in the ability of melatonin implants inserted at two different times after the winter solstice to restore reproductive activity in reduced seasonality ewes. Aust J Agric Res 2002;53:167–73.

58. Forcada F, Zarazaga L, Abecia JA. Effect of exogenous melatonin and plane of nutrition after weaning on estrous activity, endocrine status and ovulation rate in Salz ewes lambing in the seasonal anestrus. Theriogenology 1995;43:1179–93.

59. Delgadillo JA, Carrillo E, Morán J, et al. Induction of sexual activity of male Creole goats in subtropical northern Mexico using long days and melatonin. J Anim Sci 2001;79:2245–52.

60. Nowak R, Rodway RG. Effect of intravaginal implants of melatonin on the onset of ovarian activity in adult and prepubertal ewes. J Reprod Fertil 1985;74:287–93.

61. McMillan WH, Sealey RC. Do melatonin implants influence the breeding season in Coopworth ewes? In: Proceedings of meetings of the New Zealand Society of Animal Production; 1989. p. 43–6.

62. Haresign W, Peters AR, Staples LD. The effect of melatonin implants on breeding activity and litter size in commercial sheep flocks in the UK. Anim Prod 1990;50:111–21.

63. Martin GB, Tjondronegoro S, Boukhliq R, et al. Determinants of the annual pattern of reproduction in mature male Merino and Suffolk sheep: modification of endogenous rhythms by photoperiod. Reprod Fertil Dev 1999;11:355–66.

64. Chemineau P, Malpaux B, Pelletier J, et al. Emploi des implants de mélatonine et des traitements photopériodiques pour maîtriser la reproduction saisonnière chez les ovins et les caprins. INRA Prod Anim 1996;9:45–60.

65. Zarazaga LA, Gatica MC, Celi I, et al. Effect of melatonin implants on sexual activity in Mediterranean goat females without separation from males. Theriogenology 2009;72:910–8.
66. Chemineau P, Normant E, Ravault JP, et al. Induction and persistence of pituitary and ovarian activity in the out-of-season lactating dairy goat after a treatment combining a skeleton photoperiod, melatonin and the male effect. J Reprod Fertil 1986;78:497–504.
67. Wuliji T, Litherland A, Goetsch AL, et al. Evaluation of melatonin and bromocryptine administration in Spanish goats. I. Effects on the out of season breeding performance in spring, kidding rate and fleece weight of does. Small Rumin Res 2003;49:31–40.
68. Pelletier J, Thimonier J. The measurement of daylength in the Ile-de-France ram. J Reprod Fertil 1987;81:181–6.
69. Pellicer-Rubio MT, Leboeuf B, Bernelas D, et al. Highly synchronous and fertile reproductive activity induced by the male effect during deep anoestrus in lactating goats subjected to treatment with artificially long days followed by a natural photoperiod. Anim Reprod Sci 2007;98:241–58.
70. Pellicer-Rubio MT, Leboeuf B, Bernelas D, et al. High fertility using artificial insemination during deep anoestrus after induction and synchronization of ovulatory activity by the "male effect" in lactating goats subjected to treatment with artificial long days and progestagens. Anim Reprod Sci 2008;109:172–88.
71. Bister JL, Noël B, Perrad B, et al. Control of ovarian follicles activity in the ewe. Domest Anim Endocrinol 1999;17:315–28.
72. Abecia JA, Forcada F, Zuñiga O. The effect of melatonin on the secretion of progesterone in sheep and on the development of ovine embryos in vitro. Vet Res Commun 2002;26:151–8.
73. Robinson JJ, Wigzell S, Aitken RP, et al. The modifying effects of melatonin, ram exposure and plane of nutrition on the onset of ovarian activity, ovulation rate and the endocrine status of ewes. Anim Reprod Sci 1991;26:73–91.
74. Abecia JA, Palacín I, Forcada F, et al. The effect of melatonin treatment on the ovarian response of ewes to the ram effect. Domest Anim Endocrinol 2006;31:52–62.
75. Casao A, Vega S, Palacin I, et al. Effects of melatonin implants during non-breeding season on sperm motility and reproductive parameters in Rasa Aragonesa rams. Reprod Domest Anim 2010;45:425–32.
76. Casao A, Mendoza N, Perez-Pe R, et al. Melatonin prevents capacitation and apoptotic-like changes of ram spermatozoa and increases fertility rate. J Pineal Res 2010;48:39–46.
77. Vazquez MI, Forcada F, Casao A, et al. Undernutrition and exogenous melatonin can affect the in vitro developmental competence of ovine oocytes on a seasonal basis. Reprod Domest Anim 2010;45:677–84.
78. Berlinguer F, Leoni G, Succu S, et al. Exogenous melatonin positively influences follicular dynamics, oocyte developmental competence and blastocyst output in a goat model. J Pineal Res 2009;46:383–91.

Control of Important Causes of Infectious Abortion in Sheep and Goats

Paula I. Menzies, DVM, MPVM

KEYWORDS

- Abortion • *Campylobacter* • *Chlamydophila* • *Coxiella* • Goat
- Q fever • Sheep • *Toxoplasma*

Abortion in sheep flocks and goat herds at a level that significantly affects productivity is a common clinical problem. Accurate diagnosis is critical to ensure that control measures are effective. The case definition of abortion should include any of the following clinical findings and, on a flock/herd basis, many or all of these signs may be evident in many animals in the farm:

- A repeat breeding (remarking) rate of more than 10%, indicating embryo loss before day 12 gestation
- Remating (rebreeding, retupping) after a delay, indicating embryo loss after day 12 gestation
- A ewe/doe that does not lamb/kid at lambing/kidding time, despite a positive pregnancy diagnosis and no observed abortion
- Observation of a blood-tinged vaginal discharge, but no fetus or placenta found
- A preterm fetus (<142 days of gestation) and/or placenta are found
- Lambs or kids born at term (>142 days of gestation), with a proportion stillborn or born weak or moribund.

DEFINING AN ABORTION PROBLEM

In healthy flocks and herds, the proportion of ewes and does visibly aborting is generally less than 2%. This value is calculated as follows: no. of females aborting/[no. of females diagnosed pregnant or no. of females exposed to the male].

Abortion levels exceeding 5% or a clustering of abortions within a short time (eg, 2 weeks) or a given location (eg, pen or farm) suggests the need for an aggressive

The author has nothing to disclose.
Department of Population Medicine, Ontario Veterinary College, University of Guelph, Guelph, ON N1G 2W1, Canada
E-mail address: pmenzies@uoguelph.ca

Vet Clin Food Anim 27 (2011) 81–93
doi:10.1016/j.cvfa.2010.10.011
0749-0720/11/$ – see front matter © 2011 Elsevier Inc. All rights reserved.

diagnostic investigation. An abortion rate between 2% and 5% suggests that endemic disease may be present.

DIAGNOSTIC APPROACH TO AN ABORTION PROBLEM

A good history is critical in helping to focus the diagnostic investigation. Information to be collected should include proportion of animals at risk that have aborted; age, source and location on the farm of animals that have aborted; stage of gestation at abortion; animal movements and additions into the farm, including rams and bucks; previous abortion problems, including problems on farms from which brought-in animals have been sourced; vaccination history, particularly with respect to abortion vaccines, including timing of administration and dose; nutritional history, particularly salt and mineral feeding, starvation, and over-feeding of pregnant females; possible exposure to toxic or teratogenic plants or drugs; possible environmental factors, such as extreme heat, stress, or predation; clinical illness in the dam before, during, or after abortion.

To optimize the chances of a diagnosis, material from more than 1 abortion should be submitted for laboratory examination. It is critical that the placenta is included; 2 cotyledons with intercotyledonary placenta is the minimum material; whole fetuses and placenta are preferred. If specimens are to be submitted, the relevant diagnostic laboratory should be consulted for requirements of tissue types and preparation (eg, fresh, frozen, in formalin). Because many of the pathogens causing abortion have a zoonotic significance, gloves and protective clothing should be worn when handling abortive material. Contaminants, such as manure or dirt, should be gently removed from the specimens, but these should not be washed. Samples should be maintained chilled, but not frozen, and must be sent as quickly as possible. Serum from aborting and pregnant females may be useful in some cases. To properly aid in diagnosis, all aborting females should be sampled, followed by some (minimum of 10%) of the pregnant animals. Paired serum samples (in acute and in convalescent stage, 14–21 days after abortion) should be collected to identify an increasing titer.

MANAGING THE ABORTING FLOCK

Pregnant females should be removed from the aborting group and brought to a clean area. Aborting animals should be kept away from other livestock. Specific control measures may be initiated, based on a likely diagnosis, before any diagnosis is confirmed.

One should always be aware of the zoonotic risks from some of the infectious agents causing abortion. Farmers should be advised to wear gloves, boots, and protective clothing, to be changed before managing the healthy animals in the flock/herd. Face-protecting masks (such as an N95 mask) should be worn when assisting births or cleaning the barn. Pregnant women and immunocompromised people should not assist at lambings/kiddings and should not have any contact with parturient ewes or does. If the aborted animals are to be culled, they should be sold directly to slaughter once the vaginal discharge has cleared, rather than to an auction or to another flock as a breeding animal.

Each country or region may have a different prevalence of specific causes of abortion, but generally the most commonly diagnosed causal agents of abortion in sheep and goats are *Campylobacter jejuni* (sheep), *Campylobacter fetus* subsp. *fetus* (sheep), *Chlamydophila abortus* (sheep and goats), *Coxiella burnetii* (Q fever; primarily goats but also sheep) and *Toxoplasma gondii* (sheep and goats). This article addresses diseases caused by these agents, but there are many more other causes of abortion in sheep and goats, infectious (eg, *Salmonella* spp, border disease virus, *Listeria monocytogenes*, *Leptospira* spp, *Mycoplasma* spp, caprine herpes virus 1) or noninfectious (eg, iodine deficiency, plant toxins, heat shock, overnutrition). It is important to obtain a diagnosis, to make sure that proper control measures can be instituted.

SPECIFIC CAUSES OF ABORTION, AND CONTROL MEASURES

C jejuni

C jejuni is becoming the predominant species of *Campylobacter* associated with ovine abortion in the United States.[1] This organism is commonly isolated from sheep feces, but at least some strains and Penner serotypes are more abortifacient than others.[2,3] It can reside in the intestinal tract and gall bladder of sheep and goats, as well as of many other animal species including dogs, poultry, and wild birds.[4] Carrion-eating birds, such as crows and seagulls, may serve as a mode of transmission between flocks. *C jejuni* is well known as a human pathogen. It is responsible for diarrhea and occasionally septicemia, abortion, arthritis, and Guillain-Barré syndrome in humans.[5]

C jejuni abortion was traditionally believed to be responsible for sporadic outbreaks of abortion, affecting 25% or more of the pregnant flock and then subsiding. However, in light of recent work, it is likely that abortifacient strains are capable of flock-to-flock contagion, so flock immunity plays an important role in the duration and severity of the abortion outbreak.[1] After the initial abortion storm, flock immunity may limit disease.

The clinical picture of campylobacter abortion is usually not differentiated between species. Placentitis is moderate, with edema and hyperemia of the cotyledons.[6] Fetuses are aborted, usually about 3 days after death, and fetal livers may appear swollen with areas of target-shaped necrosis. Ewes may show transient diarrhea. Lambs may also be stillborn, or born weak and undersized if infected closer to term. Incubation period ranges from 8 to 60 days, most commonly being 14 to 21 days.[7] This short incubation suggests that ewes may become infected from ewes that aborted earlier in the lambing period.

In a recent study, most of the strains of *C jejuni* isolated were found to be of a single genetic clone.[1] This clone is highly resistant to tetracycline drugs, indicating that the use of this antimicrobial in its control is contraindicated. The same workers found that all 74 *C jejuni* isolates studied were susceptible to tilmicosin, florfenicol, tulathromycin, and enrofloxacin, whereas 97% were sensitive to tylosin, suggesting that those antimicrobials may be effective in managing a flock outbreak. In New Zealand, more than 1 strain of *C jejuni* has been implicated in ovine abortion, indicating the need for more work in this field to identify differences in abortifacient strains.[8]

Use of antimicrobials in the pregnant flock is usually recommended in an outbreak of *C jejuni* abortion, and, depending on how spread out lambing is and at what stage of pregnancies the disease is diagnosed, it may be effective in reducing abortions during an outbreak. However, it is critical that culture and sensitivity of the isolate be performed to determine the most appropriate antimicrobial to use. Treatment with antimicrobials, either to a large group of animals or in the feed for a prolonged time period, can be associated with increasing the risk of antimicrobial resistance, so, if possible, long-term use of antimicrobials should be discouraged.

In the United States and Canada, a commercial vaccine (Campylobacter Fetus-Jejuni Bacterin-Ovine, Colorado Serum Company) is available. The recommendation is to vaccinate the flock initially, using a primary series 60 to 90 days apart, starting before breeding, then to revaccinate annually, again before breeding. In the United States only, another vaccine (Campylobacter Fetus-Jejuni Bacterin, Hygieia Labs), which recommends specifically that the booster be given in mid- to late gestation, is available. Based on evidence listed in the product insert, it seems efficacious in preventing campylobacter abortions. In New Zealand, a similar attenuated combination product is available (Campyvax 4), with the primary series and booster vaccination being administered before breeding.

C fetus Subsp fetus

C fetus subsp fetus is frequently associated with large outbreaks of abortion that affect a significant percentage of the flock; however, it is becoming less common as a significant cause of ovine abortion in North America.[1] Outbreaks tend to be cyclical with marked abortion storms occurring every 4 to 6 years, but disease may occur every year at lower levels; this may suggest that flock immunity likely peaks after an abortion storm and then wanes to the point of the flock being highly susceptible again. However, little epidemiologic work has been done recently in North America with respect to this disease agent. Clinical presentation is usually not differentiated from that of C jejuni.

There are several serotypes of this organism associated with ovine abortion. In the USA, most of the isolates associated with abortion are A2 and C.[9] More recent work has shown that, in New Zealand, B1 is more frequently found.[10] This is important, because there is evidence that the vaccine strain should match the strain of the isolate.[11] If vaccination failure seems to have occurred, vaccination technique and vaccine handling should first be assessed, but identification of the strain should also be attempted to rule that out as a reason.

Antimicrobial resistance can occur with C fetus subsp fetus, but it seems less of an issue compared with C jejuni. However, all isolates should be tested for antimicrobial sensitivity. As with C jejuni, vaccination is the preferred method of control. The commercially available vaccines are the same as for C jejuni. There is some evidence that in New Zealand prompt vaccination in the face of an outbreak may be helpful.[12] Administration of the vaccine twice 10 days apart, when abortions occurred 6 weeks before the start of lambing, appeared to have some benefit compared with the unvaccinated animals, but was not of benefit when used in an outbreak already underway for 2 weeks.

C abortus (Ovine Enzootic Abortion)

This organism is one of the most common causes of abortion in sheep and goats in North America, the United Kingdom, and Europe. C abortus is a gram-negative intracellular organism that has 2 states: elementary bodies inside the cell and reticular bodies as the environmental form.[13,14] The clinical presentation is marked abortion in the flock, with severe placentitis on initial introduction and then enzootic levels of abortion of 5% to 10%, affecting mostly primiparous animals and new introductions in the flock. Abortion tends to occur at late term, but early fetal death and reabsorption can also occur.[15] The placenta is necrotic, with lesions affecting both cotyledons and intercotyledonary spaces; it becomes thickened and necrotic, as well as hemorrhagic, at the edges of the lesions.[16] Fetuses may be aborted necrotic, well preserved, or, rarely, mummified. Weak and stillborn lambs and kids are commonly seen. The cause of fetal death is believed to be the severe placentitis, which causes hypoxia and retardation of fetal growth.[17,18] Females infected as lambs/kids, before mating or at final stage of gestation, do not usually abort until the following pregnancy.[13] After aborting, ewes/does seem to be immune, but they can shed the organism in vaginal secretions during oestrus,[16] thus infecting other animals that may be pregnant at the time.

Transmission occurs from exposure to aborted materials, infected vaginal discharge, or from environmental contamination and ingestion.[13] Rams and bucks may be infected and transmit the organism.[16]

The development of immunity, which only occurs naturally after the ewe or doe aborts, is of great interest to researchers. Both humoral immunity, as measured by antibody levels, and cell-mediated immunity, as measured by IFN-γ production, develop as a result of the pathology associated with abortion.[18] Stimulation of a similar immune response is the basis for the development of effective vaccines.

Control of chlamydophila abortion in sheep and goats is effected either through the suppression of infection, by using antimicrobial drugs during gestation, or by stimulating a protective immune response. Control during an abortion outbreak is usually not successful because incubation of disease tends to be long (60–100 days), placentitis is usually severe, and fetal stress has already occurred for a long period before the first abortions occurring in the flock or herd.[17] However, the organism is generally susceptible to tetracycline drugs, so many control programs are based on either injections of long-acting oxytetracycline in mid- to late gestation or through medication of the feed or water. Either during an abortion outbreak (treatment) or commencing after 80 days of gestation (control) in flocks known to be infected, injections of long-acting oxytetracycline at a dose rate of 20 mg/kg bodyweight (bw) and repeated every 2 to 3 weeks may lower the abortion rate by half, but there is some disagreement whether multiple treatments are justified.[19–22] Despite administration of treatment as indicated, some ewes and does may still abort because of preexisting placental damage making fetal death inevitable; moreover, shedding at lambing is not always reduced.[19,20] Another consideration of using antimicrobials is assuring that antimicrobial residues are not present in meat and, perhaps more importantly, in the milk of dairy animals. Chlamydophila abortion is common in dairy goats in many parts of the world and, although a milk withdrawal following a single injection of 96 hours (subcutaneous injection, USA) to 7 days has been recommended in some jurisdictions, repeated injections may cause inflammation and slower elimination of the drug.[23] In countries where antimicrobials are not approved for lactating sheep or goats, the maximum residue limit (MRL) may be the detection limit, which is often lower than the published MRL for dairy cows. Therefore, it is important to test the milk before shipping and to understand local national regulations with respect to extralabel drug use in lactating dairy animals. In chronically infected flocks, feeding levels of 250 to 500 mg of the drug per animal daily, starting 60 days before the first expected lambing date has often been recommended. Higher levels are generally fed during an outbreak of abortion and lower levels are fed prophylactically; however, recommendations on dose and length of time can vary and there is no published information on true efficacy.

There are 2 types of vaccines available: inactivated and attenuated. Inactivated vaccines are usually developed from strains of _C abortus_ grown in embryonated chick eggs or, less commonly, in cell culture. At this time, only an inactivated vaccine is available in North America. The vaccination procedure is to initially vaccinate ewes 60 days before breeding and administer a second dose 30 days later (Chlamydia Psittaci Bacterin, Colorado Serum Company). Annual revaccination is required. Inactivated vaccines do not prevent shedding of chlamydial organisms at lambing.[13] Potential issues with these vaccines are loss of efficacy because of variable amounts of antigen in the vaccine or loss of antigenicity because of serial passage in in vitro cultures, as well as risks associated with vaccine production because of the zoonotic nature of the bacterium.[13,24] A temperature-sensitive mutant of _C abortus_, strain 1B, was developed for vaccine use and is currently available in Europe and elsewhere in the world. On challenge trials, this vaccine was found to protect against abortion, as well as to reduce organism shedding and confer a long-lasting protection.[25,26] It also seems to be effective in goats.[27] The vaccine is to be given once, at least 4 weeks before mating. Ewe lambs can be vaccinated at the age of 5 months. If individual ewes are revaccinated every 3 to 4 years and incoming sheep are properly vaccinated, abortion is significantly decreased in endemically infected flocks. However, because it is a live vaccine, there are warnings regarding human safety, hence it should be handled carefully. Recently, there has been a report regarding the isolation of the vaccine strain 1B from several cases of ovine abortion and it is suspected that it may sometimes be pathogenic.[28] Because current vaccines have these potential deficiencies, research continues to identify the antigens that provide the most protective response. If these can be identified and then produced using recombinant technology, the risks and disadvantages of current chlamydophila vaccines can be eliminated.[14] At this time, several subunit and inactivated vaccines have been evaluated, although none are at the commercial stage of production.[14,29]

Eradication of *C abortus* from an infected flock is difficult, so protection of an uninfected flock's status should receive attention. An accreditation program available in the United Kingdom is based on serologic examination of animals and surveillance of abortions, and is available to flocks that are likely not infected with *C abortus* and do not vaccinate (Enzootic Abortion of Ewes Accreditation, Premium Sheep & Goat Health Schemes, Scottish Agricultural Colleges). The intent is to accredit flocks as low risk and promote these flocks as a source of uninfected replacement animals for sale to other low-risk flocks. Programs like this require a serologic test with excellent sensitivity and specificity. *Chlamydophila pecorum,* frequently shed in the feces, is considered to be nonpathogenic or to cause arthritis and conjunctivitis in lambs and kids, but rarely causes abortion in small ruminants.[13] However, serologic tests may not differentiate between low titers to *C abortus* and those to *C pecorum*. Embryos obtained from infected ewes do not seem to harbor the organism and can be used to transfer valuable genetics to a clean flock.[30]

Occasionally, *C abortus* can cause significant human disease, particularly in pregnant women with contact with aborting or lambing ewes or goats.[31,32] Because of the risk of fetal death, it is important that producers and veterinarians handling infected animals take appropriate precautions.[33]

C burnetii (Q Fever)

C burnetii, the causative agent of Q fever, is an intracellular gram-negative organism that can infect a wide range of hosts, including ruminants (cattle, sheep, and goats), swine, cats, dogs, wildlife, rodents, birds, ticks, and humans.[34–40] The organism is shed in birth fluids, vaginal secretions, feces, and milk. This shedding can persists for weeks to months and the organism can survive for months to years in the environment, making infected animals a significant risk for human infection.[41,42] Sheep and goats become infected most commonly from mucous membrane contact with aborted materials but also from vaginal secretions or fluids and membranes from a normal parturition of flock mates, birth products and excretions of other species of animals, contaminated air, dust, manure, bedding, and semen from infected males.[43] Ticks may also shed the organism and contaminate the wool.

Clinically, abortion is more common in goats than in sheep; moreover, evidence indicates that goats shed many more organisms at kidding or abortion than sheep.[44] However, in both species, asymptomatic infection may be more common than reproductive disease. If the ewe or doe is pregnant and immunologically naive, then placentitis may occur and, if severe enough, abortion would occur, caused by hypoxia and starvation of the fetus. In initial outbreaks, abortion rates within a flock/herd can vary from 5% to 35%. Fetuses may be aborted in late term, and, in the same outbreak, may be stillborn or born weak. Uterine inertia and uterine rupture at the time of abortion has been reported in goats.[45] Abortion in subsequent years is less common because of flock/herd immunity, although goats can have repeated issues with reproductive failure.[46] However, it is possible to have no abortion in the flock/herd despite endemic infection.[47]

There is conflicting information on whether treatment of pregnant animals with oxytetracycline during an abortion storm has an effect on the course of disease,[48,49] and more work is needed in this regard. Shedding is not significantly affected by the prolonged use of antimicrobials in an infected flock/herd.[41,50] Application of biosecurity precautions is recommended to reduce spread of the organism, particularly to reduce risk to humans. These include burying or incinerating placentas and aborted fetuses, composting manure for at least 5 months before spreading, spreading manure only on still days, disinfection of lambing/kidding areas after careful removal of manure, wearing N95 masks when working with animals or moving manure, wearing gloves or disposable plastic sleeves when assisting with lambings/kiddings, and maintaining biosecurity regarding protective clothing.[46,49]

It is important to be able to reduce shedding, as well as abortion, to lower the risk to humans, and this is best done through the use of an available, inactivated phase I vaccine. At this time, the vaccine is not available in North America but is in common use in several countries in Europe and, of particular note, is being used in a mandatory vaccination program of dairy goats in the Netherlands.[51–53] Young stock are vaccinated twice before breeding, and annually thereafter. Animals vaccinated before exposure to the bacteria seem to be much less likely to shed. Animals infected before vaccination will continue to shed, but are much less likely to abort, thus reducing the number of organisms shed into the environment. Because of this, it may be that the disease could be eradicated from a flock/herd in 4 to 5 years, depending on replacement rate and maintenance of biosecurity measures. However, environmental contamination may persist. Other farm animals, such as parturient cats, can be an ongoing source of infection. Therefore, it is important that any vaccination program be combined with cleanup and biosecurity measures.[53]

The disease in humans (Q fever) makes this organism very important.[54] Although most people who become infected do not show any, or only mild, signs of illness, a significant proportion (20%) can develop severe illness that may result hospitalization and/or long-term disability. Disease in humans can manifest as acute atypical pneumonia, undulant fever, hepatitis, extreme myalgia and chronic fatigue syndrome, and, in chronic Q fever, endocarditis. Prompt diagnosis and treatment with an effective antimicrobial, usually doxycycline, is necessary for full recovery.[54] However, physicians are often unfamiliar with the disease and the vagueness of the signs may delay appropriate therapy. Death is a risk, particularly for elderly and immunocompromised patients.

People who work in high-risk situations must be knowledgeable regarding the signs of Q fever and the measures to reduce risk of infection from C burnetii. People may become infected from handling infected placentas and lambs/kids, from being present when sheep/goats are giving birth, and from windborne organisms from infected premises or dried organisms in the dust of barns.[55–58] In one outbreak associated with goats, the most important risk factors for humans becoming infected were contact with the placenta (odds ratio [OR] 12.32), being a smoker (OR 3.27), eating goat cheese (OR 5.27), and petting goats (OR 4.33).[59] In addition to proper biosecurity measures as discussed earlier, vaccination of humans at risk of contracting Q fever should be practiced, if possible. A commercial human vaccine is available in Australia and abattoir workers are routinely vaccinated with life-long protection.[60] A combination of animal and human vaccination with proper biosecurity measures should reduce the risk of disease, both in sheep and goats, as well as in the people who care for them or who live and work in rural communities.

T gondii (Toxoplasmosis)

T gondii is a protozoan parasite with a worldwide distribution. In many countries, it is one of the most commonly diagnosed causes of ovine abortion.[61] The sexual part of its life cycle is completed only in domestic and wild Felidae. The oocysts that are shed in their feces are infective for up to 18 months when protected from desiccation and sunlight. The asexual component of its life cycle may occur in any warm-blooded animal.[62] Naive cats, particularly kittens first learning to hunt, may become infected by ingesting food or animals containing cysts, such as rodents, birds, offal from slaughtered farm animals, and aborted fetuses and placentas. Cats will shed up to 100 million oocysts, starting 3 to 10 days after ingestion, for approximately 2 to 3 weeks.[62,63] Feces and, therefore, oocysts, are ingested by small ruminants through contamination of water, feed, or pasture. Rodents and birds may also disseminate the parasite through ingesting cat feces and then defecating oocysts. If a ewe/doe is pregnant and immunologically naive when ingesting the oocysts, the organism will infect the fetus via the trophoblast cells of the placenta approximately 14 days after ingestion.[62] A second method of infection of the fetus is through congenital infection from the dam to offspring.[64] The importance of this route of infection and its clinical consequences is still controversial, but it is claimed that lambs infected this way are more likely to suffer mortality. Other researchers state that congenital infection from the dam is a rare event and not important.[63]

Fetuses at all stages of gestation are susceptible to infection. Infection in early gestation usually results in fetal death and abortion, in which the fetus may be reabsorbed, macerated, mummified, or preserved.[63] Infection at a later stage may result in a stillbirth or weak lamb/kid. Abortion levels may vary from 5% to 100%. It is common to see mummies and stillborn kids or lambs within 1 litter, whereas other animals of the litter appear clinically healthy. Maternal immunity, timing of exposure, and dose of oocysts determine the level of abortion in a flock or herd. Ewes and does infected before pregnancy will rarely abort if reinfected.[63] Flocks affected by toxoplasma abortion often have had contact with kittens, either directly or from fecal contamination of forages, water, or grain. Presence of mummies and changes to the placental cotyledons in which there are small white foci of necrosis and calcification are suggestive of toxoplasmosis.[62] Histologic and immunohistochemical examinations will help to confirm the diagnosis. Polymerase chain reaction is usually positive.[65,66]

In flocks/herds in which toxoplasmosis has been diagnosed, often little can be done during the lambing/kidding period. Control can be instituted either through feeding of prophylactic medications during gestation or by the use of a modified live vaccine. Feeding monensin at a dose rate of 16.8 mg per head daily has been shown to reduce losses if delivered throughout gestation.[67] Decoquinate is licensed in the United Kingdom for the control of ovine abortion caused by toxoplasmosis.[68] The drug is to be included in the gestating ewe ration at a rate of 2 mg per kg bw daily for the final 14 weeks of gestation; this is twice the recommended rate of inclusion to lambs and kids for the control of coccidiosis. Inclusion rates in the feed should be calculated to deliver this dose. A similar study to evaluate the effectiveness of lasalocid in controlling toxoplasma abortion in ewes did not find protection.[69] A modified live vaccine is available in New Zealand and Europe and confers excellent immunity for at least 18 months and probably for life. The vaccine is not available in North America. The vaccine contains reconstituted freeze-dried live tachyzooites that have lost the ability to produce tissue cysts and oocysts.[61] The ewe is vaccinated at least 21 days before mating and develops a transient fever. Ewe lambs may be vaccinated after the age of 5 months. A booster vaccination is recommended after 2 years. The drawback to the vaccine is that it has a short shelf life (10 days) after reconstitution. It is also potentially zoonotic and must be handled carefully. However, the vaccine can be used in conjunction with either a modified live chlamydial vaccine or an inactivated coxiella vaccine, with no interference of immune response or risk to the ewe/doe, a program that leads to animals being immunized against 2 important causes of abortion.

Natural control of toxoplasma abortion may be practiced, either through a reduction of the risk of exposure of pregnant females to oocysts or by the intentional exposure of nonpregnant females and young stock to kittens that may be shedding oocysts, thus conferring protective immunity against reinfection during pregnancy. Reduction of exposure is achieved by removing all cats from the farm or spaying all the queens to eliminate new crops of kittens. Cats should also be prevented from defecating on hay and grain or near water. Kitty litter boxes can be kept in the barn near where the cats tend to congregate to encourage their use rather than defecating in the feed. The top layer of hay bales should be fed only to nonpregnant sheep or goats and the grain should be stored in metal containers. All these measures should help to reduce the risk of toxoplasma abortion.

Reduction of *T gondii* oocysts in the environment and in meat is important to lower the risk of toxoplasmosis in humans. Approximately 30% of adults in the United States have been found to have antibody titers to *T gondii*.[70] Pregnant nonimmune women are at the highest risk of disease. *T gondii* can cause congenital neurologic disease and blindness in human fetuses. It is an important cause of encephalitis in humans suffering from AIDS. Most humans probably become infected from consuming undercooked meat, although handling of cat feces should be considered as a source. Freezing meat to -12°C for 1 day or cooking meat to 67°C will kill tissue cysts.[70] Microwave cooking is uneven and may leave some cysts viable.[70]

SUMMARY

This article summarizes control measures for the 4 most commonly diagnosed causes of abortion in North America, New Zealand, the United Kingdom, and Europe. When dealing with an abortion outbreak in a flock or herd, diagnostic investigation is critical to assuring that any future control measures are effective and worthwhile. Biosecurity is an important consideration for any abortion control program, and should be promoted regardless of whether an abortion problem exists in the flock. Many of the infectious agents that cause abortion in small ruminants are also zoonotic pathogens, and producers should be educated to avoid risk to themselves and their families.

REFERENCES

1. Sahin O, Plummer PJ, Jordan DM, et al. Emergence of a tetracycline-resistant *Campylobacter jejuni* clone associated with outbreaks of ovine abortion in the United States. J Clin Microbiol 2008;46:1663–71.
2. Grove-White DH, Leatherbarrow AJ, Cripps PJ, et al. Temporal and farm-management-associated variation in the faecal-pat prevalence of *Campylobacter jejuni* in ruminants. Epidemiol Infect 2010;138:549–58.

3. Burrough ER, Sahin O, Plummer PJ, et al. Pathogenicity of an emergent, ovine abortifacient *Campylobacter jejuni* clone orally inoculated into pregnant guinea pigs. Am J Vet Res 2009;70:1269–76.

4. Ogden ID, Dallas JF, MacRae M, et al. *Campylobacter* excreted into the environment by animal sources: prevalence, concentration shed, and host association. Foodborne Pathog Dis 2009;6:1161–70.

5. Smith JL. *Campylobacter jejuni* infection during pregnancy: long-term consequences of associated bacteraemia, Guillian-Barré syndrome and reactive arthritis. J Food Prot 2002;65:696–708.

6. Jensen R, Miller VA, Molello JA. Placental pathology of sheep with vibriosis. Am J Vet Res 1961;22:169–84.

7. Frank FW. A comparison of some aspects of viral abortion and vibriosis of sheep. In: Proceedings of the 67th Annual Meeting US Livestock Sanitary Association. 1963. p. 308–17.

8. Mannering SA, West DM, Fenwick SG, et al. Pulsed-field gel electrophoresis of *Campylobacter jejuni* sheep abortion isolates. Vet Microbiol 2006;115:237–42.

9. Williams CE, Renshaw HW, Meinershagen WA, et al. Ovine campylobacteriosis: preliminary studies of the efficacy of the vitro serum bactericidal test as an assay for the potency of *Campylobacter* (*Vibrio*) *fetus* subsp *intestinalis* bacterins. Am J Vet Res 1976;37:409–15.

10. Mannering SA, Marchant RM, Middleberg A, et al. Pulsed-field gel electrophoresis typing of *Campylobacter fetus* subsp. *fetus* from sheep abortions in Hawke's Bay region of New Zealand. N Z Vet J 2003;51:33–7.

11. Fenwick SG, West DM, Hunter JE, et al. *Campylobacter fetus fetus* abortions in vaccinated ewes. N Z Vet J 2000;48:155–7.

12. Gumbrell RC, Saville DJ, Graham CF. Tactical control of ovine *Campylobacter* abortion outbreaks with a bacterin. N Z Vet J 1996;44:61–3.

13. Rodolakis A, Salinas J, Papp J. Recent advances on ovine chlamydial abortion. Vet Res 1998;29:275–88.

14. Longbottom D, Livingstone M. Vaccination against chlamydial infections of man and animals. Vet J 2006;171:263–75.

15. Papp JR, Shewen PE, Gartley CJ. *Chlamydia psittaci* infection and associated infertility in sheep. Can J Vet Res 1993;57:185–9.

16. Papp JR, Shewen PE. Chlamydial abortion. In: Proceedings of the American Association of Small Ruminant Practitioners. The AASRP organization; 1996. p. 83–8.

17. Navarro JA, Garcia de la Fuente JN, Sanchez J, et al. Kinetics of infection and effects on the placenta of *Chlamydophila abortus* in experimentally infected pregnant ewes. Vet Pathol 2004;41:498–505.

18. Rocchi MS, Wattegedera S, Meridiani I, et al. Protective adaptive immunity to *Chlamydophila abortus* infection and control. Vet Microbiol 2009;135:112–21.

19. Grieg A, Linklater KA. Field studies on the efficacy of a long acting preparation of oxytetracycline in controlling outbreaks of enzootic abortion of sheep. Vet Rec 1985;117:627–8.

20. Rodolakis A, Souriau A, Raynaud JP, et al. Efficacy of a long acting oxytetracycline against chlamydial ovine abortion. Ann Rech Vet 1980;11:437–40.

21. Mawhinney I, Chalmers WS, Brown D. Enzootic abortion - latest findings. In: Proceedings of the Sheep Veterinary Society. The SVS; 1998. p. 43–5.

22. Papp JR, Shewen PE. Pregnancy failure following vaginal infection of sheep with *Chlamydia psittaci* prior to breeding. Infect Immun 1996;64:1116–25.

23. Payne MA, Babish JG, Bulgin M, et al. Serum pharmacokinetics and tissue and milk residue of oxytetracycline in goats following a single intramuscular injection of a long-acting preparation and milk residues following a single subcutaneous injection. J Vet Pharmacol Ther 2002;25:25–32.

24. Keisler DH, Burke V, Copelin J, et al. A serologic survey in ewes treated with one of two Chlamydial/Campylobacter vaccines. Small Rumin Res 1989;2:345–58.

25. Rodolakis A, Souriau A. Response of ewes to temperature-sensitive mutants of Chlamydia psittaci (var ovis) obtained by NTG mutagenesis. Ann Rech Vet 1983;14:155–61.

26. Chalmers WS, Simpson J, Lee SJ, et al. Use of a live chlamydial vaccine to prevent enzootic abortion. Vet Rec 1997;141:63–7.

27. Rodolakis A, Souriau A. Response of goats to vaccination with temperature-sensitive mutants of Chlamydia psittaci obtained by nitrosoguanidine mutagenesis. Am J Vet Res 1986;47:2627–31.

28. Wheelhouse N, Aitchison K, Laroucau K, et al. Evidence of Chlamydophila abortus vaccine strain 1B as a possible cause of ovine enzootic abortion. Vaccine 2010;28(35):5657–63.

29. Jones GE, Jones KA, Machell J, et al. Efficacy trials with tissue-culture grown, inactivated vaccines against chlamydial abortion in sheep. Vaccine 1995;13: 715–23.

30. Williams AFJ, Beck NF, Williams SP. The production of EAE-free lambs from infected dams using multiple ovulation and embryo transfer. Vet J 1998;155: 79–84.

31. Jorgensen DM. Gestational psittacosis in a Montana sheep rancher. Emerg Infect Dis 1997;3:191–4.

32. Meijer A, Brandenburg A, de Vries J, et al. Chlamydophila abortus infection in a pregnant woman associated with indirect contact with infected goats. Eur J Clin Microbiol Infect Dis 2004;23:487–90.

33. Hobson D, Morgan-Capner P. Chlamydial antibodies in farmers in north-west England. Epidemiol Infect 1988;101:397–404.

34. Daoust PY. Coxiellosis in a kitten. Can Vet J 1989;30:434.

35. Htwe KK, Amano K, Sugiyama Y, et al. Seroepidemiology of Coxiella burnetii in domestic and companion animals in Japan. Vet Rec 1992;131:490.

36. Webster JP, Macdonald DW. Q fever (Coxiella burnetii) reservoir in wild brown rat (Rattus norvegicus) populations in the UK. Parasitology 1995;110:31–5.

37. Adesiyun AA, Cazabon EP. Seroprevalence of brucellosis, Q-fever and toxoplasmosis in slaughter livestock in Trinidad. Rev Elev Med Vet Pays Trop 1996;49: 28–30.

38. Boni M, Davoust B, Tissot-Dupont, et al. Survey of seroprevalence of Q fever in dogs in the southeast of France, French Guyana, Martinique, Senegal and the Ivory Coast. Vet Microbiol 1998;64:1–5.

39. Maurin M, Raoult D. Q fever. Clin Microbiol Rev 1999;12:518–53.

40. Cairns K, Brewer M, Lappin MR. Prevalence of Coxiella burnetii DNA in vaginal and uterine samples from healthy cats of north-central Colorado. J Feline Med Surg 2007;9:196–208.

41. Arricau-Bouvery N, Rodolakis A, Is Q. Fever an emerging or re-emerging zoonoses? Vet Res 2005;36:327–49.

42. Rodolakis A, Berri M, Hechard C, et al. Comparison of Coxiella burnetii shedding in milk of dairy bovine, caprine and ovine herds. J Dairy Sci 2007;90:5352–60.

43. Kruszewska D, Tylewska-Wierzbanowska S. Isolation of Coxiella burnetii from bull semen. Res Vet Sci 1997;62:299–300.

44. Rousset E, Berri M, Durand B, et al. *Coxiella burnetii* shedding routes and anti-body response after outbreaks of Q fever-induced abortion in dairy goat herds. Appl Environ Microbiol 2009;75:428–33.

45. Sandford SE, Josephson GKA, MacDonald A. *Coxiella burnetii* (Q fever) abortion storms in goat herds after attendance at an annual fair. Can Vet J 1994;35:376–8.

46. Berri M, Rousset E, Champion JL, et al. Goats may experience reproductive failures and shed *Coxiella burnetii* at two successive parturitions after a Q fever infection. Res Vet Sci 2007;83:47–52.

47. Grant CF, Ascher MS, Bernard KW, et al. Q fever and experimental sheep. Infect Control 1985;6:122.

48. Berri M, Crochet D, Santiago S, et al. Spread of *Coxiella burnetii* infection in a flock of sheep after an episode of Q fever. Vet Rec 2005;157:737–40.

49. Angelakis E, Raoult D. Review - Q fever. Vet Microbiol 2010;140:297–309.

50. Astobiza I, Barandika JF, Hurdato A. Kinetics of *Coxiella burnetii* excretion in a commercial dairy sheep flock after treatment with oxytetracycline. Vet J 2010; 184:172–5.

51. Arricau-Bouvery N, Souriau A, Bodier C, et al. Effect of vaccination with phase I and phase II *Coxiella burnetii* vaccines in pregnant goats. Vaccine 2005;23: 4392–402.

52. Enserink M. Infectious diseases. Questions abound in Q-fever explosion in the Netherlands. Science 2010;327:266–7.

53. van der Hoek W, Dijkstra F, Schimmer B, et al. Q fever in the Netherlands: an update on the epidemiology and control measures. Euro Surveill 2010;15:4–7.

54. Marrie TJ. Q fever pneumonia. Infect Dis Clin North Am 2010;24:27–41.

55. Welsh HH, Lennette EH, Abinanti FR, et al. Airborne transmission of Q fever: the role of parturition in the generation of infective aerosols. Ann N Y Acad Sci 1958; 70:528–40.

56. Yanase T, Muramatsu Y, Inouye I, et al. Detection of *Coxiella burnetii* from dust in a barn housing dairy cattle. Microbiol Immunol 1998;42:51–3.

57. Tissot-Dupont H, Torres S, Nezri M, et al. Hyperendemic focus of Q fever related to sheep and wind. Am J Epidemiol 1999;150:67–74.

58. Schimmer B, Ter Schegget R, Wegdam M, et al. The use of a geographic information system to identify a dairy goat farm as the most likely source of an urban Q-fever outbreak. BMC Infect Dis 2010;10:69–76.

59. Hatchette TF, Hudson RC, Schlech WF, et al. Goat-associated Q fever: a new disease in Newfoundland. Emerg Infect Dis 2001;7:413–49.

60. Gidding HF, Wallace C, Lawrence GL, et al. Australia's national Q fever vaccination program. Vaccine 2009;27:2037–41.

61. Dubey JP. Toxoplasmosis in sheep - the last 20 years. Vet Parasitol 2009;163: 1–14.

62. Buxton D. Protozoan infections (*Toxoplasma gondii, Neospora caninum* and *Sarcocystis* spp.) in sheep and goats: recent advances. Vet Res 1998;29:289–310.

63. Innes EA, Bartley PM, Buxton D, et al. Ovine toxoplasmosis. Parasitology 2009; 136:1887–94.

64. Hide G, Morley EK, Hughes JM, et al. Evidence for high levels of vertical transmission in *Toxoplasma gondii*. Parasitology 2009;136:1877–85.

65. MacPherson JM, Gajadhar AA. Sensitive and specific polymerase chain reaction detection of *Toxoplasma gondii* for veterinary and medical diagnosis. Can J Vet Res 1993;57:45–8.

66. Owen MR, Clarkson MJ, Trees AJ. Diagnosis of toxoplasma abortion in ewes by polymerase chain reaction. Vet Rec 1998;142:445–8.

67. Buxton D, Blewett DA, Trees AJ. Further studies in the use of monensin in the control of experimental ovine toxoplasmosis. J Comp Pathol 1988;98:225–36.
68. Buxton D, Brebner J, Wright S, et al. Decoquinate and the control of experimental ovine toxoplasmosis. Vet Rec 1996;138:434–6.
69. Kirkbride CA, Dubey JP, Libal MC. Effect of feeding lasalocid to pregnant ewes experimentally infected with *Toxoplasma gondii*. Vet Parasitol 1992;44:299–303.
70. Dubey JP. Strategies to reduce transmission of *Toxoplasma gondii* to animals and humans. Vet Parasitol 1996;64:65–70.

Control and Eradication of *Brucella melitensis* Infection in Sheep and Goats

José M. Blasco, DVM, PhD[a],*, Baldomero Molina-Flores, DVM, MSc[b]

KEYWORDS

- Abortion • *Brucella melitensis* • Brucellosis • Control
- Goat • Sheep

Brucellosis is a bacterial zoonosis caused by microorganisms belonging to *Brucella*, a genus of gram-negative bacteria that behave as facultative intracellular pathogens of ruminants, suidae, canids, and several wildlife species. Some of these bacteria are highly contagious as well as zoonotic; humans can acquire brucellosis readily from animals and their products, even though humans are not themselves contagious. Brucellosis is a complex disease, due to the variety of *Brucella* species involved that, although having species-specific disease syndromes, can sometimes cross-infect. To date, 8 species are members of the *Brucella* genus: *B abortus* (infecting mainly bovines), *B melitensis* (ovines and caprines), *B suis* (swines), *B neotomae* (desert rats), *B ovis* (ovines), *B canis* (canines), *B ceti* (cetacean), and *B pinnipedialis* (pinnipeds). Using a combination of several microbiological, serologic, and molecular tests, several biovars have been identified in some of the main *Brucella* species, including 3 biovars in *B melitensis*.[1]

B melitensis is the main etiological agent of brucellosis in sheep and goats. It is also the main agent responsible for human brucellosis, known as Malta fever. Abortion and infertility are the predominant clinical signs in small ruminants. Although there is a paucity of specific studies, it is recognized as a source of significant financial loss to both industries. Its incidence is very high in countries at the south and east of the European Union and in many low-income countries. Altogether, these affected

The authors have nothing to disclose.
[a] Unidad de Sanidad Animal, CITA/Gobierno de Aragón, Avenue Montañana 930, Zaragoza 50059, Spain
[b] ECTAD Unit for North Africa, Food and Agriculture Organization of the United Nations, FAO/SNE, 43 Avenue Kheïreddine Pacha, Tunis 1002, Tunisia
* Corresponding author.
E-mail address: jblasco@unizar.es

countries contain more than 70% of the susceptible world livestock,[2] making brucellosis internationally important. Bovine brucellosis has been successfully eradicated in many developed countries after significant investment and many years of vaccinating and culling. However, *B melitensis* infection in sheep and goats has been traditionally neglected, because small ruminant production represents generally a low-income activity practiced by landless farmers from marginal rural areas in the developing world. Due to these marginal and usually nomadic farming systems, the control and eradication of this infection is extremely difficult. The infection is practically of worldwide distribution; many countries are suffering a reemergence of the disease in sheep and goats and, accordingly, also in humans.

The global incidence of human brucellosis is not well known because of the low reporting figures, great variations existing between different geographic areas even within the same country. Whereas the reported incidence in most developed countries where infection is present is generally smaller than 1 case per 100,000 inhabitants, in endemic areas, such as some Arab countries, reports reach up to 200 cases per 100,000 inhabitants. However, because of the deficiencies in Health Services of many countries where brucellosis is endemic, there are no reliable data on the global status of the human disease. Nevertheless, a figure of 500,000 new cases per year is usually accepted as a global estimate,[3] reflecting the difficulties in recognizing a disease that, although grave, lacks pathognomonic symptoms and is thus underreported.[4]

The reasons of this high prevalence may a result of sociocultural factors, but compounded by the lack of adequate control measures being applied in small ruminant production systems. Contact with animals and occupational exposure, as well as food habits and lack of hygienic measures, represent the main risk factors for *B melitensis* infection in humans.[4] Because human-to-human transmission is rare, small ruminants are the main reservoir for human cases. Humans can be infected directly by contact with the conjunctival or oronasal mucosae of infected animals, or indirectly by the ingestion of contaminated animal products (mainly dairy products). Human brucellosis is predominantly an occupational disease; professions in direct contact with livestock (farmers, butchers, veterinarians, laboratory personnel, and so forth) are those at higher risk. As there is currently no viable method of preventing human brucellosis, to safeguard people attention must be directed toward effectively controlling the disease in sheep and goats. The diagnostic and prophylactic tools for this disease have been sufficiently validated to effectively fight *B melitensis* infection in sheep and goats, in most socioeconomic situations. What needs to be improved to assure success is the quality of the national veterinary services and administrative organizations involved. Although sheep and goats are the main reservoirs of infection for humans, in some countries bovines, buffalos, yaks, and camels can also be implicated. Unfortunately, there is a lack of knowledge on the alternatives for controlling *B melitensis* infection in these species. Accordingly, this review focuses exclusively on the different strategies that could be applied to either control or eradicate brucellosis in sheep and goats.

PREREQUISITES FOR IMPLEMENTING CONTROL OR ERADICATION PROGRAMS

When developing a national strategy for control or eradication, the veterinary services must select an approach compatible with the prevailing socioeconomic conditions and infection status. The impact of brucellosis on the livestock economy and human health and the costs of the different control or eradication strategies that could be implemented must be evaluated as part of this strategy. Aspects to consider include: knowledge of the local animal breeding practices and habits, which can vary between different regions of the country; agreement regarding the principles of the strategy with the local administration; and, in particular, the availability of adequate human resources to carry out the strategy. Finally, because of its zoonotic importance, cooperation between all related stakeholders is of paramount importance and should be promoted. Epidemiologic surveillance to detect human brucellosis in medical centers should be reinforced and notification of cases should be compulsory for both veterinary and public health services involved.

Improved collaboration between the public health and veterinary services can be encouraged, through the reinforcement or the establishment of national zoonoses committees, in which the relevant producer and consumer organizations should be also represented.[4] Provided that the national veterinary service organization is adequate, prevalence of disease and economic resources will dictate the approach. Test and slaughter (T/S) based programs are often unfeasible in developing countries because of the economic cost. In addition, countries that have successfully eradicated B melitensis offer monetary compensation to affected shepherds. Provided that the veterinary services organization, farmers' involvement, and the economic resources are adequate, the final technical elements to select a proper strategy should be the prevalence of disease and the definition of the minimal epidemiologic unit(s) of intervention. A survey should identify the percentage of infected flocks/herds, understanding that differences in prevalence would be expected between different regions placed in the same epidemiologic unit of intervention. Calculating mean prevalence figures for the whole country or particular region considered is a frequent error of decision makers, as those figures may not reflect local conditions. Accordingly, rather than taking generalist sanitary measures, decision makers should be ready to apply different strategies adequate to each of the different epidemiologic situations identified. The minimal epidemiologic unit of intervention should be a given territorial extension with similar epidemiologic situation. In some cases, this can be a couple of isolated flocks/herds in a village and in others, the whole flocks/herds of a given county, but frequently, all flocks/herds in a region or country. The implementation of any brucellosis sanitary strategies requires considerable technical training, and an awareness campaign aimed at the farmers and general population. Once all these elements have been properly defined, 2 possible alternatives exist to fight B melitensis infection in small ruminants: (1) control based on mass (whole-flock/herd) vaccination or (2) eradication based on T/S with or without vaccination. In both cases, the use of adequate vaccination procedures and diagnostic tests is of paramount importance.

DIAGNOSTIC TESTS AND VACCINES

Eradication of B melitensis in small ruminants by applying combined vaccination and T/S is unrealistic in many countries, as they do not have access to the appropriate tests. No serologic tests for B melitensis have been developed specifically, and it is widely assumed that the available tests for B abortus infection in cattle are also adequate for diagnosing B melitensis infection in small ruminants. Accordingly, the Rose Bengal (RB) and the complement fixation (CF) are the most widely used classic tests for the serologic diagnosis of brucellosis in sheep and goats.[5] Both tests detect antibodies raised against the Brucella smooth lipopolysaccharide (S-LPS). The RB test was developed originally for the diagnosis of bovine brucellosis and, despite the scant information available, it is also recommended for the screening of B melitensis infection in small ruminants.[1] The CF test is also considered suitable for the serologic diagnosis of brucellosis in small ruminants at population level.[1] However, the sensitivity of the CF test is poorer than that of both the RB and indirect enzyme-linked immunosorbent assays (ELISA).[6,7] In addition, both RB and CF tests lack specificity when testing sera from sheep and goats recently vaccinated with Rev-1, the only available vaccine against *B melitensis*.[8–10] However, specificity of all serologic tests is somewhat preserved (see later discussion), if the Rev 1 is applied by conjunctival route.[9,10] Several reports have confirmed the adequate sensitivity of the different ELISAs for the diagnosis of brucellosis in sheep. In general, the indirect ELISAs are good tests for surveillance purposes in countries in the latter phases of eradication and in which vaccination is no longer used. However, these ELISAs lack specificity when used in vaccinated animals, particularly when Rev-1 is used in adult animals. In these conditions, only the Native Hapten (NH) gel precipitation test[1,11] is useful for determining infection in vaccinated animals. Although the competitive ELISA is promising, this test lacks specificity in vaccinated animals and those infected with *Yersinia enterocolitica* O:9.[12,13]

Low-income countries would profit from improved vaccines and simple, specific, and inexpensive diagnostic tests. However, it is unlikely that these tools will be developed by richer countries, as they prefer eradication using automated surveillance tests to reduce labor costs. Therefore, interest in brucellosis research is waning in first-world countries, despite the disease imposing a severe burden elsewhere. Because of this, the World Health Organization has recently classified brucellosis among the 7 top "neglected zoonoses," a group of diseases that are simultaneously a threat to human health and a cause of poverty perpetuation.[14] The live-attenuated *B melitensis* Rev-1 vaccine is the only vaccine available, and has been proved to be effective for prevention of *B melitensis* infection in sheep and goats.[15] However, when administered by the classic subcutaneous method (individual doses of 1×10^9–2×10^9 cfu), a long-lasting serologic response is induced, which makes an eradication program based on combined T/S impractical. When the same vaccine is administered by the conjunctival method (at the same dose, but applied by conjunctival instillation in a smaller volume), the immunity conferred is similar to that induced by the classic subcutaneous method, but the serologic responses evoked are significantly reduced, making this program fully compatible with the application of an eradication program based on vaccination combined with T/S.[15] However, this type of program is still out of the reach of many countries that have only elementary veterinary services and limited economic resources. In these cases, a mass vaccination strategy is the only reasonable alternative to be applied to control brucellosis. Unfortunately, the vaccination of pregnant animals with Rev-1 administered subcutaneously can induce high numbers of abortions and the excretion of Rev-1 strain in milk.[15] Reduction of the Rev-1 dose (individual doses ranging from 10^3 to 10^6 cfu administered subcutaneously) has been reported as a method avoiding these significant adverse reactions while maintaining effective protection.[16] However, field and experimental data suggest otherwise,[15] so that the reduced doses of Rev-1 should never be recommended as an alternative to the vaccination with standard doses. Due to the risk of abortion, there is no entirely safe strategy for mass vaccination. Even conjunctival vaccination is not safe enough to be applied regardless of the pregnancy status of the animals.[15] It is recommended that Rev-1 not be used in mid-gestation animals, the main critical period for abortion as a consequence of vaccination.[15] However, this is impractical under field conditions, and some of the risks have to be assumed if the objective is to control the disease. Conjunctival vaccination of animals before the start of the mating season, during the late stages of the lambing season, or during lactation seems to be the safest approach to performing a whole-flock/herd vaccination program.[15] Another small but potential risk with the modified-live vaccine (proven minimal after >50 years of widespread use worldwide) is that this strain can infect humans[17] and is resistant to streptomycin, an antibiotic that in combination with doxycycline constitutes the most effective treatment of brucellosis in humans.[18] Accordingly, some minimal individual biosafety measures (protection glasses and gloves) and awareness campaigns addressed to people involved in vaccination procedures should be implemented to lessen the infection risks in humans. In the case of accidental infection with Rev 1, a combined doxycycline-gentamicin (or doxycycline-rifampin) treatment should be administered.[17,18]

The diagnostic interference generated by vaccination hampers T/S eradication programs. The diagnostic epitopes involved are located in the O-polysaccharide section (a homopolymer of N-formylperosamine) of the B melitensis S-LPS immunodominant surface antigen, the genetics of which have been recently elucidated.[19] Research to improve the classic vaccines by removing these S-LPS epitopes (ie, to develop rough—R—vaccines) has been conducted. Among the live rough Brucella strains obtained by classic attenuation methods, is the B abortus RB51 vaccine. However, its efficacy and safety with regard to bovine brucellosis is questioned[20,21] and it is not effective against B melitensis or B ovis infections in sheep.[20] Finally, human infections due to RB51 have also been described[22]; this mutant is resistant to rifampin, an antibiotic widely used in the treatment of human brucellosis.[18] Therefore, RB51 should never be recommended for vaccinating small ruminants. Other research efforts in developing R vaccines resulted in candidates of low overall efficacy.[20,23] Whereas R candidate vaccines do not interfere with the classic serologic tests (RB and CF), this cannot be said for ELISA. Using the S-LPS or its hydrolytic polysaccharides as antigens, it has been proved that an important proportion of ewes vaccinated with R candidates were detected to be seropositive in an indirect ELISA.[23] This result is not unexpected, because R mutants elicit antibodies to the core epitopes also present in the wild-type S-LPS and its hydrolytic polysaccharides. Core epitopes are not readily accessible on the whole S brucellae (used as antigen in the classic RB and CF tests), but they can become exposed on adsorption to ELISA plates and, therefore, prevent a clear-cut distinction of the antibody responses to S and R brucellae. This problem is likely to affect all R vaccines, including RB51, because the authors have found that a significant proportion of cows that aborted as a consequence of vaccination with RB51 develop antibodies reacting in ELISA tests.[21] As a conclusion, the potential advantages claimed for R vaccines have been seriously questioned and there is increasing evidence showing that these vaccines interfere in S-LPS–based ELISAs; flaws include lack of safety in pregnant animals, possible excretion in the milk of vaccinated animals, potential for human infection, and reduced efficacy compared with the classic Rev-1 and S19 vaccines against brucellosis in small ruminants and cattle.[20]

Other approaches to develop new-generation vaccines, such as the construction of recombinant strains deleted in relevant diagnostic proteins or DNA-based vaccines, are being also investigated.[24] In fact, a Rev-1 vaccine strain deleted in the gene coding for BP26 protein (that can be used as a differential marker) resulted in the same protective efficacy as Rev-1 in sheep.[25] Its efficacy was also evidenced against B ovis infection in rams, but evaluation of the performance of the BP26-based differential diagnostic test is limited.[26] Up to now, none of these new-generation vaccines have been found to provide an improvement over efficacy and safety of the classic Rev-1 vaccine. Therefore, Rev-1 should continue to be the reference vaccine for prevention of brucellosis in sheep and goats.[24] Independent of their origin, the Rev-1 vaccine and the diagnostic tests to be used should be always submitted for quality control to internationally recognized laboratories, and should fulfill the minimal requirements described by the World Organization for Animal Health.[1]

CONTROL STRATEGIES

Independent of the prevalence of infection, a whole flock/herd vaccination of all susceptible sheep and goats is the only reasonable strategy to control brucellosis in many low-income countries. To avoid the risk to pregnant animals, the focus should be on vaccinating young replacement animals (3–4 months old) exclusively. The hypothesis is that if 100% of young replacements (representing usually 20%–25% of the total population, depending on the animal species and breeding systems considered) are vaccinated yearly, the whole population would be fully immunized after only a moderate period of time (4–5 years). To be successful, all young replace-ments (both males and females) should be vaccinated and, ideally, also identified for successful follow-up. However, because of practical difficulties in vaccinating 100% of replacements, this strategy fails to control brucellosis even in developed countries[15] and it is generally inapplicable in the developing world. In the characteristic extensive husbandry conditions of small ruminants, several veterinary visits would be required to locate and vaccinate 100% of these animals. This practical problem, coupled with the difficulty of localizing all flocks/herds in nomadic breeding systems, results in frequent failures in adequate vaccination coverage. Therefore, the mass vaccination of all susceptible animals irrespective of age is the only suitable strategy to control brucellosis in sheep and goats in many countries. This mass vaccination could be complemented with an individual ear tagging (or alternative identification procedure) of vaccinated animals to facilitate appropriate follow-up of animals in subsequent years. However, ear tagging is not considered permanent, is expensive, and can predispose animals to fly-strike.

To be effective, any whole-flock/herd vaccination program should be maintained over time. The ideal follow-up procedure to minimize Rev-1 side effects could be vaccinating exclusively the young replacements every year and for at least 5 to 6 years following the first mass vaccination campaign, which should include ear tagging. The characteristic annual replacement figures for small ruminants in extensive breeding systems usually range from 20% to 25%. Therefore, the next year after the one when the first mass vaccination program takes place, only 20% to 25% of the popu-lation would be new and susceptible to the disease. Because of a flock/herd immunity effect, transmission to this relatively low percentage of unvaccinated replacements— already low risk as they are not pregnant—is much smaller, making the need for an annual mass vaccination unnecessary. By contrast, 2 years after mass vaccination, around 40% to 50% of the entire flock/herd population would be fully unprotected and would contain a high proportion of animals at risk (pregnant and lactating). There-fore, a practical and cost-effective recommendation would be to repeat the mass vaccination of the entire flock/herd animals by using Rev-1 every 2 years.[15] To mini-mize the Rev-1 side effects, the ideal window of opportunity (ie, before the start of the mating season, during the late stages of the lambing season, or during lactation) should be selected. This approach is especially feasible when taking into account the characteristic seasonal breeding of sheep and goats. In fact, many mass vaccina-tion campaigns, covering several million of sheep and goats in many countries, have been applied using this strategy and very few adverse effects have been reported.

ERADICATION PROGRAMS

Vaccination itself is a suitable measure to control brucellosis, but additional measures are required for eradication. Once the disease is controlled, and provided that the veterinary services and economic resources of the concerned country have been also improved, eradication could become feasible. Eradication could be achieved through implementation of a very complex and expensive program based on the combination of vaccination of young replacements (3–4 months old, both males and females, and exclusively by the conjunctival method) with the T/S of adult animals found to be seropositive. The basic principle for eradication is avoiding the introduction of infected animals into healthy flocks/herds. Accordingly, as complementary tools, the effective control of all animal movements and the adequate individual identification would be implemented in the selected epidemiologic unit of intervention. The control of animal movements is probably one of the most problematic issues faced by the veterinary services involved in any brucellosis eradication program. The successful application of this complex combined eradication program for at least one entire generation (5–6 years) could lead to a generalized brucellosis-free status in the epidemiologic unit involved. In a final eradication step, ban of Rev-1 vaccination and application of an exclusive T/S program (applying either partial of full depopulation of infected flocks/herds) could lead to complete eradication of the disease and granting of official brucellosis-free status for the epidemiologic unit considered.

Once brucellosis has been controlled by Rev-1–based mass vaccination, a combined eradication program could be selected. Because the serologic interference caused by Rev-1 in vaccinated adult animals is of higher intensity and duration than that induced in young replacements,[12] the interpretation of serologic results during the passage from mass vaccination to a combined eradication program is critical to avoid the unnecessary culling of healthy but seropositive animals. With this in consideration, 2 effective possibilities could be recommended when finishing a mass vaccination control strategy and starting a combined eradication program.

The first possibility could be to avoid the serologic screening of the mass-vaccinated animals for a period of at least 2 years after finishing mass vaccination. Vaccinated adults, particularly those having contact with field *B melitensis* strains, are at risk of developing persistent antibody responses. To prevent these specificity issues, it is recommended that during the 2 first years after stopping mass vaccination, veterinary services (1) maintain the conjunctival vaccination of the whole replacements, and/or (2) individually identify the entire sheep and goat population and establish a system for controlling animal movements. Effective control of the animal movement is very expensive and requires suitable identification, perfect administrative organization of the veterinary services involved, and the active collaboration of farmers. Once this recommended period of 2 years is finished, it is expected that the serologic background of the vaccinated population will be reduced significantly. Then the individual testing (RB test as screening test) of all adult animals, that is, older than 12 to 16 months (with, at least, the first pair of permanent incisors erupted), and culling of those detected as positive in the CF test (≥30 IU) could be recommended as complementary to the aforementioned interventions (1) and (2). The flocks/herds having at least one CF-positive animal should be retested as many times as necessary, until 2 negative consecutive whole-flock CF tests result. This outcome would allow the certification of the flock/herd as "brucellosis-free."

The second possibility could include, in addition to the interventions (1) and (2), testing and culling of seropositive animals soon after mass vaccination is finished. As indicated, the serologic background of adult vaccinated animals living in infected contexts is complex, and none of the S-LPS–based immunologic tests available (ie, RB, CF, or ELISA) is 100% sensitive nor specific. However, as mentioned previously, the NH gel precipitation test has superior sensitivity and specificity in vaccinated animals.[1,11,12] Accordingly, 6 to 12 months after the last mass vaccination has been performed, NH gel precipitation testing and culling of seropositive animals could be implemented in those older than 12 to 16 months. Not only would this eliminate infected animals but would lower the challenge to vaccinated animals (anamnestic response), making their serologic responses easier to interpret. This NH testing should be repeated as frequently as possible in each flock/herd identified as infected, until at least 2 consecutive negative tests are obtained. Then the testing schedule could be performed using the classic RB and CF testing already indicated. This strategy could be applied for several years, until arriving at null prevalence and obtaining a generalized brucellosis-free status in the epidemiologic unit of intervention. This brucellosis-free status is the most recommendable technical strategy, because the disease is eradicated yet, simultaneously, the population is immunized, thus being able to facing new infections caused by accidental reintroduction from neighboring epidemiologic units still infected.

When a brucellosis-free situation is maintained for many years, an exclusive test and slaughter program with banning of vaccination could be applied with the objective of a country or region obtaining the brucellosis "officially-free" status. This status is required for international animal trade[1] and is considered erroneously by many veterinarians as the highest sanitary standard. However, it is difficult to understand why the veterinary services from many countries where B melitensis has not been eradicated are in favor of the generalized officially-free rather than the brucellosis-free status, even in the absence of farmers exporting live animals to international markets. Vaccination should be banned only when a generalized brucellosis-free status has been firstly obtained in the whole epidemiologic unit involved, and this situation has been maintained for many years. Premature cessation of vaccination is the most frequent error of decision makers during the late stages of a B melitensis eradication campaign. As a general rule, the Rev-1 vaccine should be never abandoned until 4 requisites are fulfilled simultaneously: (1) existence of a generalized need of farmers to access international markets, (2) the prevalence is null in the whole epidemiologic unit, (3) this eradication situation is maintained in absence of new cases during at least one entire generation (4–6 years), and (4) risks of transmission or reintroduction of infection from infected neighboring epidemiologically related units are negligible. Once Rev-1 vaccination is stopped, the detection and immediate culling of positive animals in an adequate repetitive context by means of the proper diagnostic tests (ie, association RB + CF, indirect ELISAs + CF, or indirect ELISAs alone), could allow the generalized officially-free status. During these final eradication steps, it is recommended that test results have a collective rather than an individual interpretation. The entire stamping out of flocks/herds detected as infected is frequently more practical and effective than the partial culling of only the seropositive animals identified. As prevalence drops, even a test with acceptable specificity will have a low predictive value of a positive test (PVPT), meaning that most test-positive individuals are actually healthy. By way of example, with a test with 99% sensitivity and 99% specificity and a disease prevalence of 20% (1 in 5 animals infected), the PVPT is 96%, meaning that of 100 positive tests 96 animals will actually be infected. But at a prevalence of 1%, the PVPT is 50%, meaning half of all test-positive animals will be healthy. This problem has increased significantly in many officially-free countries as a consequence of the false-positive serologic responses caused by Y enterocolitica O:9 and other bacteria sharing cross-reactive epitopes with the Brucella S-LPS.[5]

When the disease has been eradicated, a surveillance program has to be implemented for early detection of new outbreaks or reintroduction. Passive surveillance systems based, for example, on the compulsory declaration of abortions by farmers are not sensitive enough and have proved ineffective for the early detection of disease. Accordingly, an active surveillance system is preferred that can be based on the regular serologic screening of a representative sample of the population (RB or indirect ELISAs could be suitable tests for this purpose). Use of generalist and empiric sampling rules (as an example, some European Union countries test only 25% of adult females in a 3-year interval to maintain the officially-free status) should be avoided. It is more recommendable to test regularly (once a year should be a minimum) a representative sample of the population considered, the composition of the sample being calculated using adequate epidemiologic software, by taking into consideration the number of flocks/herds, the average number of animals per flock/herd, the threshold level of expected prevalence, and the confidence level of the expected results.

SUMMARY

B melitensis is the main responsible causal agent of brucellosis in sheep and goats and is the primary cause of brucellosis in human beings in many countries. Several strategies to control and eradicate this infection in small ruminants have been proposed and used by national and international animal health organizations. This article reviews the different control and eradication strategies used in small ruminants in different socioeconomic and epidemiologic situations.

REFERENCES

1. OIE. Manual of diagnostic tests and vaccines for terrestrial animals. 6th edition. Paris: OIE; 2008. p. 1343.
2. FAO. Global livestock production and health atlas. Rome (Italy): FAO; 2006. Electronic edition. Available at: http://kids.fao.org/glipha/. Accessed May 5, 2010.
3. Pappas G, Papadimitriou P, Akritidis N, et al. The new global map of human brucellosis. Lancet Infect Dis 2006;6:91–9.
4. WHO. The control of neglected zoonotic diseases: a route to poverty alleviation. In: Proceedings of a Joint WHO/DFID-AHP/FAO/OIE Meeting. Geneva (Switzerland): 20 and 21 September, 2005.
5. MacMillan A. Conventional serological tests. In: Nielsen K, Duncan JR, editors. Animal brucellosis. Boca Raton (FL): CRC Press; 1990. p. 153–98.
6. Blasco JM, Garin-Bastuji B, Marín CM, et al. Efficacy of different Rose Bengal and complement fixation antigens for the diagnosis of *Brucella melitensis* in sheep and goats. Vet Rec 1994;134:415–20.
7. Blasco JM, Marín C, De Bagués MP, et al. Evaluation of allergic and serological tests for diagnosing *Brucella melitensis* infection in sheep. J Clin Microbiol 1994; 32:1835–40.
8. Fensterbank R, Pardon P, Marly J. Comparison between subcutaneous and conjunctival route of vaccination of Rev-1 strain against *B. melitensis* infection in ewes. Ann Rech Vet 1982;13:295–301.
9. De Bagués MPJ, Marín CM, Blasco JM, et al. An ELISA with *Brucella* lipopolysaccharide antigen for the diagnosis of *B. melitensis* infection in sheep and for the evaluation of serological responses following subcutaneous or conjunctival *B. melitensis* Rev-1 vaccination. Vet Microbiol 1992;30:233–41.
10. Díaz-Aparicio E, Marín C, Alonso B, et al. Evaluation of serological tests for diagnosis of *B. melitensis* infection of goats. J Clin Microbiol 1994;32:1159–65.
11. Díaz R, Garatea P, Jones L, et al. Radial immunodiffusion test with a *Brucella* polysaccharide antigen for differentiating infected from vaccinated cattle. J Clin Microbiol 1979;10:37–41.
12. Marín C, Moreno E, Moriyón I, et al. Performance of competitive and indirect ELISAs, gel immunoprecipitation with native hapten polysaccharide and standard

serological tests in diagnosis of sheep brucellosis. Clin Diagn Lab Immunol 1999;6: 269–72.

13. Muñoz PM, Marín CM, Monreal D, et al. Efficacy of several serological tests and antigens for diagnosis of bovine brucellosis in the presence of false-positive serological results due to *Yersinia enterocolitica* O:9. Clin Diagn Lab Immunol 2005;12:141–51.

14. Maudlin I, Weber S. The control of neglected zoonotic diseases: a route to poverty alleviation. Geneva (Switzerland): WHO; 2006. p. 54.

15. Blasco JM. A review of the use of *B. melitensis* Rev-1 vaccine in adult sheep and goats. Prev Vet Med 1997;31:275–81.

16. Al Khalaf SA, Mohamad BT, Nicoletti P. Control of brucellosis in Kuwait by vaccination of cattle, sheep and goats with *Brucella abortus* strain 19 or *Brucella melitensis* strain Rev-1. Trop Anim Health Prod 1992;24:45–9.

17. Blasco JM, Díaz R. *Brucella melitensis* Rev 1 vaccine as a cause of human brucellosis. Lancet 1993;342:805.

18. Ariza J, Bosilkovski M, Cascio A, et al. Perspectives for the treatment of brucellosis in the 21st century: the Ioannina recommendations. PLoS Med 2007;4:1872–8.

19. González D, Grilló MJ, de Miguel MJ, et al. Brucellosis vaccines: assessment of *Brucella melitensis* lipopolysaccharide rough mutants defective in core and O-polysaccharide synthesis and export. PLoS One 2008;3:e2760.

20. Moriyón I, Grilló MJ, Monreal D, et al. Rough vaccines in animal brucellosis: structural and genetic basis and present status. Vet Res 2004;35:1–38.

21. Mainar-Jaime RC, Marín CM, De Miguel MJ, et al. Experiences on the use of RB51 vaccine in Spain. In: Proceedings of the Brucellosis 2008 International Conference, London (United Kingdom): Veterinary Laboratory Agency; 2008. p. 40.

22. Villarroel M, Grell M, Saenz R. Isolation and identification of *Brucella abortus* RB51 in human: first report in Chile. Arch Med Vet 2000;32:89–91.

23. Barrio MB, Grilló MJ, Muñoz PM, et al. Rough mutants defective in core and O-polysaccharide synthesis and export induce antibodies reacting in an indirect ELISA with smooth lipopolysaccharide and are less effective than Rev-1 vaccine against *Brucella melitensis* infection of sheep. Vaccine 2009;27:1741–9.

24. Blasco JM. Existing and future vaccines against brucellosis in small ruminants. Small Rumin Res 2006;62:33–7.

25. Jacques I, Verger JM, Larocau K, et al. Immunological responses and protective efficacy against *Brucella melitensis* induced by bp26 and omp31 *B. melitensis* Rev.1 deletion mutants in sheep. Vaccine 2007;25:794–805.

26. Grilló MJ, Marín CM, Barberán M, et al. Efficacy of bp26 and bp26/omp31 *B. melitensis* Rev.1 deletion mutants against *Brucella ovis* in rams. Vaccine 2009;27:187–91.

Treatment and Control of Peri-Parturient Metabolic Diseases: Pregnancy Toxemia, Hypocalcemia, Hypomagnesemia

Christos Brozos, DVM, PhD[a], Vasia S. Mavrogianni, DVM, PhD[b],
George C. Fthenakis, DVM, Msc, PhD[b],*

KEYWORDS

- Goat • Hypocalcemia • Hypomagnesemia
- Metabolic diseases • Pregnancy toxemia • Sheep • Treatment

In general, peri-parturient metabolic diseases in ewes and does—pregnancy toxemia, hypocalcemia, and hypomagnesemia—are caused by the failure of animals to have their nutritional requirements met during late pregnancy and/or early lactation. These disorders can be significant causes of peri-parturient mortality of ewes and does.[1–3] Decreased intake of the respective nutrients, usually in association with increased requirements of the animals, contributes to development of the pathologic conditions. Various factors can predispose the animals to these diseases. The early stages of the pathologic conditions are characterized by reduced appetite, which leads to further reduction of the intake of nutrients, in turn precipitating development of the disease and increasing morbidity. This article provides guidelines on the treatment and control of 3 peri-parturient diseases in ewes and does, namely pregnancy toxemia, hypocalcemia, and hypomagnesemia.

PREGNANCY TOXEMIA

Pregnancy toxemia ("twin-lamb disease") is a metabolic disorder of pregnant small ruminants, caused by an abnormal metabolism of carbohydrates and fats, which

The authors have nothing to disclose.
[a] School of Veterinary Medicine, Aristotle University of Thessaloniki, Thessaloniki, Greece
[b] University of Thessaly, PO Box 199, 43100 Karditsa, Greece
* Corresponding author. University of Thessaly, PO Box 199, 43100 Karditsa, Greece.
E-mail address: gcf@vet.uth.gr

occurs at the final stage of pregnancy. The disease occurs more frequently in ewes than in does; lean (body condition score <2 in the 5-point scale) or obese (body condition score ≥4) animals, as well as animals carrying 2 or more fetuses, are at higher risk of developing the disease. The disease is characterized by development of hypoglycemic encephalopathy. Animals show anorexia, depression, neurologic signs, and blindness, followed by recumbency and coma.[4] The salient paraclinical findings are hypoglycemia and hyperketonemia/hyperketonuria of affected animals.

Treatment of Clinically Ill Female Animals

Treatment of the disorder should be based on 2 general principles: (a) administration of energy sources and (b) removal of factors that increase energy requirements of affected animals. The efficacy of the treatment depends on early instigation which, in turn, relies on timely and correct diagnosis of the disease. However, even in cases of early instigation of treatment, this may still fail. In animals with signs of the terminal stage of the disease (neurologic signs, blindness, recumbency), treatment often leads to transient improvement of the general condition of the animal, which could subsequently deteriorate, with eventual death of the animal. In such cases, for welfare reasons euthanasia of affected animals would be recommended, even before instigation of treatment. Substandard welfare of sick animals adds to the financial constraints of treatment, which can be expensive but frequently fruitless. In fact, Sargison[5] has reported that, despite a full course of treatment of toxemic ewes, only one-third of the animals would likely survive.

In hospitalized animals, intensive care involves indwelling intravenous catheterization, followed by administration of glucose (5–7 g) every 3 to 4 hours until full recovery.[1]

In veterinary practice situations, emergency pharmaceutical treatment consists of oral administration of propylene glycol (600 mg/mL). Rook[1] recommended administration of 100 to 200 mL twice daily, whereas other investigators recommend 60 mL twice daily,[6,7] which is considered less likely to cause side effects. A better approach would be to start treatment with 2 doses, each 150 to 200 mL, on the first day, thereafter reducing it to 60 mL per dose. The regime should be followed for up to 6 days, depending on the improvement of the animal's condition. Alternatively, glycerol (60 mL/animal, twice daily for 3–6 days) may be administered. Sodium propionate, liquid molasses, sodium lactate, or ammonium lactate may also be used as glucose sources, but they are not metabolized as quickly as propylene glycol. High doses of all these substances can disrupt normal function of the animal's ruminal flora, thus predisposing to ruminal acidosis. Oral administration of a concentrated dextrose plus electrolytes solution at a dose of 160 mL/animal, 3 to 4 times daily for 3 to 6 days, has also been found to be effective.[8,9]

Administration of recombinant bovine somatotropin at 0.15 mg/kg body weight (BW)[7] or single administration of a slow-release formulation at 160 mg/kg BW[10] has been shown to be of some benefit. Administration of insulin (intramuscular administration of protamine zinc insulin, 20–40 IU/animal daily, every 2 days until recovery) restores glucose uptake and has been suggested as an adjunct to the energy treatments described here, to increase recovery rates of seriously ill ewes[1,11]; in financial terms, however, its use would be justified only in animals of high reproductive value. Flunixin meglumine (intramuscular administration at 2.5 mg/kg BW for up to 3 days) can also be of help as an adjunct therapy to the aforementioned protocols.[12]

Administration of broad-spectrum anthelmintic(s) for effective treatment of gastrointestinal nematodes and liver trematode parasites should be considered. In such a case administration of levamisole is not recommended, as it has been associated with causing abortion in animals during late pregnancy.[13]

In ewes and does at early stage of the disease, it is possible to attempt induction of parturition for removal of fetus(es), in order to decrease energy requirements of the pregnant animal. Induction of parturition can be attempted in ewes after the 140th day and in does after the 143rd day of gestation without compromising fetal development. Various protocols have been proposed for induction of parturition in small ruminants. Of these, administration of 15 to 20 mg of dexamethasone (ewes/does), 10 mg of betamethasone (ewes), or 2.5 mg of flumethazone (ewes/does) is the most appropriate scheme, leading to parturition of ewes within 40 to 45 ($\pm$10–15) hours or of does within 48 to 72 h.[14,15] As often in toxemic ewes and does, endogenous concentration of corticosteroids may be increased[6,9]; simultaneous administration of 0.375 mg cloprostenol in ewes or 15 mg prostaglandin $F_{2\alpha}$ in does would increase the efficacy of the regime. Induction should be followed by intravenous administration of 20% dextrose solution (dose: 200–300 mL/animal) or 50% dextrose solution (dose: 80–120 mL/animal) twice daily until parturition is completed. Animals should be monitored at regular intervals, because the regime often leads to dystocia and retention of fetal membranes.

In ewes and does at advanced stage of the disease, removal of fetus(es) should be performed by cesarean section. In such cases, prognosis is generally poor; survival rate of operated female animals does not exceed 60% and can be even smaller if the fetus(es) had died in utero and was (were) autolyzed.[16,17] Therefore, euthanasia of affected pregnant ewes or does should always be considered before starting surgery. If surgery is decided on, then throughout the operation dextrose solution should be administered intravenously to the animal.

Immediately after induced parturition or after surgery, animals should be administered a broad-spectrum antibacterial agent (as injectable solution), a nonsteroid anti-inflammatory agent (eg, flunixin meglumine), and oxytocin (5 IU daily for 3 days) to facilitate expulsion of fetal membranes and to prevent metritis.[18,19] After removal of fetuses, the general condition of the animal usually is improved. Often, however, it may deteriorate again, especially if the fetus had died in utero In such a case, intravenous dextrose administration in combination with electrolytes must be continued until full recovery of the animal.

Care for Newborn Lambs or Kids Born from Sick Female Animals

Newborn lambs/kids from ewes/does with pregnancy toxemia require increased care. These animals usually have a suboptimal birth weight, are stressed, and may be premature. If their cardiac or respiratory function is weak, their body should be massaged to induce respiration. Doxapram hydrochloride (5–10 mg/animal) should be administered by intravenous or subcutaneous injection or by sublingual dropping.[20] If the dam cannot produce an adequate amount of colostrum, the newborns should be given colostrum from another female in the flock/herd or from the "colostrum bank" of the farm at a dose of 50 mL/kg BW, 4 times in the first 24 hours of life. Subsequently it should be evaluated whether the ewe or doe would be able to produce enough milk for feeding the newborns; if this is not considered to be possible, artificial feeding should be undertaken.

Care for Other Animals in the Affected Flock/Herd

Pregnancy toxemia should always be considered to be a flock/herd problem.[1,2] Therefore, appropriate measures must be taken for the clinically healthy animals. Risk factors, both at individual level (eg, age, poor teeth, lameness, or other disease) and flock/herd level (eg, feeder space, protection from inclement weather, poor quality forage, and so forth) should be evaluated at the time of attending any ill animals.

A metaphylactic treatment course to other ewes/does on the farm can be considered, based on the appraisal of the healthy flock/herd.

Initially, a broad-spectrum anthelminthic treatment course should be administered to all animals if a diagnosis of gastrointestinal parasitism can be supported (eg, quantitative fecal egg count). Ideally, pregnant animals should then be grouped, according to (a) their body condition score and (b) the stage of pregnancy. This grouping helps improve feeding appropriate to the needs of each group, and prevents wasteful feeding to animals bearing one fetus or to animals in early pregnancy.[9] However, if this is not possible then high-energy supplementary feed should be provided to all pregnant animals on the farm. For convenience, these feeds (eg, vegetable fat or molasses) can be given as a "top-dress" feeding, up to 50 g/animal daily, supplementary to concentrate feed and high-quality hay. In intensively managed dairy sheep, administration of a propionic salt (sodium or calcium), at a dose of 20 g/animal daily during the last month of pregnancy is also beneficial.

The situation in the flock/herd should be reevaluated every fortnight. Animals at risk of developing pregnancy toxemia can be identified for individual feeding, to prevent development of the disease; this can be achieved by measuring β-hydroxybutyrate concentration in the blood of pregnant ewes and does during the last month of pregnancy. If the number of fetuses carried has not been identified, the value of 0.8 mmol/L should be considered to distinguish animals at risk of developing the disorder. Otherwise, if the number of fetuses carried has been determined, β-hydroxybutyrate concentration should be measured in the blood of animals carrying multiple fetuses only; in this case, the cutoff value to be used for identifying animals at risk is 1.1 mmoL/L.[9,21] If financial or labor constraints preclude examination of all animals as described, then examination of 10% to 15% of animals will provide valuable information. If blood measurement is not feasible, semiquantitative measurement in urine by using dipsticks can be advocated, but results should be considered cautiously. Animals found to have increased concentration of β-hydroxybutyrate in blood (over the aforementioned thresholds) or urine should be separated from other animals and monitored closely. If early signs of the disease are observed, individual treatment should be instigated immediately.

PERI-PARTURIENT HYPOCALCEMIA

Hypocalcemia ("parturient paresis," "lambing sickness") is an acute or subacute pathologic condition, which occurs more often shortly before or after parturition. The salient features of the disorder include reduced serum concentrations of calcium, progressive paralysis of smooth and striated muscles, recumbency, and lack of conscience.[22] The incidence of the disease is associated with imbalanced nutrition and/or improper handling and housing. In older animals, the ability of absorption and mobilization of stored calcium is reduced; thus, these animals are more susceptible to the condition.[23] In contrast to "milk fever" in cows, which always occurs at calving, hypocalcemia in ewes and does can develop from several weeks before until the first 2 weeks after parturition when the fetal skeletons are mineralizing. Incidence of the disease is usually less than 5%, only occasionally rising up to 20%. On the other hand, in intensively managed dairy flocks/herds the disease is more frequent after lambing, coinciding with the time of peak milk production. Calcium concentration in ewes' milk is almost double that in cows' milk[24]; because there are individuals producing over 3 L of milk daily, there is a high and prolonged demand of calcium during the first stage of lactation.[25]

At early stages of the disease, animals become isolated from the flock/herd and have a temporary stiff gait, with muscle tremors; potentially, they can become hyperesthetic. Soon afterwards, they become hyposensitive and weak, and remain recumbent. Depleted muscle contractions result in constipation and decreased rumen motility, leading to development of bloat.[26,27] As disease progresses depression can occur, usually ending in coma. Ears are typically cold, although rectal temperature usually remains within the normal range.[22,28]

Hypocalcemia may coexist with pregnancy toxemia. Differential diagnosis between the 2 diseases is difficult on a farm level, and can be accurately performed only by measuring concentrations of calcium and β-hydroxybutyrate in the blood of affected animals.

Uncomplicated hypocalcemia responds immediately (within 5 minutes) to intravenous administration of calcium; this can also be used to confirm the diagnosis.[29] Intravenous administration of 30 to 60 mL of 20% calcium borogluconate solution usually is sufficient. A combination product containing phosphorus, magnesium, and/or potassium with dextrose can also be used and may be preferred. Calcium solution should be heated to 35°C to 40°C before administration. Administration must be performed slowly over 5 to 7 minutes, while the clinician monitors the animal's heart rate and rhythm; administration should be stopped at once if there is evidence of arrhythmia. Subsequently, an additional dose of 60 mL of calcium borogluconate, without dextrose, can be administered subcutaneously to ensure a more prolonged absorption. During subcutaneous administration, and as calcium solutions are irritant, the quantity to be administered should be divided into 2 equal volumes and injected at 2 different sites of the body. In view of the potential dangers associated with intravenous administration of calcium solutions, preference of the subcutaneous route over the intravenous route has been advocated.[30] However, dangers are minimized if appropriate precautions are taken, while intravenous administration offers the advantage of immediate response by the animal.

Calcium administration can be repeated after 24 hours, especially in high-yielding dairy animals, to avoid relapse of the disease. In such a case, an amount of 50 mL is administered subcutaneously, divided into 2 equal volumes and injected at 2 different sites of the body. The total amount of 170 mL (60+60+50 mL) is the maximum recommended to be administered in a ewe or doe. If no response is evident, the diagnosis should be reevaluated.[31,32]

In cases of prepartum hypocalcemia complicated with pregnancy toxemia, it is preferable to avoid intravenous administration, as calcium solutions can be fatal in animals with impaired liver function.[30,33]

For grazing animals, attention to calcium content of feeds during diet formulation and avoidance of unnecessary stressors usually suffice to reduce the risk of animals developing the disease.[32,34,35] Cereal pastures and hays have very low levels of calcium, so supplementation is required. Stressors such as transportation can precipitate the disease. Special attention should be given to feedstuffs containing oxalates, which precipitate formation of nonabsorbent compounds with calcium. Among feedstuffs commonly provided to small ruminants, beet pulp (oxalate content in dry matter: 1%–2%), alfalfa leaves (oxalate content 0.1%–1%), sugar beet leaves (oxalate content 2%–5%), and sesame meal (oxalate content 0.1%–0.25%) are the ones with the highest content of oxalates.[36] Thus, their increased inclusion in compound feeds for pregnant or lactating ewes and does should be avoided. The source of calcium supply is important; in general, inorganic calcium is more digestible than calcium contained in feedstuffs.[37]

There are no detailed data concerning prevention of the disease in dairy ewes and does. Perhaps an effective preventive strategy against the disease can be built on knowledge from dairy cows, in which the disease has been studied thoroughly.[38] This knowledge should include control of body condition,[39] regulation of calcium,[40] magnesium,[41] and phosphorus[42] content in the feed, monitoring of cation/anion balance in the feed,[43] and regular monitoring of calcium concentration in the animal's blood.[44]

HYPOMAGNESEMIA

Magnesium deficit, leading to hypomagnesemia, is primarily an issue in animals grazing young, rapidly growing pasture with reduced magnesium content, especially during the spring or autumn. The disease is rare in ewes and does raised under intensive conditions, as nutrition of these animals is based on feeding concentrates to support increased production. The etiology of the disorder is complex, with numerous interacting factors influencing magnesium content in the diet, as well as its availability and absorption.[45] Increased potassium (eg, from alfalfa hay or haylage) and/or reduced sodium content in the diet, coupled with increased milk yield are the main risk factors for the disease.[46–48] Adult ewes and does have a limited ability to mobilize magnesium body reserves; thus, they are dependent on daily intake to meet their requirements.[49] Clinical signs are caused by spontaneous activation of neurons in the central nervous system by the decreased magnesium concentrations in blood, leading to tetany.[50]

Recumbent animals with seizures require immediate treatment and should be considered as emergency cases; their condition may deteriorate and they can die within hours of development of the neurologic signs. Administration of magnesium and calcium salts, separately or as a combination solution, is the recommended treatment, as often there is concurrent hypocalcemia.[51] Intravenous administration of a solution containing 4% to 5% magnesium chloride and 20% calcium borogluconate (50 mL) is ideal, but combinations of 2 different products, according to commercial availability, can also be considered. Recovery is generally quick, but subsequent relapses are common; therefore, additional subcutaneous administration, 12 to 24 hours later, is advisable.[30] When clinical cases occur in a flock/herd, it is advisable to provide clinically healthy animals on the farm with magnesium oxide at a dose of 7 g/animal, given per os,[52] to avoid further clinical incidents in the farm.

Prevention is best accomplished by providing mineral supplements, rich in magnesium content, to the animals before lambing and the beginning of grazing in lush spring pastures. As most of these mineral supplements are not palatable, adequate feed consumption should be regularly monitored and ensured. Decreasing potassium intake by animals may prevent the inhibitory effect on magnesium absorption, but this is not practical or applicable in grazing animals.[50] Sodium deficiency has the same consequences as increased potassium intake and, thus, can be a significant risk factor for grazing animals. Lick blocks containing magnesium and sodium chloride can help prevent sodium deficiency and promote magnesium intake.[53]

SUMMARY

This article reviews treatment and control of pregnancy toxemia, hypocalcemia, and hypomagnesemia, the important peri-parturient diseases of small ruminants. Treatment of pregnancy toxemia benefits from early instigation, that is, on timely diagnosis, and is based on administration of energy sources to sick animals. Removal of fetuses, by induced parturition or cesarean section, should also be performed. Individual cases within a farm require close monitoring of other animals present, as well as measures to avoid development of further clinical cases. Treatment of hypocalcemia is based on administration of calcium solution. Finally, hypomagnesemic animals need urgent treatment with calcium and magnesium solutions.

REFERENCES

1. Rook JS. Pregnancy toxaemia of ewes, does, and beef cows. Vet Clin North Am Food Anim Pract 2000;16:293–317.
2. Mavrogianni VS, Brozos C. Reflections on the causes and the diagnosis of peri-parturient losses of ewes. Small Rumin Res 2008;76:77–82.
3. Farquharson B. A whole farm approach to planned animal health and production for sheep clients in Australia. Small Rumin Res 2009;86:26–9.
4. Menzies PI, Bailey D. Diseases of the periparturient ewe. In: Youngquist RS, editor. Current therapy in large animal theriogenology. Philadelphia: WB Saunders; 1997. p. 639–43.
5. Sargison ND. Recent advances in the diagnosis, prognosis and treatment of ovine pregnancy toxaemia. In: Proceedings of Meetings of the Sheep Veterinary Society. Edinburgh: Sheep Veterinary Society; 1995. p. 27–32.
6. Andrews A. Pregnancy toxaemia in the ewe. In Pract 1997;19:306–12.
7. Andrews AH. Recombinant bovine somatotropin and propylene glycol following glucose injection in treating pregnancy toxaemia. Large Anim Pract 1998;19:31–3.
8. Buswell JF, Haddy JP, Bywater RJ. Treatment of pregnancy toxaemia in sheep using a concentrated oral rehydration solution. Vet Rec 1986;118:208–9.
9. Sargison ND. Pregnancy toxaemia. In: Aitken ID, editor. Diseases of sheep. 4th edition. Oxford (UK): Blackwell Publishing; 2007. p. 359–63.
10. Scott PR, Sargison ND, Penny CD. Evaluation of recombinant-bovine somato-tropin in the treatment of ovine pregnancy toxaemia. Vet J 1998;155:197–9.
11. Henze P, Bickhardt K, Fuhrmann H, et al. Pregnancy toxaemia (ketosis) in sheep and the role of insulin. J Vet Med A 1998;45:255–66.
12. Zamir S, Rozov A, Gootwin E. Treatment of pregnancy toxaemia in sheep with flunixin meglumine. Vet Rec 2009;165:265–6.
13. Braun W. Non-infectious prenatal pregnancy loss in the doe. In: Youngquist RS, editor. Current therapy in large animal theriogenology. Philadelphia: WB Saunders; 1997. p. 548–50.
14. Aurich JE, Aurich C. Induction of parturition in domestic animals. Prakt Tierarzt 1994;75:742–6.
15. Ingoldby L, Jackson P. Induction of parturition in sheep. In Pract 2001;23:228–31.
16. Scott PR. Ovine caesarian operations—a study of 137 field cases. Br Vet J 1989; 145:558–64.
17. Brounts SH, Hawkins JF, Baird AN, et al. Outcome and subsequent fertility of sheep and goats undergoing cesarean section because of dystocia: 110 cases (1981–2001). J Am Vet Med Assoc 2004;224:275–9.
18. Mavrogianni VS, Amiridis GS, Gougoulis DA, et al. Efficacy of difloxacin for the control of postpartum uterine infections of ewes. J Vet Pharmacol Ther 2007; 30:583–5.
19. Orfanou DC, Fragkou IA, Athanasiou LV, et al. Use of oxytocin to control post-partum metritis in ewes. In: Proceedings of the 7th International Sheep Veterinary Congress. Stavanger (Norway): 7th International Sheep Veterinary Congress; 2009. p. 154–5.
20. Monin P. Modifications of ventilator reflexes. An efficient therapy for apneas of prematurity. Biol Neonate 1994;65:247–51.
21. Braun JP, Trumel C, Bézille P. Clinical biochemistry in sheep: a selected review. Small Rumin Res 2010;92:10–8.
22. Pugh DG. Sheep and goat medicine. Philadelphia: Saunders; 2002. p. 468.

23. Goff JP. Pathophysiology of calcium and phosphorus disorders. Vet Clin North Am Food Anim Pract 2000;16:319–37.

24. Moreno-Rojas R, Zurera-Cosano G, Amaro-Lopez MA. Concentration and seasonal variation of calcium, magnesium, sodium and potassium in raw cow, ewe and goat milk. Int J Food Sci Nutr 1994;45:99–105.

25. Polychroniadou A, Vafopoulou A. Variations of major mineral constituents of ewe milk during lactation. J Dairy Sci 1985;68:147–50.

26. Care AD, Abbas SK, Harmeyer J, et al. The relaxant effects of parathyroid hormone (1–34) and parathyroid hormone-related protein (1–34) on ovine reticulo-ruminal smooth muscle in vivo. Exp Physiol 1999;84:665–75.

27. Cockcroft PD, Whiteley P. Hypocalcaemia in 23 ataxic/recumbent ewes: clinical signs and likelihood ratios. Vet Rec 1999;144:529–32.

28. Scott PR. Sheep medicine. London: Manson Publishing; 2007. p. 336.

29. Scott PR. Differential diagnosis of common metabolic disorders in sheep. In Pract 1995;17:266–9.

30. Behrens H, Ganter M, Hiepe TH. Lehrbuch der Schafkrakheiten 4. vollstandig neubearbeitete Auflage. Berlin: Parey; 2001. p. 499.

31. Sykes AR. Deficiency of mineral macro-elements. In: Aitken ID, editor. Diseases of sheep. 4th edition. Oxford (UK): Blackwell; 2007. p. 363–77.

32. Roger PA. Problems of the post-partum ewe. In Pract 2009;31:122–9.

33. Bickhardt K, Henze P, Ganter M. [Clinical findings and differential diagnosis in ketosis and hypocalcaemia of sheep]. Dtsch Tierarztl Wochenschr 1998;105: 413–9 [in German].

34. Wilson GF. Stimulation of calcium absorption and reduction in susceptibility to fasting-induced hypocalcaemia in pregnant ewes fed vegetable oil. N Z Vet J 2001;49:115–8.

35. Dove H. Balancing nutrient supply and nutrient requirements in grazing sheep. Small Rumin Res 2010;92:36–40.

36. Spais AB, Florou-Paneri P, Christaki E. Feeds and feeding. Thessaloniki (Greece): Synchroni Paedia; 2002. p. 364.

37. Dias RS, Kebreab E, Vitti DM, et al. Application and comparison of two models to study effects of calcium sources in sheep. Anim Feed Sci Technol 2008;143: 89–103.

38. Mulligan FJ, O'Grady L, Rice DA, et al. A herd health approach to dairy cow nutrition and production diseases of the transition cow. Anim Reprod Sci 2006;96: 331–53.

39. Ostergaard S, Sorensen LT, Houe H. A stochastic model simulating milk fever in a dairy herd. Prev Vet Med 2003;58:125–43.

40. Sorensen JT, Ostergaard S, Houe H, et al. Expert opinions of strategies for milk fever control. Prev Vet Med 2002;55:69–78.

41. Roche JR. The incidence and control of hypocalcaemia in pasture-based systems. Acta Vet Scand 2003;97(Suppl):141–4.

42. Lean IJ, DeGaris PJ, McNeil DM, et al. Hypocalcemia in dairy cows: meta-analysis and dietary cation anion difference theory revisited. J Dairy Sci 2006;89: 669–84.

43. Goff JP. Macromineral disorders of the transition cow. Vet Clin North Am Food Anim Pract 2004;20:471–94.

44. Oetzel GR. Monitoring and testing dairy herds for metabolic disease. Vet Clin North Am Food Anim Pract 2004;20:651–74.

45. Robson AB, Field AC, Sykes AR, et al. A model of magnesium metabolism in young sheep. Magnesium absorption and excretion. Br J Nutr 1997;78:975–92.

46. Dua K, Care AD. Impaired absorption of magnesium in the aetiology of grass tetany. Br Vet J 1995;151:413–26.
47. Underwood EJ, Suttle NE. The mineral nutrition of livestock. New York (NY): CABI Publishing; 1999. p. 614.
48. Phillips CJC, Mohamed MO, Chiy PC. The critical dietary potassium concentration for induction of mineral disorders in non-lactating Welsh Mountain sheep. Small Rumin Res 2006;63:32–8.
49. Martens H, Schweigel M. Magnesium homeostasis and grass tetany. In: Rayssiguier Y, Mazur A, Durlach J, editors. Advances in magnesium research: nutrition and health. London: John Libbey; 2001. p. 475–81.
50. Martens H, Schweigel M. Pathophysiology of grass tetany and other hypomagnesemias. Vet Clin North Am Food Anim Pract 2000;16:339–68.
51. Foster A, Livesey C, Edwards C. Magnesium disorders in ruminants. In Pract 2007;29:534–9.
52. National Research Council. Nutrient requirements of sheep. 6th edition. Washington, DC: National Academy Press; 1985.
53. Martens H, Rohr K, Daenicke R, et al. Orale magnesiumsupplementation bei Kuhen nach der Umstellung von einer Winterrration auf getrocknetes Fruhjahrsgras. Dtsch Tierarztl Wochenschr 1981;88:261–9.

Principles of Mastitis Treatment in Sheep and Goats

Vasia S. Mavrogianni, DVM, PhD[a],*, Paula I. Menzies, DVM, MPVM[b],
Ilektra A. Fragkou, DVM, PhD[a], George C. Fthenakis, DVM, MSc, PhD[a]

KEYWORDS

- Control • Dry-ewe treatment • Goat • Mastitis • Sheep
- Staphylococcus • Treatment

Mastitis is the term for inflammation of the mammary gland, which may be caused by various microorganisms, including bacteria, viruses, and fungi, as well as injury. This article is limited to treatment of bacterial mastitis. The disease is characterized by presence of bacteria and increased leukocyte counts in mammary secretion and by pathologic changes in the mammary tissue. *Staphylococcus aureus* and *Mannheimia haemolytica* are two frequent causative agents of clinical mastitis. *S aureus* is responsible for approximately 40% of cases of clinical mastitis in ewes suckling lambs and approximately 80% of cases in dairy ewes; the organism is the most common cause of clinical mastitis in dairy goats. *M haemolytica* is responsible for approximately 40% of cases of clinical mastitis in ewes suckling lambs. Other bacterial agents causing clinical mastitis in lactating ewes and does are coagulase-negative *Staphylococci* (which, moreover, are the most frequent causal agents of subclinical mastitis), *Escherichia coli*, and *Streptococci*. Several species of mycoplasma can cause mastitis in sheep and goats, specifically *Mycoplasma agalactiae*, the cause of contagious agalactia syndrome (sheep and goats); *Mycoplasma mycoides* subsp *mycoides* large-colony type (goats); and *Mycoplasma putrefaciens* (goats). In dry ewes/does, the primary causal agents of mammary abnormalities are *Arcanobacterium pyogenes* and staphylococci.[1,2]

   Mastitis is one of the most important diseases in sheep flocks and goat herds. It raises significant welfare concerns, is difficult to control, and has significant economic impact. In most cases, it is the outcome of bacterial invasion into the mammary gland through the teat rather than hemotogenous. Subsequently, bacteria multiply and produce toxins; thus, an inflammatory reaction follows. Reports of the disease have appeared from all countries of the world.[1,2]

The authors have nothing to disclose.
[a] University of Thessaly, PO Box 199, 43100 Karditsa, Greece
[b] Department of Population Medicine, Ontario Veterinary College, University of Guelph, 2541 Stewart Building (#45), Guelph, ON N1G 2W1, Canada
* Corresponding author.
E-mail address: vmavrog@vet.uth.gr

Vet Clin Food Anim 27 (2011) 115–120
doi:10.1016/j.cvfa.2010.10.010
0749-0720/11/$ – see front matter © 2011 Elsevier Inc. All rights reserved.

PRINCIPLES OF TREATMENT OF MASTITIS DURING LACTATION

In small ruminants, no detailed protocols for treatment of mastitis, as have been developed in cows,[3] are available. There is one established rule for the treatment of mastitis, however: the combination of speed and efficacy. Treatment should start immediately after detection of the first signs of the disease and should be performed using effective antimicrobial agents.[4] Development of disease and subsequent damage to the gland is rapid; histologic lesions in the mammary gland are evident within 2 days after infection.[5] Consequently, early instigation of treatment is important, to minimize mammary lesions and to restore health of the affected ewes and does. Thus, treatment should be applied with the first clinical signs. Although clinical cure takes place, sometimes bacteriologic cure cannot be achieved. Subsequently, bacteria present in the mammary gland may cause decreased production, develop mammary abscesses, or cause a recrudescence of clinical disease.[5]

Effective antimicrobial agents should be used for treatment. Ideally and to preserve susceptibility of pathogens to the available drugs, treatment is performed using a narrow-spectrum drug specifically effective against the causal agent of each particular case. Administration of the drug should follow the identification of the causal agent and the establishment of its susceptibility profile.[6] This may not be always possible, however, because of two conflicting factors: (1) the necessity for early instigation of treatment and (2) the time required to perform a full bacteriologic examination (including bacterial isolation, identification, and susceptibility testing). Therefore, treatment can start blindly by means of a broad-spectrum product effective against the major causal agents of the disease. Apart from the obvious reason (ie, cure of the affected ewe or doe), effective treatment is also important as a means of minimizing sources of infection for other animals in the flock.[6]

Nevertheless, even if treatment starts blindly, collection of samples (before administration of any antimicrobial agent) for identification of the causative agent and establishment of the antibiotic susceptibility pattern should be performed. After repeated samplings, a flock/herd profile can be established for susceptibility patterns of causative bacteria.[7] For this, the evaluation of at least 10 isolates of each bacterial species is required,[8] which provides useful information regarding antimicrobial susceptibility status of isolates. This epidemiologic information can be used[9] to provide targeted blind treatments in the future. In such cases, dosage for the antibiotic to be used thereafter should achieve an intramammary concentration exceeding the minimum inhibitory concentration for that antibiotic in greater than or equal to 90% of the isolates already tested. This approach is useful for the treatment of S aureus and M haemolytica (ie, organisms transmitted between the animals) but has little merit in mastitis caused by E coli, because environmental sources of those isolates are diverse.[7]

In principle, treatment should be performed by using intramammary antibiotic tubes, although injectable administration can also be used either alone or as an adjunct to intramammary administration. There are no data comparing the efficacy of the two routes of administration. Moreover, there are few products for intramammary administration licensed specifically for ewes or does. Hence, if the intramammary route is selected, products licensed for use in cows have to be used. In that case, the procedures for extra-label use of veterinary drugs should be adhered to (see the article by Virginia R. Fajt elsewhere in this issue for further exploration of this issue). Often also, the recommended dosing regimens are not adequate for complete cure of the affected animal; thus, extending the treatment for 2 to 3 days beyond the manufacturer's recommendations may need to be considered to achieve a complete bacteriologic cure. This can have a profound effect on persistence of antimicrobial residues in the milk, so it is important to test milk before adding back to the bulk tank or at least to maintain an extended period of milk withdrawal (7 days according to European Union regulations)

When infusing intramammary tubes to ewes and does, various mistakes can occur and may lead to treatment failure. The most common mistakes are (1) inadequate cleansing of the teat orifice before insertion of the tube, which can lead to introduction of new bacteria, fungi, or yeasts into the teat, potentially leading to more severe disease[3]—the area around the teat orifice should be thoroughly cleaned and disinfected with an alcohol solution before insertion of the antibiotic tube—and (2) administration of half an intramammary tube (when using tubes for cows), in the belief that because the mammary gland of ewes/does is smaller than that of cows', it requires a smaller amount of antibiotic—however, this only leads to underdosing, with two consequences: failure of treatment and promotion of resistance development among causal bacteria. The authors have also witnessed the practice of intramammary infusion of antibiotic preparations produced for systemic (intramuscular or subcutaneous or intravenous) administration; such practices, apart from being ineffective, may also be risky for the animal, because excipients of a preparation made for systemic administration may be harmful when infused into the mammary gland, which is a delicate organ.

Systemic administration of injectable antibiotics is indicated (1) when the course of the disease is rapid or if the disease is accompanied by systemic signs, in which case the ensuing bacteremia cannot be treated by intramammary administration of antibiotics alone; (2) in cases of longstanding, subacute mastitis, when inflammatory debris clogs the duct system of the mammary gland, thus impeding full diffusion of intramammary antibiotics; and (3) in treating cases of mammary abscesses, which cannot be effectively treated with intramammary antibiotic administration. In cows, concurrent administration of intramammary and injectable administration of antibiotics has increased cure rate of animals treated[8,10] but also has increased costs. Of the commonly used antimicrobial agents, sulfonamides, penicillins, aminoglycosides, and first-generation cephalosporins do not penetrate readily into the mammary gland after injectable administration, whereas macrolides, trimethoprim, tetracyclines, and fluoroquinolones distribute well into an inflamed mammary gland.[4,11]

Treatment failure in mastitis is a common event. The principal reasons for treatment failure are as follows: (1) delayed start of treatment; (2) use of an improper/ineffective drug (ie, a drug that is not suitable/effective against the causal agents of that particular mastitis case); (3) use of inappropriate route of administration (eg, inability of antimicrobial agent infused into the mammary gland to reach bacteria in a case of abscessation within the parenchyma); (4) interruption of the treatment with the first signs of clinical improvement—improvement of clinical signs does not imply killing of all bacteria, which can lead to a subsequent recrudescence of the disease; (5) administration of less than the prescribed dose (ie, a full intramammary tube) at each treatment point; (6) use of expired products, which have reduced efficacy; (7) use of products that have been contaminated as a result of inappropriate storage or usage conditions; and (8) contamination of the mammary gland while inserting the intramammary tube to an inadequately cleansed teat orifice—this can result in simultaneous entrance of other organisms that can cause mastitis.

The use of nonsteroidal anti-inflammatory agents as supportive treatment in mastitis has been advocated to alleviate the clinical signs of the disease and improve the welfare standards of the animal.[12] For this, flunixin meglumine has been found to contribute to improvement of clinical signs, particularly of the mammary gland, and to returning body temperature to normal both in ewes[13] and does.[14] In severe cases of the disease, intravenous dextrose administration in combination with electrolytes can be advocated and continued until full recovery of the animal.

ADMINISTRATION OF ANTIMICROBIAL AGENTS AT DRYING OFF

Administration of antimicrobial agents at drying off of ewes/does is not a treatment as such, because the treated animals are not always ill. It is an important part of control programs against mastitis, however. Administration of antimicrobial agents at drying off has two objectives: (1) to eliminate existing intramammary infections, which may cause recrudescence of clinical disease during the dry period, and (2) to prevent new infections during the dry period, when ewes/does are particularly susceptible.

There is a positive effect of the administration of antimicrobial agents at drying off with reduced intramammary infections during the dry period, reduced cases of clinical mastitis developing immediately post lambing, and increased milk production.[15–17] The parenteral administration of tilmicosin (ie, an antimicrobial agent with very good pharmacokinetic properties in the mammary gland) has also been found to result in a similar beneficial effect in meat sheep.[18]

In contrast to treatment of clinical mastitis during lactation, there are no time limitations to perform the administration of antimicrobial agents and, because sheep/goats are seasonal breeders, often ewes/does are dried off in groups. This allows the time to collect samples from animals to be dried off for microbiologic examination and a susceptibility profile. This is of great help to selecting the most appropriate antimicrobial agent to use for optimum results.

DETECTION OF INHIBITORS IN MILK

Because intramammary and parenteral antimicrobial products are not approved for use in sheep and goats in most of the world and because milk withdrawal periods cannot be extrapolated from those required for dairy cattle with dependability,[19–24] veterinarians and farmers must use test kits to detect inhibitors in the milk before shipping for human consumption. Although these tests when used under farm or veterinary clinic environments are not comparable in accuracy to regulatory laboratory conditions, their use may help avoid costly mistakes. Some of these kits have been evaluated for use in small ruminants. Some studies have found that false-positive results may occur, particularly toward the end of the lactation period,[25] whereas some found that detection limits were higher than the maximum residue limits set by the regulatory agency.[26–28] The latter situation is of more concern than the former. Other studies, however, have found that the tests seemed accurate.[29,30]

When selecting a test, it is advisable to make sure that it has been properly evaluated for use in small ruminants and meets the regulatory standards of that country. For example the Charm SL Beta-lactam Test has been evaluated by the Food and Drug Administration and found suitable for use in raw, commingled goat milk. For veterinarians working in other jurisdictions, however, maximum residue limits may differ; hence, the tests may not be adequate. In the long term, the only solution is for pharmaceutical companies to seek a license for a milk withdrawal period in sheep and goats for commonly used drugs. Until then, the risk of presence of inhibitors—or other commonly used therapeutic agents—in the milk of dairy small ruminants is large, making production and consumption of products from it a constant risk for manufacturing failure (eg, cheese or yogurt making) or a public health issue.

SUMMARY

This short article indicates the principles for treatment of mastitis in ewes/does and explains reasons why treatment may occasionally fail. Moreover, it presents the principles for administration of antimicrobial agents at drying off of the animals. Finally, it addresses the risk of antimicrobials present in milk when improper withdrawal periods are used and the issues around testing for inhibitors before putting the milk into in a farm's tank.

REFERENCES

1. Menzies PI, Ramanoon SZ. Mastitis of sheep and goats. Vet Clin North Am Food Anim Pract 2001;17:333–48.
2. Contreras A, Sierra D, Sanchez A, et al. Mastitis in small ruminants. Small Rumin Res 2007;68:145–53.
3. Roberson JR. Establishing treatment protocols for clinical mastitis. Vet Clin North Am Food Anim Pract 2003;19:223–34.
4. Erskine RJ, Wagner S, DeGraves FJ. Mastitis therapy and pharmacology. Vet Clin North Am Food Anim Pract 2003;19:109–38.
5. Fthenakis GC, Jones JET. The effect of inoculation of coagulase-negative staphylococci into the ovine mammary gland. J Comp Pathol 1990;102:211–9.
6. Kiossis E, Brozos CN, Petridou E, et al. Program for the control of subclinical mastitis in dairy chios breed ewes during lactation. Small Rumin Res 2007;73:194–9.
7. Constable PD, Morin DE. Treatment of clinical mastitis: using antimicrobial susceptibility profiles for treatment decisions. Vet Clin North Am Food Anim Pract 2003;19:139–55.
8. Sears PM, McCarthy KK. Management and treatment of staphylococcal mastitis. Vet Clin North Am Food Anim Pract 2003;19:171–85.
9. Green LE. Epidemiological information in sheep health management. Small Rumin Res 2010;92:57–66.
10. Kirk JH. Diagnosis and treatment of difficult mastitis cases. Agri Pract 2001;12:5–8.
11. Ziv C. Practical pharmacokinetic aspects of mastitis therap—2. Practical and therapeutic applications. Vet Med Small Anim Clin 1980;75:469–74.
12. McKellar QA. The health of the sheep industry and the medicines to maintain it. Small Rumin Res 2006;62:7–12.
13. Fthenakis GC. Field evaluation of flunixin meglumine in the supportive treatment of ovine mastitis. J Vet Pharmacol Ther 2000;23:405–7.
14. Mavrogianni VS, Alexopoulos C, Fthenakis GC. Field evaluation of flunixin meglumine in the supportive treatment of ovine mastitis. J Vet Pharmacol Ther 2004;27:373–5.
15. Chaffer M, Leitner G, Zamir S, et al. Efficacy of dry-off treatment in sheep. Small Rumin Res 2003;47:11–6.
16. Gonzalo C, Tardáguila JA, De La Fuente LF, et al. Effects of selective and complete dry therapy on prevalence of intramammary infection and on milk yield in the subsequent lactation in dairy ewes. J Dairy Res 2004;71:33–8.
17. Shwimmer A, Kenigswald G, Van Straten M, et al. Dry-off treatment of Assaf sheep: Efficacy as a management tool for improving milk quantity and quality. Small Rumin Res 2008;74:45–51.
18. Croft A, Duffield T, Menzies P, et al. The effect of tilmicosin administered to ewes prior to lambing on incidence of clinical mastitis and subsequent lamb performance. Can Vet J 2000;41:306–11.
19. Buswell JF, Knight CH, Barber DML. Antibiotic persistence and tolerance in the lactating goat following intramammary therapy. Vet Rec 1989;125:301–3.
20. Buswell JF, Barber DM. Antibiotic persistence and tolerance in the lactating sheep following a course of intramammary therapy. Br Vet J 1989;145:552–7.

21. Karzis J, Donkin EF, Petzer IM. Intramammary antibiotics in dairy goats: withdrawal periods of three intramammary antibiotics compared to recommended withdrawal periods for cows. Onderstepoort J Vet Res 2007;74:217–22.
22. Karzis J, Donkin EF, Petzer IM. Withdrawal periods and tissue tolerance after intramammary antibiotic treatment of dairy goats with clinical mastitis. Onderstepoort J Vet Res 2007;74:281–8.
23. Pengov A, Kirbis A. Risks of antibiotic residues in milk following intramammary and intramuscular treatments in dairy sheep. Anal Chim Acta 2009;637:13–7.
24. Athanasiou LV, Orfanou DC, Fragkou IA, et al. Proposals for withdrawal period of sheep milk for some commonly used veterinary medicinal products: a review. Small Rumin Res 2009;86:2–5.
25. Molina MP, Althaus RL, Balasch S, et al. Evaluation of screening test for detection of antimicrobial residues in ewe milk. J Dairy Sci 2003;86:1947–52.
26. Molina MP, Althaus RL, Molina A, et al. Antimicrobial agent detection in ewes' milk by the microbial inhibitor test brilliant black reduction test—BRT AiM. Int Dairy J 2003;13:821–6.
27. Montero A, Althaus RL, Molina A, et al. Detection of antimicrobial agents by a specific microbiological method (Eclipse 100) for ewe milk. Small Rumin Res 2005;57:229–37.
28. Sierra D, Contreras A, Sánchez A, et al. Detection limits of non-β-lactam antibiotics in goat's milk by microbiological residues screening tests. J Dairy Sci 2009;92:4200–6.
29. Contreras A, Paape MJ, Di Carlo AL, et al. Evaluation of selected antibiotic residue screening tests for milk from individual goats. J Dairy Sci 1996;80: 1113–8.
30. Hozová B, Minarovičová L. Verification of suitability of selected detection systems for estimating antibiotic residues in goat's milk. Czech J Food Sci 2001;19: 207–12.

Control of Important Clostridial Diseases of Sheep

Christopher J. Lewis, BVetMed, DSHP, MRCVS

KEYWORDS

- Clostridia • Goat • Sheep • Sudden death • Toxins
- Trigger factors • Vaccines

Clostridial diseases have affected sheep ever since these animals were first domesticated. James Hogg,[1] the Ettrick shepherd, writing in 1807 described diseases that were clearly those we now recognize as caused by clostridia. The early part of the last century saw flocks decimated by clostridial disease. Huge losses occurred wherever sheep were farmed. In Scotland, lamb dysentery and braxy predominated, in Wales, black disease and in England, pulpy kidney and enterotoxemias were common. Disease caused by clostridia can be broadly divided into 4 groups: those affecting the alimentary system (the enterotoxemias), those affecting the parenchymatous organs, those causing myonecrosis and toxemia, and those causing neurologic disorders (**Table 1**). While this is a convenient generalization, many members of the clostridial family can be implicated as causing diseases in more than one group. Ten species of clostridia are involved in disease processes in sheep.

The clostridia are anaerobic rod-shaped bacteria, usually with rounded ends. The bacteria vary in length from 3 to 10 μm and in width from 0.5 to 1.5μm. All clostridial species have the ability to form spores, all with their own specific morphology. Clostridia stain gram-positive, but pleomorphism can occur and, in particular in old cultures, they will stain gram-negative. Most organisms require a trigger factor to induce rapid multiplication; in the process they release powerful exotoxins, which damage and destroy vital organs of the host. Some clostridia produce toxins and are also invasive. Variability exists between strains of the same species in their ability to produce toxin. In some cases, certain strains may be nontoxin producers whereas others produce large quantities of lethal toxin. This variation complicates diagnosis, and the presence of the bacteria alone does not indicate that it is responsible for the ensuing death. The gross postmortem lesions and the detection of the respective toxin are keys to successful diagnosis.

The author has nothing to disclose.
Sheep Veterinary Services, Fields Farm, Green Lane, Audlem, Cheshire, CW3 0ES, United Kingdom
E-mail address: christopher@knightellington.plus.com

Vet Clin Food Anim 27 (2011) 121–126
doi:10.1016/j.cvfa.2010.10.009
0749-0720/11/$ – see front matter
vetfood.theclinics.com

Table 1
Clostridial diseases of sheep

Organism	Associated Disease	Comment
The enterotoxemias		
C perfringens type A	Enterotoxemia	Increasingly incriminated in young lambs; worldwide significance
C perfringens type B	Lamb dysentery and hemorrhagic enteritis	Worldwide prevalence, except in New Zealand and Australia
C perfringens type C subtype 1	"Struck"	Prevalent in the UK in adult sheep; prevalent in Australia in lambs
C perfringens type C subtype 2	Necrotic enteritis	Only reported in USA
C perfringens type D	"Pulpy kidney disease"	All ages of sheep affected; worldwide significance
C septicum	"Braxy"	Prevalent in the UK and Scandinavia, occurring in weaned lambs and shearlings during the autumn; no clinical disease reported in New Zealand, despite similar climatic conditions
C sordellii	Abomasitis and toxemia syndrome	Acute abomasitis in lambs and toxemia in older sheep; prevalent in the UK and New Zealand
Clostridial diseases affecting parenchymatous organs		
C novyi type B	"Black" disease	Mainly occurring in adult sheep; worldwide prevalence
C haemolyticum (C novyi type D)	Bacillary hemoglobinuria	Sporadic occurrence in the UK and Ireland
Clostridial diseases presented with myonecrosis and toxemia		
C chauvoei	Blackleg, blackquarter, postparturient gangrene, malignant edema	Worldwide prevalence, but more significant in hotter climates
C novyi type B	Big head and malignant edema	More frequent in rams in hotter climates
C perfringens type A	Malignant edema	Rare; usually in multiple infections
C septicum	Malignant edema	Rare in Europe; well documented in Australia and USA
C sordelii	Malignant edema	Prevalent in USA and New Zealand
Clostridial neurotropic diseases		
C botulinum type C and type D	Botulism	Prevalent in South Africa and Australia, under drought conditions; in the UK, consequent to consumption of poultry litter
C tetani	Tetanus	Worldwide prevalence, mainly in lambs
C perfringens type D	Focal symmetric encephalomalacia	Worldwide prevalence

Isolation of clostridia requires strict anaerobic techniques with a variety of media, particularly so when 2 or more species are present; some species can overgrow and mask others. Once isolated, the identity of the individual is confirmed by either gas chromatography or fluorescent antibody techniques.

The enteric clostridia are best identified by polymerase chain reaction techniques,[2] which are able to identify toxins by genotyping.[3] However, not all laboratories are able to use these techniques and, in the case of some of these clostridia, identification can be made by the use of an enzyme-linked immunosorbent assay (ELISA).[4,5]

All pathogenic clostridia cause disease by production of powerful toxins as they rapidly multiply under favorable conditions. Most of these bacteria produce toxins specific to their species and, in many cases, they produce 2 or more toxins.[6] Each disease is specific, and each has differing etiological and trigger factors.[5]

THE CLOSTRIDIAL DISEASES
The Enterotoxemias

The enterotoxemias are caused by various types of *Clostridium perfringens*. In all the major sheep-breeding countries, they are the commonest clostridial diseases of sheep. The 5 distinct types of *C perfringens* are distinguished by the toxins they produce. Types B, C, and D are of major significance but, with the use of improved diagnostic tools, type A is now recognized as more than an occasional pathogen. The major toxins of importance are α(alpha)-toxin, β(beta)-toxin, and ϵ(epsilon)-toxin.[7] The role of ι(iota)-toxin still remains unclear.[8] Recently, *C perfringens* type B has been shown to produce a further toxin, $\beta2$-toxin, which is considered to be a significant factor in causing diseases in pigs and horses; however, its possible effect in sheep is unclear.[9]

The 2 most commonly encountered enterotoxemias are lamb dysentery caused by *C perfringens* type B and pulpy kidney disease (also called enterotoxemia in the United States) caused by *C perfringens* type D.

Lamb dysentery is seen in lambs younger than 3 weeks of age. Bacteria are ingested by the lamb and under as yet ill-understood conditions, multiply rapidly producing large quantities of both β- and ϵ-toxin. β-Toxin is highly sensitive to and is inactivated by trypsin, a powerful inhibitor of which is contained in colostrum. Disease outbreaks tend to occur toward the end of lambing in the better fed lambs.

In pulpy kidney disease, bacteria are often found as natural inhabitants of the small intestine. Soil or manure contaminated with spores, which usually persist for a year, are a common external source. The disease is associated with a sudden change of diet or a sudden change to a higher plane of nutrition, particularly of concentrates or lush pasture rich in easily fermentable carbohydrates. This change results in conditions conducive to rapid multiplication of the bacteria, with the production of large quantities of nontoxic protoxin; this is converted by trypsin to the lethal necrotizing ϵ-toxin. Large quantities of toxin need to be accumulated in the intestine before it can be absorbed.[10]

C perfringens type A has comparatively recently been associated with fatal disease in sheep. Most sheep harbor a flora of *C perfringens* type A, many of which live as commensals because they do not produce toxins. Certain strains do produce large quantities of α-toxin. α-Toxin can now be identified by ELISA in a similar manner that which identifies both β- and ϵ-toxins, thus enabling a diagnosis to be established when both β- and ϵ-toxin are not present. In clinical terms cases closely resemble enterotoxemia caused by *C perfringens* type B, although the age range is wider.

C perfringens type C contains 2 subtypes, 1 and 2.[11] Subtype 1 produces the classic "struck," a disease of adult animals, confined mainly to local areas of the United Kingdom but also likely to be distributed worldwide, although few investigations have been performed into the causes of sudden death in extensively farmed sheep. In addition, the β-toxin is labile and rapidly decomposes. Subtype 2 causes necrotic enteritis of young and growing lambs.

Two other diseases are considered enterotoxemias: "braxy," caused by *C septicum*, and abomasitis and toxemia, caused by *C sordellii*.

Braxy, or "bradshot," is a disease of autumn and winter, usually in first-year sheep grazing frosted pastures. Braxy has been recorded in young lambs, born early in the year and turned out onto frosted grazing. It appears that the ingestion of frosted forage precipitates a primary abomasitis, as a consequence of which the abomasum is rapidly colonized by *C septicum*, which produces 4 lethal toxins. Diagnosis is by culture or by fluorescent antibody techniques of impression smears.[12]

Abomasitis and toxemia syndrome occur in all ages of sheep, but most dramatically in lambs aged 4 to 10 weeks and fed on a carbohydrate-rich creep feed. The responsible organism was comparatively recently identified as *C sordelli*.[13] Subsequently it has been reported from cases of the disorder in New Zealand and Australia. Unlike many of the clostridia, it can cause disease in any age of sheep and is seen in conditions similar to those producing pulpy kidney in weaned lambs. It is also recognized as a cause of sudden death in ewes either just before or after lambing. This syndrome is frequently confused with hypomagnesemia or hypocalcemia.

Clostridial Diseases Affecting Parenchymatous Organs

Two diseases are caused by 2 closely related members of the clostridial family *C novyi*. Type B causes "black" disease and *C haemolyticum*, originally *C novyi* type D, causes bacillary hemoglobinuria. By far the most important is black disease. Consequent to an insult to the liver, usually caused by liver fluke migration, an area of necrosis is produced at which the bacteria flourish, producing huge quantities of lethal toxin, leading to rapid death. Black disease has a worldwide distribution and, after pulpy kidney disease, is probably the most commonly encountered clostridial disease. Bacillary hemoglobinuria is far more sporadic, occurring in the United Kingdom, Ireland, and the wetter areas of South America. It is probably underdiagnosed, due to its sporadic nature and confusion with black disease. It appears that infection with *Cysticercus tenuicollis* may be the main trigger factor.

Clostridial Diseases Presented with Myonecrosis and Toxemia

Five members of the clostridial family have been incriminated in causing malignant necrosis, while also being incriminated in other specific disease entities. *C chauvoei* falls within this group but also causes other specific diseases. *C chauvoei* is found wherever sheep are farmed but, unlike the other clostridia, its mode of action is invasive as well as producing 4 potent toxins. It is associated with "blackleg," postparturient gangrene, navel-ill and, more recently, cardiac necrosis.[14] The organism usually enters through a wound or following trauma. A characteristic of blackleg is the very rapid bloating and decomposition of the carcass. *C chauvoei* causes considerable economic losses, particularly in hotter climates.

Malignant necrosis, often referred to as malignant edema, is rapidly fatal following wound contamination by 5 members of the clostridial family. It is particularly prevalent in mobs of rams run together, where fighting often occurs. There is frequently edema, and in some cases crepitus present around the eyes and head and upper neck. Malignant necrosis can be associated with injection of irritating substances, particularly if asepsis is not adhered to. The condition tends to be sporadic, except in areas of large groups of sheep kept in hotter climates.

Clostridial Neurotropic Diseases

Tetanus, botulism, and focal symmetric encephalomalacia are the clostridial diseases in which the nervous system is affected.

Tetanus is a highly fatal disease, seen mainly in younger sheep, and is found worldwide. Contamination of wounds is frequently the route of entry, as the spores survive for many years in the environment. Unlike most of the clostridial diseases, aggressive treatment in the early stages may be rewarding, but is very expensive and would be reserved for very valuable animals. Hygiene is important in reducing contamination.

Botulism is caused by toxins produced in feedstuffs by *C botulinum* and then ingested. Seven toxigenic types are recognized, but only types C and D cause disease in sheep, with C being by far the most common. Botulism has been traditionally associated with drought conditions in South Africa and Australia; more recently, it has become far more prevalent in the United Kingdom, where sheep graze pastures top-dressed with poultry manure containing carcasses of birds.[15] Big-bale silage can also be a problem when it contains dead rodents. The disease has also been associated with feeding of bakery waste or drinking from stagnant ponds where ducks have succumbed to the disease.

Focal symmetric encephalomalacia is caused when only small quantities of *C perfringens* type D toxins have been absorbed. While true pulpy kidney disease is an extension, in some flocks where animals only exhibit nervous signs, these are thought to be associated with differing strains of the causative organism.

TREATMENT AND CONTROL

Except in the early cases of tetanus, clostridial diseases fail to respond to treatment, because too much tissue damage has occurred by the time symptoms are observed. The potent toxins produced lead to the very rapid onset of disease and subsequently to death. Incidence may be reduced by reducing the influence of trigger factors, but these measures alone are unlikely to prevent the disease.

Control is by vaccination, as all clostridia are ideal candidates for this approach. Modern vaccines contain inactivated toxoids; the only exception is *C chauvoei* vaccines, which require the inclusion of some cellular material. The purified toxins of all clostridia are highly antigenic. Although monovalent vaccines can be used for specific conditions, there is an increasing tendency to produce polyvalent vaccines tailored to either the age range of sheep or geographic areas.

Prevention of diseases affecting lambs soon after birth is achieved by ensuring that the dams have a high level of circulating antibody at lambing time. Ewes have the ability to concentrate these antibodies in the colostrum and thus provide high amount of antibodies to their lambs, leading to their effective passive protection.[16]

As the clostridial toxoids are inactivated, it requires 2 doses of each vaccine administered 4 to 6 weeks apart to establish protective concentrations of antibodies. These concentrations wane over a period of a year, thus annual booster vaccinations are required. Ideally, booster vaccinations should be performed in ewes about 4 to 3 weeks before the start of the lambing season. In flocks where the total lambing season extends over 2 months (consequent to a long mating period earlier in the season) and with a high incidence of lamb dysentery, one should consider revaccination of ewes that would not have lambed up to 8 weeks after the vaccination.

SUMMARY

Clostridia cause many different diseases, all characterized by sudden death, most occurring worldwide. Their mode of action is to produce one or more potent toxins when multiplying under favorable conditions. Considerable variation exists between different strains of the same organism. Specific trigger factors are required to induce toxin production. Excellent control is obtained by the use of toxoid vaccines. Protection is passed to the lamb via the colostrum.

REFERENCES

1. Hogg J. The shepherd's guide. reproduction of the book published in. London: BVA Publications; 1807.
2. Roode JL, Cole ST. Molecular genetics and pathogenesis of *Clostridium perfringens*. Microbiol Rev 1991;55:621–48.
3. Petit L, Gilbert M, Popoff MR. C. perfringens: toxin type and genotype. Trends Microbiol 1999;7:104–10.
4. Martin PK, Naylor RD, Sharpe RT. Detection of *Clostridium perfringens* beta toxin by enzyme linked immunosorbent assay. Res Vet Sci 1997;63:101–2.
5. Malone FE, Hartley HM, Skuce RA. Bacteriological examinations in sheep health management. Small Rumin Res 2010;92:78–83.
6. Lewis CJ. Clostridial diseases. In: Aitken ID, editor. Diseases of sheep. 4th edition. Oxford (UK): Blackwell Publishing; 2007. p. 156–67.
7. Sterne M. Clostridial infections. Vlaams Diergen Tijds 1983;52:414–25.
8. Gilbert M, Jolivet-Renaud C, Popoff MR. Beta 2 a novel toxin produced by *C. perfringens*. Gene 1997;203:65–73.
9. Garmory HS, Chanter N, French NP, et al. Occurrence of *Clostridium perfringens* beta 2 toxin amongst animals determined using genotyping and subtyping PCR analysis. Epidemiol Infect 2000;124:61–7.
10. Bullen JJ. Role of toxins in host-parasite relationships. In: Ajil SJ, Kadis S, Monte TC, editors. Microbial toxins. New York: Academic Press; 1970. p. 223–76.
11. Niilo L. *Clostridium perfringens* Type C enterotoxaemia. Can Vet J 1988;29:658–64.
12. Buxton A, Fraser G. Animal microbiology. Oxford (UK): Blackwell; 1997.
13. Lewis CJ, Naylor RD. Sudden death in sheep associated with *Clostridium sordellii*. Vet Rec 1998;142:417–21.
14. Glastonbury JRW, Searson JE, Links IJ, et al. Clostridial myocarditis in lambs. Aus Vet J 1998;65:208–9.
15. Burgt van der GM. An outbreak of suspected botulism in sheep. In: Proceedings of the 6th International Sheep Veterinary Congress. Hersonissos (Greece): The Hellenic Ministry of Rural Development and Food; 2005. p. 151.
16. Cooper BS. The transfer from ewe to lamb of clostridial antibodies. N Z Vet J 1967;15:1–7.

Control of Paratuberculosis in Sheep and Goats

Ramon A. Juste, DVM, PhD[a],*, Valentin Perez, DVM, PhD[b]

KEYWORDS

• Crohn's disease • Goat • Mycobacterium • Paratuberculosis
• Sheep • Vaccination

Paratuberculosis, or Johne disease, is a disease caused by a regional intestinal inflammation associated with infection by *Mycobacterium avium* subsp *paratuberculosis* (MAP). Although it was generally assumed that the disease should present similarly in all domestic ruminant species, there is abundant evidence that small ruminant paratuberculosis is different from the disease in cattle both in the clinical form and in the strains of MAP involved.[1–6] Even among small ruminants, clinical forms and strains differ substantially between sheep and goats.[7–10] These differences do not seem unique to paratuberculosis but extend to other mycobacterial infections, in particular tuberculosis, which rarely causes disease in sheep. This different susceptibility of each species has conditioned the approach to control of paratuberculosis, in the sense that sheep paratuberculosis has been smoothly dealt with by vaccination, whereas interferences with tuberculosis diagnosis in goats have caused widespread rejection of vaccination strategies in countries where the vaccine is available.

Control of paratuberculosis has been the subject of field and experimental research as well as of a large variety of management and quality assurance programs.[11–14] Surprisingly, the strategy that has been successful for more than 80 years in the field tends to be systematically overlooked by mainstream microbiologic and epidemiologic researchers, who are more focused on eradication and concepts of biosecurity than on practical short term–oriented compromises.

This article reviews some relevant epidemiologic and pathogenetic features of paratuberculosis in small ruminants and then presents and discusses the available information on the characteristics of paratuberculosis control strategies and their experimental and field outcomes.

Ramón A. Juste leads a project for paratuberculosis vaccine improvement, which is supported by a company that is a spin-off of NEIKER and a vaccine-producing commercial company.
[a] Department of Animal Health, NEIKER and a Vaccine-producing Commercial Company (CZV, SL), Berreaga 1, 48160 Derio, Bizkaia, Spain
[b] Department of Animal Health, Faculty of Veterinary Medicine, University of León, Campus de Vegazana s/n, 24071 León, Spain
* Corresponding author.
E-mail address: rjuste@neiker.net

HISTORICAL AND COMPARATIVE VIEWS

Paratuberculosis was first described in one cow in Germany in 1895 by Johne and Frothingham.[15] According to Chiodini,[16] the first reports in small ruminants were made 16 years later, in 1911, by Stockman in sheep and, nearly 30 years later, in 1924, in goats. Since then, small ruminant paratuberculosis has regularly appeared in the veterinary literature even though at a much lower frequency than cattle paratuberculosis.

The introduction of paratuberculosis, maedi, and sheep pulmonary adenocarcinoma into Iceland have taught the veterinary profession much on epidemiology, microbiology, pathogenesis, and disease control of those pathogens. Most of this knowledge is due to the insight of a physician, not a veterinarian, the regrettably short-lived Bjorn Sigurdsson, who proposed the new concept of slow infection, identified the first member of the infamously well-known family of lentiviruses, and designed specific control measures.[17] The infection of sheep, maedi, then almost unknown, was completely eradicated in a few years, thanks to a heroic stamping-out effort of farmers and government. The more ubiquitous paratuberculosis was controlled but not eradicated with a vaccination program, which 60 years later is still a regular practice for replacement sheep.[18,19]

Paratuberculosis reached Iceland in the 1930s, after a small group of Karakul rams was introduced from a veterinary school in Germany. The animals seemed healthy both before export to Iceland as well as while in extended quarantine in Iceland. Only a few years after they had arrived at their destination farms, however, a new disease was observed by the farmers who had received the rams. Its study by Sigurdsson provided a new concept of disease that challenged the current knowledge of infectious diseases and laid the grounds for the discovery of a new set of animal and human infections.

Maedi-visna was accompanied by paratuberculosis in one-fourth of the imported sheep and because eradication by testing and culling experiences was perceived as ineffective, control efforts were soon focused on the success obtained by vaccination in cattle in different countries. Thus, Sigurdsson[20–22] developed a new version of the oil and pumice powder adjuvant live vaccine, which had been successful in the French field experience reported a few years previously by Vallée and colleagues.[23] Application of this vaccine to young replacement ewe lambs for several years led to 94% reduction in the presence of paratuberculosis in slaughtered animals several years later and allowed the maintenance of sheep production at proper levels. This was the first report on the control of paratuberculosis in sheep and the second history of field vaccination against paratuberculosis; it was successful and is still going on as a routine for preparation of replacement ewes.[19]

MAP infection has become a highly contentious issue regarding the cause of human inflammatory bowel disease (IBD), the main form of which is known as Crohn disease. It was at approximately the same time as sheep paratuberculosis was first described that a Scottish surgeon, Dalziel, pointed out the pathologic similarities of ruminant and human regional inflammatory disease.[24] Since then, many efforts have been made to properly describe the role of MAP in human IBD, but there is still much debate on whether or not there is causal association or only association. There is a significant accumulation of epidemiologic, microbiologic, immunologic, genetic, pathologic, and comparative physiopathologic evidence showing an association of MAP infection in ruminants with human IBD.[25–32] Even though these associations do not necessarily imply causality under standard infectious disease paradigms, the perspective of a slow infection model where only a small fraction of the exposed and infected population ever becomes clinical cases would allow seeing more clearly a common causative role of MAP in natural IBD throughout different species. Reversing the perspective, rejection of MAP causality in human IBD seriously compromises the criteria applied to paratuberculosis causality in animals, because the association between MAP and paratuberculosis in ruminants has almost the same weakness regarding the failure to isolate acid-fast bacilli in some cases and lack of a consistent specific immune response. Even the strongest argument, experimental infection with MAP, has not always been successful in animals.[33–35]

EPIDEMIOLOGY OF SMALL RUMINANT PARATUBERCULOSIS

Sheep paratuberculosis is generally caused by a group of strains that are difficult to isolate[9,36] and present more variability than those strains causing bovine paratuberculosis.[10] These types are defined as ovine (S) strains using clinicoepidemiologic criteria,[37] or types I and II according to authors that focus mostly on their microbiologic and molecular characteristics.[38,39] Although there is a certain exchange between hosts and strains, the general rule is that sheep have S strains and other hosts have C strains, or, as recent information indicates, other types of strains, like the bison or Indian types.[40,41] Goats seem to share sheep and cattle strains.[10,42]

Sheep paratuberculosis is widespread and is a serious threat to sheep production, because it tends to remain hidden, showing only indirect production effects. Many sheep-producing countries, with the partial exception of the United Kingdom and the USA, have adopted control programs based on vaccination to avoid these losses. Paratuberculosis has been a problem in goats, but it has received less attention than in other species, probably due to its more marginal numbers in countries with a more developed cattle industry.

It is assumed that like bovine paratuberculosis, infection is acquired by small ruminants in the early weeks of life from the bacteria excreted through feces by the dam or other females in the farm.[43]

PATHOGENESIS

Once in the intestinal lumen, MAP enters the intestine through the M cells of the Peyer patch dome, especially at the caudal jejunal and ileocecal levels. Then, it is taken up by macrophages that move to the interfollicular T-cell rich zone.[44–46] The first signs of inflammation are seen there, at approximately 45 days' postinfection, characterized by the focal accumulation of macrophages forming small granulomas, surrounded by a lymphocytic infiltrate.[4,47] At this stage, infected animals can remain in a subclinical state of latency for long periods, causing only these focal lesions in the intestinal lymphoid tissue as infection progresses to cause diffuse and severe granulomatous enteritis associated with clinical signs. According to the composition and extension of this inflammatory process, different immunopathologic forms have been described: focal forms (latency forms), related to intense peripheral cellular immune responses (Th1 response), or diffuse lesions, mostly associated with high peripheral humoral responses (Th2 response).[48–50] Attempts to define paratuberculosis immunopathologic forms have been reported since the 1950s, more often in sheep than in cattle.[5–7]

CONTROL STRATEGIES

Because vaccination was such an early success and there were no concerns about tuberculosis diagnosis, use of vaccines in sheep has been almost the only widely used strategy for paratuberculosis control. The main exception was a socially painful and short-lived attempt at eradication in the late 1990s in Australia.[51,52] This program required that any flock confirmed positive was completely destroyed in the belief that only a few flocks were infected and that the agent was a strict pathogen that could not survive outside its domestic hosts.[14,53–58] Introduction of a commercial killed vaccine was quickly demonstrated a more efficient method, and the eradication program shifted to control of the infection and prevention of clinical losses, which has found wide acceptance after showing high efficacy.[57]

In Spain, paratuberculosis was first reported in sheep in the 1970s, in the northern regions of Castilla and Léon,[59] and, 7 years later, in Aragon.[60] A quick intervention by the Spanish Ministry of Agriculture, promoting the development as well as importation of a live vaccine, together with education and free availability of vaccines for ewe lambs, quickly kept ovine paratuberculosis in check. Currently, a killed vaccine is an option for farmers who have to assume the charge of the costs. There are only a few studies published, however, on the results of paratuberculosis vaccination in sheep in Spain.[61–66] There is even less written evidence of goat vaccination, in spite of the vaccine having been freely available and the presence of abundant anecdotal evidence by farmers and veterinarians.[61,62]

Apart from the first report by Sigurdsson[20] and recent work in Australia,[55,57,67] there are only isolated reports on the use of paratuberculosis vaccines in other countries, including New Zealand,[68] Cyprus,[69] and the United Kingdom.[70] Most of the use of paratuberculosis vaccines is not recorded in the veterinary literature, even though millions of doses are used every year, according to commercial sources.

The story of control in goats is quite different. Even though it was once thought that goats behaved like sheep regarding tuberculosis and, thus, were considered relatively resistant to paratuberculosis, goats are highly susceptible to both tuberculosis and paratuberculosis. In spite of that, vaccination against paratuberculosis in goats has been applied with the same criteria as in sheep. This has caused a large amount of confusion in some regions, where both infections are present, because it has been possible neither to evaluate vaccine efficacy properly nor control tuberculosis efficiently.

Goat vaccination against paratuberculosis seems currently in use in Spain, the Netherlands, France, Norway, and India, at least, according to commercial sources, even though, as discussed previously, formal publication of results in the veterinary literature is scarce.

Vaccination in Norway is interesting because that was the country where the first large-scale field study on paratuberculosis control in goats was performed. It started with an effort based on hygiene and management measures that failed to decrease the incidence of the disease and was replaced with vaccination. Immunization with a vaccine made with two British-origin strains was made obligatory and, according to a 1985 report, it resulted in a 98% reduction in postmortem finding of lesions, which, during a period of 16 years, reduced incidence from 53% to 1%.[71] A later change in the vaccination policy making it voluntary seemed to result in a rebound of incidence.

In the United States, there is a registered vaccine for use in cattle, which, according to the minor species cascade principle, should provide a base for veterinary prescription in small ruminants as an individual clinical act. Specific state legislation might establish specific restrictions, however. In general, there are some countries, states, or regions that do not allow any use of paratuberculosis vaccines in any species. This is meant to prevent deviation of the vaccines to species submitted to tuberculosis control programs. In these circumstances, the only economically profitable strategy should be the improvement of biosecurity and management measures to reduce the chances of exposure of animals in their more susceptible lifetime points. Individual serologic testing or pooled fecal detection is advisable in those operations where high individual value or when upscaling can yield a positive economic balance compared to the increased costs of testing and culling strategies.

VACCINE EFFICIENCY

The first paratuberculosis vaccine was an attenuated (live) vaccine with oil and pumice powder adjuvants,[72] a type of vaccine that has been widely used.[73] In the 1960s it was shown that inactivated (killed) vaccines had the same efficacy as the attenuated ones[20,74–76]; therefore, for biosecurity considerations, it steadily replaced the use of attenuated vaccines. Neither inactivation nor vaccine strain seems to have substantial effects on the protection conferred by vaccination. The use of cell fractions[76,77] or administration by the oral route,[78] however, dramatically reduced the efficacy of vaccination. Recent research using genetic engineering tools might bring new improved approaches based on modified organisms or specific antigens.[79–84]

The mechanisms of protection elicited by vaccination are not well known. It is widely accepted that vaccination neither fully prevents nor clears paratuberculosis infection. It is assumed that vaccination modifies the immunopathologic processes that lead to the persistent progressive regional intestinal inflammation responsible for clinical disease in such a way that immunized individuals are able to arrest the progression of the infection and the ensuing lesions. This results in reduction of the excretion of MAP and significant decrease in the severity of clinical signs and economic losses.[85] It is not clear that reduced excretion of MAP can, in the long term, completely prevent infection in vaccinated farms, but it seems likely that a low level of infection can persist indefinitely and make establishing paratuberculosis vaccination necessary as a permanent routine in replacer raising. Whether or not that is caused by the persistence of MAP in neighboring nonvaccinating farms or wildlife or in the vaccinated animals themselves remains to be determined. In regard to environmental contamination, it should be taken into account that vaccination seems to reduce more the overall contamination than the prevalence. According to a study by van Schaik and coworkers,[86] performed in cattle, it is possible to calculate that although the prevalence reduction was 13.3%, the overall contamination reduction was 66.6% thanks to the decrease in the number of heaviest shedders. Persistence of low-level infection might be a risk in absolute terms, but it raises the question of whether or not, in the absence of a complete control of MAP in the environment or in other farms, the combination of vaccine and low-intensity challenge might help keep high the immune status in the vaccinated farms.

Reports on paratuberculosis vaccination in sheep have appeared in the literature since 26 years after the first formal description of paratuberculosis in cattle. There have been 49 trials reported in 21 articles on the results of vaccination in sheep, with different variables taken into consideration; these can be summarized in 3 categories: clinical signs/mortality, presence of lesions, and isolation of the causal agent. In 94% of cases, positive effects of vaccination have been reported. In goats, the number of trials is even smaller: 24 trials reported in 9 articles. In this case, positive effects of vaccination have been reported in 92% of cases (Bastida F and Juste RA, unpublished data, 2010).

CONTROL OR ERADICATION

The simplicity and robustness of Koch postulates, which allowed the early success of some countries in the eradication of tuberculosis by a testing and culling strategy, led the veterinary community to think that the only reasonable goal in the control of most infectious diseases was full eradication. This has proved an optimistic perspective, because many microorganisms can survive in hidden reservoirs and because the perspective on animal welfare, ecological balance, biodiversity, drug and antibiotic usage, and sustainable production is forcing a change of paradigm in the approach to animal disease control. Thus, considerations about the role of natural population regulation factors have shown that killing individuals is part of the ecological balance and that it can be achieved not only by superior predators but also by microscopic agents that, in the end, are also part of the general biodiversity of any system. The loss of animals in programs based on testing and culling of nonzoonotic infections and the wasting-associated rapid turnover of animals based on productivity are not always socially acceptable; thus, more sustainable strategies are demanded. When approaching the control of nonzoonotic, chronic, slow infections that are widespread and prevalent but are not highly contagious, long-term strategies that exploit natural resistance in the populations both by stimulating effective immune responses in the short term or by selecting individuals with a higher genetic resistance to infection in the long run should be considered.

There are few doubts about the economic profitability of vaccination versus any other strategy, including doing nothing. A few years ago, this was shown in a simulation model.[87] Even though it was a simple computer simulation developed for sheep, it allowed modification for considering other susceptible species managed as a flock/herd. It predicted that test and cull would lead to eradication in half the time that

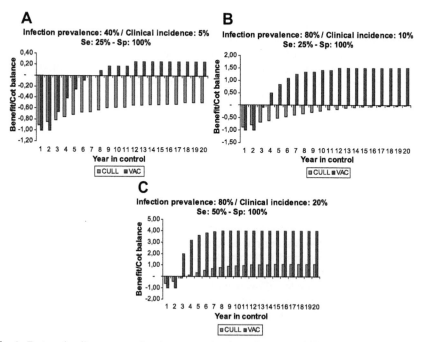

Fig. 1. Test-and-cull versus vaccination strategies; benefit-to-cost balance according to Juste and Casal at 2 different levels of initial disease impact and different test sensitivities (A) in low clinical incidence with a low-sensitivity test, (B) in moderate clinical incidence with a low-sensitivity test, and (C) in high clinical incidence with a medium-sensitivity test. Cull, culled animals; Se, test sensitivity; Sp, test specificity; Vac, vaccinated animals. (*Data from* Juste RA, Casal J. An economic and epidemiologic simulation of different control strategies for ovine paratuberculosis. Prev Vet Med 1993;15:101–5.)

vaccination would. When economic costs were included in the analysis, however, it was evident that the best strategy was vaccination, because it yielded approximately 3 to 4 times better benefit-to-cost ratios than did testing and culling (**Fig. 1**).

PREVENTION OR THERAPY

Another aspect that has received little attention in the fight against paratuberculosis with vaccines is when to vaccinate. Although the general recommendation has been to give the vaccine within the first days of life, to immunize the animals before infection, there have been reports in sheep and goats that suggest that later vaccination could be more advisable, because it is easier for management reasons (there is more time available for selection of replacements and vaccinations can be grouped) as well as because the immune system is in a more advanced maturation stage.[88] The real goal of vaccination is to prevent clinical cases, which is achieved by modifying the course of pathogenesis of the disease rather than preventing infection and colonization in the animal; hence, it seems more appropriate to use the vaccine in older animals. In this sense, there are some reports using vaccination in adult sheep from flocks with paratuberculosis, presumably already infected, with satisfactory results in terms of regression of lesions and reduction of clinical cases/losses.[61,62] This is different from cattle where a milder immune response can be a bonus, because it makes less likely later interferences with tuberculosis testing schedules.

It is obvious that animals are surrounded by MAP from birth and that only a few might be vaccinated before exposure. The later vaccine administration program strongly suggests that vaccination has more a therapeutic than a preventive effect, as confirmed by the positive results obtained when vaccinating adults.

SUMMARY

Control of paratuberculosis in small ruminants can be easily achieved by vaccination. Vaccination prevents clinical cases and thus may lead to increased production at a highly profitable benefit-to-cost ratio. Because bacterial shedding is greatly reduced, vaccination can help control the general contamination risks. There are no restrictions to vaccination in sheep, but potential interference with diagnosis of tuberculosis must be taken into account in goats. Other control strategies have failed, because of either high costs or lack of efficacy on a large scale.

REFERENCES

1. Corpa JM, Garrido JM, García Marín JF, et al. Classification of lesions observed in natural cases of paratuberculosis in goats. J Comp Pathol 2000;122:255–65.
2. González J, Geijo MV, García-Pariente C, et al. Histopathological classification of lesions associated with natural paratuberculosis infection in cattle. J Comp Pathol 2005;133:184–96.
3. Pérez V, García Marín JF, Badiola JJ. Description and classification of different types of lesion associated with natural paratuberculosis infection in sheep. J Comp Pathol 1996;114:107–22.
4. Verna AE, Garcia-Pariente C, Munoz M, et al. Variation in the immuno-pathological responses of lambs after experimental infection with different strains of Mycobacterium avium subsp. paratuberculosis. Zoonoses Public Health 2007; 54:243–52.

5. Buergelt CD, Hall C, McEntee K, et al. Pathological evaluation of paratuberculosis in naturally infected cattle. Vet Pathol 1978;15:196–206.

6. Stamp JT, Watt JA. Johne's disease in sheep. J Comp Pathol 1954;64:26–38.

7. Rajya BS, Singh CM. Studies on the pathology of Johne's disease in sheep: III. Pathologic changes in sheep with naturally occurring infections. Am J Vet Res 1961;22:189–203.

8. Paliwal OP, Rajya BS. Evaluation of paratuberculosis in goats: pathomorphological studies. Indian J Vet Pathol 1982;6:29–34.

9. de Juan L, Alvarez J, Romero B, et al. Comparison of Four Different Culture Media for Isolation and Growth of Type II and Type I/III Mycobacterium avium subsp. paratuberculosis Strains Isolated from Cattle and Goats. Appl Environ Microbiol 2006;72:5927–32.

10. Sevilla I, Garrido JM, Geijo M, et al. Pulsed-field gel electrophoresis profile homogeneity of Mycobacterium avium subsp. paratuberculosis isolates from cattle and heterogeneity of those from sheep and goats. BMC Microbiol 2007;7:18.

11. Rossiter CA, Lein DH, Shin S. Objectives and current status of the NYS paratuberculosis eradication and certification program. In: Chiodini RJ, Kreeger JM, editors. Proceedings of the III International Colloquium on Paratuberculosis. Providence (RI): IAP; 1991. p. 25.

12. Collins MT. Diagnosis of paratuberculosis. Vet Clin North Am Food Anim Pract 1996;12:357–71.

13. Collins MT. Paratuberculosis: review of present knowledge. Acta Vet Scand 2003; 44(3–4):217–21.

14. Kennedy DJ. The Australian national Johne's disease market assurance program. In: Chiodini RJ, Collins MT, editors. Proceedings of the V International Colloquium on Paratuberculosis. Madison (WI): IAP; 1996. p. 16.

15. Johne HA, Frothingham L. Ein eigenthümlicher fall von tuberculose beim Rind. Deut Zeits Tiermed Vergl Pathol 1895;21:438–54.

16. Chiodini RJ. The history of paratuberculosis (Johne's disease). A review of the literature 1985–1992. Providence (RI): International Association of Paratuberculosis; 1993. p. 658.

17. Sigurdsson B, Palsson PA. Visna of sheep; a slow, demyelinating infection. Br J Exp Pathol 1958;39:519–28.

18. Sigurdsson B, Gunnarsson E. Paratuberculosis in sheep, cattle, goats and reinder in Iceland. A result of an import of a flock of sheep from Germany 1933. The controlof the disease. In: Merkal RS, editor. Proceedings of the I International Colloquium on Paratuberculosis. Ames (IA): NADC; 1983. p. 238–43.

19. Gunnarsson E, Fridriksdottir V, Sigurdarson S. Control of paratuberculosis in Iceland. Acta Vet Scand 2003;44:255.

20. Sigurdsson B. A killed vaccine against paratuberculosis (Johne's disease) in sheep. Am J Vet Res 1960;21(1):54–67.

21. Sigurdsson B, Tryggvadottir AG. Immunization with heat-killed Mycobacterium paratuberculosis in mineral oil. J Bacteriol 1949;58:271–8.

22. Sigurdsson B, Tryggvadottir AG. Immunization with heat-killed Mycobacterium paratuberculosis in mineral oil. J Bacteriol 1950;59:541–3.

23. Vallée H, Rinjard P, Vallée M. Sur la prémunition de l'entérite paratuberculeuse des bovidés. Rev Gen Med Vet 1934;43:777–9.

24. Dalziel TK. Chronic interstitial enteritis. Br Med J 1913;2:1068–70.

25. Golan L, Livneh-Kol A, Gonen E, et al. Mycobacterium avium paratuberculosis invades human small-intestinal goblet cells and elicits inflammation. J Infect Dis 2009;199:350–4.

26. Greenstein RJ. Is Crohn's disease caused by a mycobacterium? Comparisons with leprosy, tuberculosis, and Johne's disease. Lancet Infect Dis 2003;3:507–14.

27. Naser SA, Ghobrial G, Romero C, et al. Culture of Mycobacterium avium subespecies paratuberculosis from the blood of patients with Crohn's disease. Lancet 2004;364:1039–44.

28. Uzoigwe JC, Khaitsa ML, Gibbs PS. Epidemiological evidence for mycobacterium avium subspecies paratuberculosis as a cause of Crohn's disease. Epidemiol Infect 2007;135:1057–68.

29. Yamamoto-Furusho JK, Korzenik JR. Crohn's disease: innate immunodeficiency? World J Gastroenterol 2006;12:6751–5.

30. Juste RA, Elguezabal N, Garrido JM, et al. On the prevalence of M. avium subspecies paratuberculosis DNA in the blood of healthy individuals and patients with inflammatory bowel disease. PLoS One 2008;3:e2537.

31. Juste RA, Elguezabal N, Pavon A, et al. Association between Mycobacterium avium subsp. paratuberculosis DNA in blood and cellular and humoral immune response in inflammatory bowel disease patients and controls. Int J Infect Dis 2008;13:247–54.

32. Juste RA, Portu J, Aldamiz M, et al. Seroreactivity of Crohn's disease patients to mycobacterial antigens: original data and analytical review of the literature. An Vet (Murcia) 2007;23:91–103.

33. Watkins C, Schock A, May L, et al. Assessing virulence of vaccine strains of Mycobacterium avium subspecies paratuberculosis in a calf model. Vet Microbiol 2010;146:63–9.

34. Pérez V. In: Estudio de la paratuberculosis en la especie ovina [PhD thesis]. University of Zaragoza; 1992.

35. Chávez GG. In: Estudio comparativo de las lesiones y de la respuesta inmunológica observadas en corderos infectados experimentalmente con Mycobacterium paratuberculosisy Mycobacterium avium subsp. silvaticum [PhD thesis]. University of Zaragoza; 1993.

36. Juste RA, Marco JC, Saez de Ocariz C, et al. Comparison of different media for the isolation of small ruminant strains of Mycobacterium paratuberculosis. Vet Microbiol 1991;28:385–90.

37. Collins DM, Gabric DM, de Lisle GW. Identification of two groups of mycobacterium paratuberculosis strains by restriction analysis and DNA hybridization. J Clin Microbiol 1990;28:1591–6.

38. Stevenson K, Hughes VM, de Juan L, et al. Molecular characterization of pigmented and nonpigmented isolates of Mycobacterium avium subsp. paratuberculosis. J Clin Microbiol 2002;40:1798–804.

39. de Juan L, Mateos A, Dominguez L, et al. Genetic diversity of Mycobacterium avium subspecies paratuberculosis isolates from goats detected by pulsed-field gel electrophoresis. Vet Microbiol 2005;106:249–57.

40. Sevilla I, Singh SV, Garrido JM, et al. PCR-REA genotype of paratuberculosis strains isolated from different host species and geographic locations. Rev sci tech Off int Epiz 2005;24:1061–6.

41. Singh SV, Singh PK, Singh AV, et al. Comparative efficacy of an indigenous 'inactivated vaccine' using highly pathogenic field strain of Mycobacterium avium subspecies paratuberculosis 'Bison type' with a commercial vaccine for the control of Capri-paratuberculosis in India. Vaccine 2007;25:7102–10.

42. de Juan L, Alvarez J, Aranaz A, et al. Molecular epidemiology of Types I/III strains of Mycobacterium avium subspecies paratuberculosis isolated from goats and cattle. Vet Microbiol 2006;115:102–10.

43. Chiodini RJ, Van Kruiningen HJ, Merkal RS. Ruminant paratuberculosis (Johne's disease): the current status and future prospects. Cornell Vet 1984;74:218–62.
44. Momotani E, Whipple DL, Thiermann AB, et al. Role of M cells and macrophagos in the entrance of Mycobacterium paratuberculosis into domes of ileal Peyer's patches in calves. Vet Pathol 1988;25:131–7.
45. Momotani R, Whipple DL, Thiermann AB, et al. Role of intestinal M-cells and macrophages in the mycobacterium paratuberculosis infection in calves. In: Thorel MF, Merkal RS, editors. Proceedings of the II Interantional Colloquium on Paratuberculosis. Maisons-Alfort (France): Laboratoire Central de Recherches Vétérinaires; 1998. p. 150–6.
46. García Marín JF. Patogenia de la tuberculosis caprina. In: Juste RA, editor. Paratuberculosis ovina. Ovis Madrid: Luzan 5; 1996. p. 23–31.
47. Juste RA, García Marín JF, Peris B, et al. Experimental infection of vaccinated and non-vaccinated lambs with Mycobacterium paratuberculosis. J Comp Pathol 1994;110:185–94.
48. Pérez V, Tellechea J, Badiola JJ, et al. Relation between serologic response and pathologic findings in sheep with naturally acquired paratuberculosis. Am J Vet Res 1997;58:799–803.
49. Pérez V, Tellechea J, Corpa JM, et al. Relation between pathologic findings and cellular immune responses in sheep with naturally acquired paratuberculosis. Am J Vet Res 1999;60:123–7.
50. Stabel JR. Host responses to Mycobacterium avium subsp. paratuberculosis: a complex arsenal. Anim Health Res Rev 2006;7:61–70.
51. Tobin F, Wood I, Doyle C. The Victorian Ovine Johne's disease Eradication Program—Impact on sheep producers. In: Juste RA, Geijo MV, Garrido JM, editors. Proceedings of the VII International Colloquium on Paratuberculosis. Madison (WI): IAP; 2002. p. 450–4.
52. Hood B, Seedsman T. Psychosocial investigation of individual and community rsponses to the experience of Ovine Johne's Disease in rural Victoria. Aust J Rural Health 2004;12:54–60.
53. de Lisle GW. Can Johne's disease be eradicared from sheep in Australia? Aust Vet J 1997;75:336.
54. Denholm LJ, Ottaway SJ, Marshall DJ. Control of ovine Johne's disease in New South Wales. In: Chiodini RJ, Collins MT, editors. Proceedings of the V International Colloquium on Paratuberculosis. Madison (WI): IAP; 1996. p. 18.
55. Eppleston J, Reddacliff LA, Windsor PA, et al. Efficacy of a killed Mycobacterium paratuberculosis vaccine for the control of OJD in Australian sheep flocks. In: Manning EJB, Nielsen SS, editors. Proceedings fo the VIII International Colloquium on Paratuberculosis. Madison (WI): IAP; 2005. p. 43.
56. Kennedy DJ, Allworth B. Ovine Johne's disease—progress and challenges. Aust Vet J 2001;79:482–3.
57. Reddacliff L, Eppleston J, Windsor P, et al. Efficacy of a killed vaccine for the control of paratuberculosis in Australian sheep flocks. Vet Microbiol 2006;115:77–90.
58. Sergeant ES. Ovine Johne's disease in Australia—the first 20 years. Aust Vet J 2001;79:484–91.
59. Aller B, Fernández-Díez M, Escudero-Díez A. Paratuberculosis ovina. Sup Cient Bol Inf Cons Gen Col Vet Esp 1973;196:11–8.
60. Badiola JJ, García de Jalón JA, Cuervo LA. Paratuberculosis ovina. An Fac Vet Zaragoza 1980;14–15:14–5.

61. Corpa JM, Pérez V, Sanchez MA, et al. Control of paratuberculosis (Johne's disease) in goats by vaccination of adult animals. Vet Rec 2000;146:195–6.
62. García Marín JF, Tellechea J, Gutiérrez M, et al. Evaluation of two vaccines (killed and attenuated) against small ruminant paratuberculosis. In: Chiodini RJ, Collins MT, editors. Proceedings of the V International Colloquium on Paratuberculosis. Madison (WI): IAP; 1996. p. 22.
63. García Marín JF, Tellechea J, Gutiérrez M, et al. Histopathological evaluation of a killed vaccine against paratuberculosis in sheep. In: Proceedings of 13th Congress of the European Society of Veterinary Pathology; 1995. p. 57.
64. Aduriz JJ. In: Epidemiología, diagnóstico y control de la paratuberculosis ovina en la Comunidad Autónoma del País Vasco [PhD thesis]. University of Zaragoza; 1993.
65. Aduriz JJ, Juste RA, Saez de Ocariz C, et al. Paratuberculosis in sheep flocks: II. vaccination. In: Chiodini RJ, Kreeger JM, editors. Proceedings of the III International Colloquium on Paratuberculosis. Providence (RI): IAP; 1991. p. 27.
66. Geijo MV, Garrido JM, Aduriz G, et al. Paratuberculosis vaccination response in cattle, sheep and goats. In: Juste RA, Geijo MV, Garrido JM, editors. Proceedings of the VII International Colloquium on Paratuberculosis. Madison (WI): IAP; 2002. p. 31.
67. Windsor PA, Eppleston J, Whittington RJ, et al. Efficacy of a killed Mycobacterium avium subsp. paratuberculosis vaccine for the control of OJD in australian sheep flocks. In: Juste RA, Geijo MV, Garrido JM, editors. Proceedings of the VII International Colloquium on Paratuberculosis. Madison (WI): IAP; 2002. p. 98.
68. de Lisle GW. Johne's disease in New Zealand: the past, present and a glimpse into the future. N Z Vet J 2020;50(Suppl 3):53–6.
69. Crowther RW, Polydorou K, Nitti S, et al. Johne's disease in sheep in cyprus. Vet Rec 1976;98:463.
70. Cranwell MP. Control of Johne's disease in a flock of sheep by vaccination. Vet Rec 1993;133:219–20.
71. Saxegaard F, Fodstad FH. Control of paratuberculosis (Johne's disease) in goats by vaccination. Vet Rec 1985;116:439–41.
72. Vallée H, Rinjard P, Vallée M. Sur la prémunisation de l'entérite paratuberculeuse due au bacille de Johne. Bull Acad Med 1941;125:195–8.
73. Wilesmith JW. Johne's disease: a retrospective study of vaccinated herds in Great Britain. Br Vet J 1982;138:321–31.
74. Huitema H. Johne's disease in cattle and vaccination. Bull Off Int Epizoot 1967; 15:1–6.
75. Brotherston JG, Gilmour NJL, Samuel JM. Quantitative studies of Mycobacterium johnei in the tissues of sheep. II Protection afforded by dead vaccines. J Comp Pathol 1961;71:300–11.
76. Hurley SS. Efficacy of bacterins. In: Proceedings of the I International Colloquium on Paratuberculosis. Ames (IA); 1983. p. 289–90.
77. Larsen AB, Moyle AI, Himes EM. Experimental vaccination of cattle against paratuberculosis (Johne's disease) with killed bacterial vaccines: a controlled field study. Am J Vet Res 1978;39:65–9.
78. Gilmour NJL, Halhead WA, Brotherston JG. Studies on immunity to Mycobacterium johnei in sheep. J Comp Pathol 1965;75:165–73.
79. Koets A, Hoek A, Langelaar M, et al. Mycobacterial 70 kD heat-shock protein is an effective subunit vaccine against bovine paratuberculosis. Vaccine 2006; 24(14):2550–9.

80. Kathaperumal K, Kumanan V, McDonough S, et al. Evaluation of immune responses and protective efficacy in a goat model following immunization with a coctail of recombinant antigens and a polyprotein of mycobacterium avium subsp. paratuberculosis. Vaccine 2009;27(1):123–35.

81. Sechi LA, Mara L, Cappai P, et al. Immunization with DNA vaccines encoding different mycobacterial antigens elicits a Th1 type immune response in lambs and protects against Mycobacterium avium subspecies paratuberculosis infection. Vaccine 2006;24(3):229–35.

82. Bull TJ, Gilbert SC, Sridhar S, et al. A novel multi-antigen virally vectored vaccine against Mycobacterium avium subspecies paratuberculosis. PLoS One 2007; 2(11):e1229.

83. Roupie V, Leroy B, Rosseels V, et al. Immunogenicity and protective efficacy of DNA vaccines encoding MAP0586c and MAP4308c of Mycobacterium avium subsp. paratuberculosis secretome. Vaccine 2008;26(37):4783–94.

84. Huntley JF, Stabel JR, Paustian ML, et al. Expression library immunization confers protection against Mycobacterium avium subsp. paratuberculosis infection. Infect Immun 2005;73(10):6877–84.

85. Juste RA, Alonso-Hearn M, Molina E, et al. Significant reduction in bacterial shedding and improvement in milk production in dairy farms after the use of a new inactivated paratuberculosis vaccine in a field trial. BMC Res Notes 2009;2:233.

86. van Schaik G, Kalis CHJ, Benedictus G, et al. Cost-benefit analysis of vaccination against paratuberculosis in dairy cattle. Vet Rec 1996;139:624–7.

87. Juste RA, Casal J. An economic and epidemiologic simulation of different control strategies for ovine paratuberculosis. Prev Vet Med 1993;15:101–5.

88. Corpa JM, Perez V, Garcia Marin JF. Differences in the immune responses in lambs and kids vaccinated against paratuberculosis, according to the age of vaccination. Vet Microbiol 2000;77:475–85.

Pharmaceutical Control of Endoparasitic Helminth Infections in Sheep

Neil D. Sargison, BA, VetMB, PhD, DSHP, FRCVS

KEYWORDS

- Anthelmintics • Endoparasites • Helminths
- Pharmaceutics • Sheep

Sheep are hosts to numerous genera and species of helminth parasites. For most of these parasites, a balance has evolved between them and their sheep hosts, whereby the host provides the environment and nutrients required by the parasitic population, while the parasite does not compromise the host to an extent that will threaten the survival of its future generations. Circumstances that upset this evolutionary balance can give rise to production-limiting disease, for example, when sheep are exposed to a previously unrecognized or new helminth species, as illustrated by the fact that the common large intestinal nematode species, *Oesophagostomum venulosum*, is not considered pathogenic, whereas the closely related, but rare species, *Oesophagostomum columbianum*, is highly pathogenic.[1] The balance between sheep hosts and helminth parasites has evolved over millions of years, but has been upset in relatively recent times by domestication and farming practices that favor the parasites by the inadvertent selection of more susceptible hosts or by the creation of environments that enable the establishment of larger populations of free-living stages of the parasites. This upset to the evolutionary host-parasite balance affects different parasite species to differing extents, enabling some nematode, trematode, or cestode species to be potentially production limiting while others are not.

Helminth parasites, such as *Haemonchus contortus*, *Bunostomum trigonocephalum*, and *Fasciola hepatica*, limit sheep production, due to the direct effects of their blood feeding behavior, while the pathogenic effects of most helminth species arise

The author has nothing to disclose.

University of Edinburgh, Royal (Dick) School of Veterinary Studies, Large Animal Practice, Easter Bush Veterinary Centre, Roslin, Midlothian, EH25 9RG, UK

E-mail address: neil.sargison@ed.ac.uk

as a consequence of host innate and adaptive immune responses.[2] In fact, the parasites may have evolved to stimulate these responses in order to create the optimal environment for their own nutrition and survival, while differences in components of the host immune responses influence the extent to which the parasites limit production.[3] This has been shown by the demonstration of higher cumulative live-weight gains in corticosteroid-immunosuppressed sheep compared with control animals exposed to the same daily challenge of *Teladorsagia circumcincta* or *Trichostrongylus colubriformis*.[4,5] Furthermore, sheep that are naturally immune to gastrointestinal nematode parasites may suffer production loss despite harboring relatively low parasite burdens, whereas those that prioritize their protein resources toward survival, rather than immune responses that ensure maximal productivity, may harbor relatively high and epidemiologically relevant parasite burdens with relatively little effect on their productivity, and are resilient to the effects of helminth parasitism.[6,7]

The major production-limiting nematode parasite species affecting sheep in temperate climates are *Teladorsagia circumcincta*, *H contortus*, *Trichostrongylus vitrinus* or *Trichostrongylus colubriformis*, and *Nematodirus battus*. These parasites limit the productivity of susceptible animals because of their direct feeding activities that remove nutrients from the ingesta, and due to indirect effects on the immune response in their hosts, damaging the absorptive lining of the gastrointestinal tract or, in the case of *H contortus*, feeding on blood. The net pathophysiological effects of these activities are inefficient feed utilization, inducing a state of relative protein deficiency, fluid and electrolyte or macroelement imbalances, and anemia, leading to clinical signs such as reduced appetite, poor weight gains, diarrhea, and death.[8–10] Overall, the greatest economic importance of nematode parasites is suboptimal productivity arising from continuous low-level exposure to infective larvae.[11] Sheep can also be affected by several trematode parasites, in particular *F hepatica*, *Fasciola gigantica*, *Fascioloides magna*, *Dicrocoelium dendriticum*, and *Paramphistomum* spp. The feeding and migratory activities of these parasites are direct causes of production loss, because they remove blood and nutrients and cause tissue damage. Cestode parasites, such as *Taenia multiceps*, *Taenia hydatigena*, and *Taenia ovis*, or *Echinococcus granulosus*, for which sheep are intermediate hosts, cause disease through the development and space-occupying nature of their second-stage coenurus, cysticercus, or hydatid larval cysts, respectively. The cestode tapeworm parasite, *Monezia expansa*, which has sheep as its final host, passively absorbs nutrients from the intestinal digesta and has few, if any, adverse effects on productivity.[12] Helminth parasitism also causes production loss, due to the considerable cost incurred by its treatment and management.

Gastrointestinal helminth parasites are arguably the most important causes of suboptimal productivity in sheep, albeit that they often occur concurrently with other problems. The principal reason for keeping farmed sheep is to convert primary forage, herbage, or cereal crops into a marketable product. The efficiency of conversion of feed to meat is greater in sheep that achieve maximal growth rates than in ill-thrifty animals, because there is a daily feed requirement for maintenance that must be met before growth can occur, irrespective of the time taken to reach slaughter weight. Furthermore, sheep that are slow to finish are more susceptible to compounding effects of production-limiting diseases than rapidly growing animals, which may leave the farm before the main risk period for these problems. Therefore, the profitability of global sheep farming is heavily influenced by the efficiency of feed conversion to meat; control of gastrointestinal helminth parasites is a prerequisite for economically sustainable production.

PHARMACEUTICAL CONTROL OF NEMATODE PARASITES

Under conditions where naïve lambs are grazed on pasture that is heavily contaminated with infective parasitic nematode L_3, frequent treatment with a conventional, short-acting anthelmintic may improve animal performance for a few days, but production losses are inevitable. Although such lambs that are exposed to a high level of infective larval challenge can achieve satisfactory growth rates after the onset of acquired immunity, their cumulative weight gains never match those of animals which were only exposed to a small challenge.[10] Very low levels of infective larval challenge may have negligible effects on productivity while enabling the development of immunity, important in store lambs or future replacement breeding sheep, which will spend more than one season on pasture. The underlying principles of nematode control are, therefore, to limit the exposure of naïve animals to infective L_3 on pasture,[11] while allowing sufficient challenge to enable the development of protective immunity.

Pasture contamination in the spring with L_3 of sheep nematode parasites (predominantly with *T circumcincta* in temperate regions) arises both from overwintered infective L_3 on pasture and from nematode eggs shed by recently-lambed ewes.[13] The egg output of lactating ewes, referred to as the "periparturient rise," derives from nematodes that have overwintered within the ewes as inhibited L_4 larvae, and from completion of the life cycle of overwintered L_3 ingested from pasture after lambing.[14] The relative importance of these sources of pasture larval contamination differs from year to year with different winter weather conditions and sheep grazing management; also, it varies between different regions and depends on the nematode genera involved. When ingested by naïve lambs, these infective L_3 give rise to adult nematodes, which accumulate over the summer months and contribute to subsequent pasture larval contamination, potentially leading to disease.

Exposure of naïve animals to infective L_3 on pasture can be minimized (a) by finishing lambs quickly, before pasture L_3 burdens become production limiting (this strategy has positive knock-on effects, with lower overwinter larval survival and challenge during the subsequent spring), (b) by grazing susceptible sheep or cattle only on "safe" pasture, thereby evading infective L_3 challenge (see the article by Gareth F. Bath elsewhere in this issue for further exploration of this topic), or (c) by using anthelmintic drugs to suppress pasture larval contamination. In fact, most commercial sheep farms are unable to provide sufficient safe pasture for the purpose of nematode parasite control in all susceptible sheep, without compromising the efficiency of crop and cattle production. Most nematode control regimes, therefore, rely to different extents on the use of pharmaceutical drugs with the primary objective of suppressing pasture L_3 contamination.[15] Effective pharmaceutical drugs are, and will always be, essential for the treatment of clinical cases of parasitic gastroenteritis.

Before the introduction of effective broad-spectrum anthelmintic drugs, control of nematode parasites depended on frequently impracticable evasive management strategies and on the use of crude drugs such as sodium arsenite, tetrachloroethylene, carbon tetrachloride, carbon bisulfide, copper sulfate, and nicotine sulfate, which were potentially equally toxic to the parasites and to their sheep hosts. Nematode parasites, therefore, made intensive sheep production uneconomic in many regions. The introduction of phenothiazine in the 1940s[16] was followed by the first tubulin-binding benzimidazole drug, thiabendazole, in the early 1960s,[17] the first ganglion-blocking imidazothiazole drug, levamisole, in the early 1970s,[18] the first macrocyclic lactone, ivermectin, in the early 1980s,[19] and the amino-acetonitrile derivative (AAD) drug, monepantel, in 2010.[20] These broad-spectrum anthelmintic drugs initially enabled profitable sheep production on livestock farms, which had become economically unsustainable. In addition, the salicylanilide-derivative drug, closantel, has a narrow spectrum of activity against *H contortus*.[21] Various highly successful nematode parasite control strategies subsequently evolved, based on the understanding that production losses due to nematode parasites arise primarily from the hosts' immune responses to L_3 challenge. Not surprisingly, most farmers became dependent on frequent routine anthelmintic treatments of their sheep, including the common practice of dosing before a move onto "clean" grazing.

Problems with the Use of Anthelmintic Drugs for the Control of Nematode Parasites

It would have been naïve to have expected the routine use of anthelmintic drugs with the aim of suppressing pasture larval contamination to be sustainable, due to the enormous potential of the helminth parasites to adapt to environmental challenges that has been afforded by millions of years of evolution. During recent years, suboptimal sheep productivity resulting from parasitic gastroenteritis has become commonplace, despite the adoption of blueprint nematode parasite control programs. These problems have arisen due to a combination of factors, including: (a) effects of concurrent disease or management on anthelmintic drug pharmacokinetics, exemplified by the common failure of benzimidazole drugs to kill *N battus* in scouring lambs when the anthelmintic bioavailability may be reduced due to rapid flow of digesta through the intestines[22]; (b) the evolution of parasites in response to climate change,[23] exemplified by the opportunities afforded to *H contortus* by wetter and milder spring and autumn weather in northern Europe[24] and the changing seasonal pattern of nematodirosis in the United Kingdom[25]; (c) changes in farm and grazing management resulting from changing economics of sheep production[26]; and (d) the emergence of anthelmintic resistance. *T circumcincta* or *H contortus* resistance to benzimidazole, imidazothiazole, and/or macrocyclic lactone anthelmintics is now commonplace in many countries. Once resistance to an anthelmintic group has emerged within an individual sheep flock, parasitic gastroenteritis can no longer be controlled using any of the drugs belonging to that anthelmintic group, and long-term reversion to susceptibility within flocks has not been demonstrated. Multiple anthelmintic resistance is, therefore, a serious threat to economically sustainable sheep production,[27] because it necessitates fundamental, often expensive, changes to animal management and compromises for the control of nematode parasites if it is allowed to reach a high enough level.

On most sheep farms, the first indications of anthelmintic resistance are the failure of lambs to reach finished weights by late autumn, which may be combined with scouring and even deaths due to parasitic gastroenteritis, despite preventive anthelmintic treatments. However, many farmers fail to recognize the significance of these problems in their flocks or attribute them to other causes, such as weather conditions or sheep genetics. Furthermore, anthelmintic resistance can result in clinically inapparent, suboptimal growth rates for some time before these overt signs of disease are seen.[28] The economic impact of anthelmintic resistance is further complicated by the fact that provided nutrition is good, healthy and productive sheep can be maintained on a farm with a minimum anthelmintic efficacy of 80%, although this figure is not sustainable because the resistant nematodes will make ever more significant contributions to following generations.[29]

The emergence of anthelmintic resistance is an inevitable consequence of good nematode control, not a result of bad farming practice.[30] To date there is no evidence to show that anthelmintic-resistant nematodes are any more pathogenic than nonresistant nematodes, so resistance itself is not production limiting. In addition, although anthelmintic resistance complicates effective nematode parasite control, in most cases gastrointestinal nematodes can still be adequately managed.

The launch of the AAD anthelmintic group[20] and the realistic probability that other novel anthelmintic groups or combinations could be introduced in the foreseeable future might help to reduce the impact of anthelmintic resistance in the short term, but also highlights the challenge of how to maintain the practical efficacy of both new and existing drugs. Unfortunately, the molecular and population genetic basis of anthelmintic resistance is poorly understood, so best advice concerning its management is largely empirical. Practical inefficacy of an anthelmintic drug group, due to resistance in nematode parasites, might arise on a sheep farm in 1 or more of 3 ways: (a) by gene flow in nematodes introduced with newly arrived animals, (b) following repeated exposure of nematodes to subtherapeutic drug concentrations, or (c) by selection of preexisting resistant nematodes by affording them a competitive advantage over susceptible nematodes.[31] Once resistance alleles have emerged, effective exposure of nematode populations within their sheep host to anthelmintic drugs kills most of the susceptible nematodes and confers a selective advantage to those nematodes having resistance alleles. Feces produced by the sheep or cattle host during the subsequent prepatent period contain mostly eggs of the surviving resistant nematodes, which consequently contribute to a greater proportion of succeeding generations. The evolution of resistance is thus determined by the extent to which survivors of the drug treatment contribute their genes to future generations. The rate of selection for resistance is therefore dependent on the number of genes involved, the dominance, partial dominance, or recessiveness of the alleles, and on the intensity of the selection pressure. The intensity of the selection pressure is influenced by the frequency and timing of anthelmintic treatments and by the drug efficacy, which is in turn influenced by the dose rate, its inherent efficacy, and the pharmacodynamics and pharmacokinetics within the host. The rate of selection for anthelmintic resistance is also influenced by the life expectancy and fecundity of adult nematodes, the parasite generation interval, the ability or otherwise for the parasite to self-fertilize, and the proportion of the susceptible population exposed to the anthelmintic compared with that on pasture.[31,32] The likelihood should be considered that alleles conferring anthelmintic resistance are already present in most sheep flocks, albeit at a low and clinically insignificant level. It is therefore important to ensure that these resistant alleles are not afforded any survival advantage as a result of nematode control practices.

Anthelmintic Treatment of Introduced Animals

The frequency of alleles conferring anthelmintic resistance within a nematode population may change because of the introduction of alleles conferring resistance or susceptibility with introduced animals. The impact of this would depend on the number of animals introducing resistance, the fecundity of the resistant nematodes, and the subsequent grazing management of these animals. In the absence of any sensitive, rapid, and accurate diagnostic test for anthelmintic resistant nematodes in individual sheep, all introduced sheep and goats (the major sheep parasitic nematode species also infect goats) should be assumed to be a source of multiple anthelmintic resistant nematodes. Therefore, it is intuitive best practice that all introduced sheep and goats should be treated with an effective anthelmintic on arrival[33–35] and yarded for 48 hours to ensure that any viable nematode parasite eggs have been voided, before they are turned onto pastures that might be grazed by sheep within the life span of any hatched L_3. Ideally, introduced animals should then be turned onto likely contaminated pasture, so that any resistant nematode parasites that survive anthelmintic treatment make up only a very small proportion of the otherwise susceptible population *in refugia*. Entry of stray sheep or goats should be prevented, and basic biosecurity should be imposed to ensure that sheep or goat feces are not brought onto the farm. The need for quarantine anthelmintic treatments applies equally to all introduced animals, including those returning from grazings away from home as well as purchased animals.

The choice of anthelmintic for quarantine treatment is not straightforward. In the United Kingdom, T circumcincta resistance to benzimidazole, imidazothiazole, and avermectin anthelmintics and to combinations of avermectin and benzimidazole or levamisole anthelmintics is widespread,[36–39] so the logical option is to recommend the use a sequentially administered combination[40] of monepantel and moxidectin, which when given by injection has the added benefit of quarantine treatment for sheep scab[41] (extended meat withdrawal periods are seldom problematic in recently introduced animals).

Ensuring that Nematodes are Exposed to an Effective Anthelmintic Drug Concentration

Underdosing due to inaccurate judgment of sheep body weights and faulty dosing guns is commonplace. Although this may have little immediate economic effect on animal production, it inevitably selects for anthelmintic resistance.[42] Poor drenching technique, miscalculation of the correct dose volume, and use of inaccurate weighing scales compounds the problem.[43] The effect of underdosing may also arise following incorrect storage of anthelmintic drugs, use of expired product, mixing incompatible drugs or chemicals before dosing, or use of products of dubious origin.[44,45]

The efficacy of drugs against nematode parasites can be altered by the effects of management on the physiology of their host. The efficacy of benzimidazole and oral macrocyclic lactone anthelmintics is dependent on the duration of nematode exposure to a therapeutic drug concentration, and can be enhanced by prolongation of the drug's plasma concentration profile.[46] Australian studies have shown that this can be achieved by reducing feed intake through yarding for 24 hours before drenching,[47] thereby slowing the rate of flow of digesta-bound anthelmintic drug from the rumino-reticulum to the abomasum and site of absorption in the proximal small intestine, and may reduce selection for anthelmintic resistance.[48] However, New Zealand studies have shown that when sheep have been grazed on lush green pasture before yarding for a period of 24 hours, oral dosing can stimulate closure of the reticular groove, diverting the dose into the abomasum rather than the rumino-reticulum,[49] which can potentially reduce the efficacy of benzimidazole or macrocyclic lactone anthelmintics.[50] While the incidence of rumino-reticulum bypass in lambs, which have been yarded for 24 hours, can be reduced by using low-volume drench formulations,[48,51] the scenario highlights that strategies developed for use in a particular sheep grazing management system may not be applicable to others.

Sheep and goats both serve as natural hosts for many of the same pathogenic nematode parasites, and cross-infection of multiple drug-resistant strains from goats to sheep has long been considered a significant risk to sheep.[52,53] Intrinsic differences exist between host immune responses to nematode parasites and between the pharmacokinetics of anthelmintic drug absorption and elimination in goats and sheep (see the article by Hoste and colleagues elsewhere in this issue for further exploration of this topic),[54–56] imposing a significantly higher selection pressure for anthelmintic resistance in goats. Resistance in individual parasitic nematode species to each class of anthelmintic drug has been reported globally in goats, several years before the first field report in sheep. For example, T circumcincta resistance to ivermectin was first reported in goats in Scotland[57] 9 years before the first report in sheep.[36]

Provision of a Refuge of Anthelmintic Susceptible Nematodes

Anthelmintic treatments of introduced animals and ensuring that nematodes are exposed to effective anthelmintic drug concentrations are important, but relatively straightforward in terms of management advice to reduce the risk of selection for resistance. However, the probability should be considered that nematodes are already present in all sheep flocks, which have alleles of genes that might confer resistance both to the current and to future anthelmintic drug groups. The major challenge is, therefore, to avoid further selection by affording the resistant nematodes a competitive advantage over susceptible nematodes. It is imperative that sustainable strategies are adopted for the control of nematode parasites, using grazing management and strategically targeted anthelmintic treatments to achieve a balance between maintaining adequate reservoirs of anthelmintic-susceptible nematodes *in refugia*[58,59] and limiting pasture contamination with infective larvae.[11] The practical application of *refugia*-based strategies, including selectively targeted anthelmintic treatments of sheep and goats, is described by Gareth F. Bath; and Hoste and colleagues elsewhere in this issue in articles covering therapeutics and control of diseases of sheep and goats.

The rate of selection for anthelmintic resistance by a nematode parasite species is influenced by the proportion of its total population exposed to the drug.[31] The greater the proportion of the nematode population exposed to the drug in its sheep host as compared with that on pasture at the time of anthelmintic treatment, the faster the selection for resistance. Thus, the rate of selection for anthelmintic resistance is inversely proportional to the percentage of the total parasite population that is in a refuge from anthelmintic exposure at the time of treatment.[58–60] If the proportion of free-living nematode parasites with the potential to complete their development to adults at the time of anthelmintic treatment is large, then the offspring of resistant nematodes are diluted and the opportunity for expansion of a resistant population is reduced. Conversely, if the nematode population *in refugia* is small, then the offspring of resistant nematodes will constitute a larger proportion of the next generation.[61] When the proportion of resistant nematodes in the population is low, then any measure that reduces the size of the susceptible population will favor those with resistant genes. Reduction of the size of the susceptible population will occur within the host subsequent to anthelmintic treatment, but also occurs on pasture, following suppressive anthelmintic treatment regimes or a move to safe grazing, conferring a selective advantage for the resistant worms.

The concept of maintaining a pool of susceptible parasites to control resistance has its origins in the management of crop pests.[62] For parasites to be considered to be part of a refuge (*in refugia*), they must be susceptible to the particular anthelmintic being used at the time, capable of being ingested by a suitable host and able to establish and mate so as to contribute their genes to subsequent generations.[58] The vast majority of eggs passed onto pasture do not develop to L_3 on pasture or establish to adults within the host, so are by definition not *in refugia*. It is also important to take into account seasonal variation in nematode species; for example, if the nematodes on pasture are predominantly *Trichostrongylus* spp, then they are ineffective as a refuge for *Teladorsagia* spp Similarly, seasonal variations between different populations of the same parasite species may also prove to be relevant.

The concept that failure to ensure a population of susceptible nematodes *in refugia* at the time of anthelmintic treatment selects strongly for resistance is supported by practical experience. For example, in winter rainfall areas of Western Australia, anthelmintic treatments at ecologically critical times during periods of drought,[63] when few L_3 would have survived on the pasture, would have enabled those resistant nematode parasites remaining in the sheep to make up a greater proportion of the overall surviving population following egg development to infective larvae when subsequent weather conditions permitted,[64] accounting for the rapid development of macrocyclic lactone resistance.[65] In the United Kingdom, rapid selection for moxidectin resistance has been demonstrated following treatment of hill ewes shortly after a move to clean grazing.

Various strategies have been developed to slow the emergence of anthelmintic resistance, with the theoretical objective of ensuring that only a small proportion of the total nematode population is exposed to the anthelmintic drug. These recommendations include: (a) extending the interval between anthelmintic treatments[66]; (b) avoiding unnecessary treatments, for example, of lambs when they are grazed on safe pasture or, in parts of the world where breeding period starts in the autumn, of ewes before mating[67]; and (c) targeting anthelmintic treatments at those animals that are predicted to be most affected by nematode parasitism or to contribute most toward pasture contamination.[68–70] The aims of these approaches are (a) to ensure a balance between a reasonable level of parasite control, (b) to reduce anthelmintic treatment costs and, importantly, (c) to ensure that a population of susceptible nematodes is maintained in refugia.[71] The objective of nematode control is to limit exposure of susceptible sheep to infective larvae on pasture. Therefore, strategies that only expose a small proportion of the total nematode population to the anthelmintic drug inevitably involve a compromise between achieving adequate nematode parasite control and reducing the rate of selection for anthelmintic resistance. Hence, approaches based on maintaining a susceptible nematode population in refugia are counterintuitive, because the fundamental aim of conventional anthelmintic treatment regimes is to minimize the L_3 challenge from pasture, which is an important part of the in refugia population. Conflicting approaches involving maintaining a reservoir of susceptible nematode L_3 in refugia and achieving good parasite control are only likely to be adopted if their theoretical basis is understood, or they are shown to be valid in terms of both achieving an acceptable level of nematode control and reducing the rate of selection for resistance.

In fact, nematode control does not necessitate eradication, which in any case is not achievable and would not enable the important development of host immunity. The conventional principle of nematode control was to either use evasive strategies, such as interchange grazing management with cattle or cereal crops, or to use anthelmintic drugs to suppress nematode egg output and thus to suppress pasture contamination; or to use an integrated combination of both. When used effectively, none of these strategies enable the establishment of a susceptible nematode population in refugia. Unfortunately, this problem cannot be addressed by simply reducing the overall number of anthelmintic treatments, because treatments of different cohorts of animals at different times of year exert different selection pressures for resistance, depending on the in refugia population at the time of treatment (and in the case of moxidectin, during the period of persistent protection) and on the immune status of the host.[72] Instead, farmers need to view nematode control as a continuum, challenging the effects of anthelmintic treatments at different times of the year. For example, concentrating less on the control of the periparturient rise in ewes, in the knowledge that the strategy may necessitate additional lamb anthelmintic treatments, may prove to be less selective for anthelmintic resistance, depending on the in refugia populations considered to be present at the time of each treatment.[73]

High-risk practices in relation to anthelmintic resistance must be identified and their use limited.[73] For example, modeling,[74] epidemiologic,[75] and observational[72] studies in New Zealand indicate that treatment of periparturient ewes with long-acting anthelmintics exerts a strong selection pressure for resistant genotypes of the larval challenge to their lambs, increasing the rate at which resistance develops. This situation has arisen when the size of the population of nematodes *in refugia* at the time of treatment is small.[76] Selection for anthelmintic resistance by the use of macrocyclic lactone anthelmintics in adult sheep may be compounded if the immune response of those animals limits rates of reinfection; this delays dilution of surviving resistant nematodes with unselected parasites ingested from pasture during the persistent period, and allows more time for the surviving resistant nematodes to mate with each other and produce more potentially homozygous resistant progeny.[73] However, it is important not to extrapolate from rational recommendations concerning the use of persistent anthelmintics to control of the periparturient rise in New Zealand to other countries, where sheep production patterns and management may differ. The size of the *in refugia* nematode population around the time of lambing may be small on New Zealand farms,[76] because grazing management aimed at enabling set-stocking of easy-care lambing ewes means that the lambing pastures are routinely rested for a longer period of time before lambing than occurs in other parts of the world. Furthermore, milder winter weather in New Zealand may result in lower rates of overwinter survival of L_3 than occurs in countries with harsh winter conditions. The concept of ensuring a susceptible nematode population *in refugia* at the time of anthelmintic treatment and during the period of persistent activity of moxidectin is fundamental, but on many sheep farms it is difficult to reconcile with the goal of good nematode parasite control, which is to limit the exposure of susceptible sheep to infective larval challenge. Adopting the simplistic approach that the treatment of ewes with moxidectin should be avoided would be unhelpful, because it ignores the fundamental requirement to control nematode parasites. Instead the size of the unselected, susceptible nematode population *in refugia* must first be estimated, based on knowledge of previous grazing management and monitoring of parasitic challenge, for example by using fecal worm egg counts (FWECs). The use of moxidectin to control ewes' periparturient rise in nematode egg output should then be avoided in situations such as hill flocks where the size of the susceptible nematode population *in refugia* may be low; however, partial flock treatments can be recommended in low-ground flocks under circumstances where the extent of overwinter survival of infective larvae is high and control of the ewes' periparturient rise in nematode egg output is fundamental for effective nematode parasite control in their lambs.

Selection for Anthelmintic Resistance by the Use of Injectable Macrocyclic Lactones as Systemic Endectocides

The risks of emergence of anthelmintic resistance may be compounded in countries with an unacceptably high prevalence of sheep scab that necessitates the frequent, routine use on many farms of systemic endectocides.[41] The use of a persistent macrocyclic lactone endectocide during the autumn for the management of sheep scab might select strongly or resistance, for example, if ewes are moved onto relatively safe grazing during the period of persistent protection against nematodes and that grazing is subsequently used during the following spring for naïve lambs. It has become commonplace for some farmers to treat their sheep flocks with a macrocyclic lactone endectocide injection up to 4 times per year, between September and May, in often unsuccessful attempts to control sheep scab.[77] There is now concern that this level of endectocide use increases the selection pressure on anthelmintic-resistant parasitic nematodes.

The macrocyclic lactone anthelmintics can be administered to sheep both orally and systemically, but are only fully effective against *Psoroptes ovis* or *Sarcoptes scabiei* mites when administered parenterally by injection. The pharmacokinetics of oral and injectable macrocyclic lactone drugs differ. The most efficient method of administration in terms of drug bioavailability is by injection,[78] leading to higher systemic drug concentrations, which closely parallel concentrations at target tissues,[79,80] and a longer period of activity against reinfection.[81] However, macrocyclic lactones appear to be more effective against both susceptible and resistant parasitic nematodes when given orally rather than by the subcutaneous route.[82,83] This apparent conflict between the pharmacologic observations of higher tissue concentrations and field observations of lower efficacy of injectable macrocyclic lactone anthelmintics is probably related to the importance of initial exposure of nematodes in the abomasum and proximal small intestine within a few hours of oral administration of the drug.[84] Conversely, the treatment of animals harboring macrocyclic lactone–resistant nematodes with an injectable macrocyclic lactone formulation will allow resistant nematodes to survive and could promote the development of resistance. Furthermore, a significant proportion of the nematodes present in adult sheep hosts during the autumn and winter when systemic endectocide treatments for sheep scab control are regularly administered may be hypobiotic, hard-to-kill EL_4,[85] increasing the risk of selection for anthelmintic resistance.

Annual Drench Rotation

The use of a different broad-spectrum anthelmintic group each year has been widely promoted,[31,35,86] although epidemiologic evidence and field data to support this strategy are not currently apparent.[29] Although annual drench rotation is not contraindicated and may indeed be shown to be beneficial, the perceived need to adhere to an annual anthelmintic group rotation may interfere with good nematode parasite control practice, for example, involving the choice of anthelmintic drug for quarantine treatment of introduced sheep or for periparturient ewes. Rather than adhering strictly to the annual rotation of anthelmintic groups, consideration should be given to ensuring that the most appropriate drug is used for each anthelmintic treatment.

Periodic use of narrow-spectrum salicylanilide-derivative anthelmintics, such as closantel, has been recommended to slow the evolution of anthelmintic resistance in the hematophagous parasite *H contortus*, in regions where hemonchosis predominates.[21]

CONTROL OF TREMATODE PARASITES

The principal objective of a control program for fasciolosis is to minimize the metacercarial challenge to susceptible final hosts. The complex life cycle of the flukes affords different opportunities for such control, including (a) the use of anthelmintic drugs to suppress fluke egg output and pasture metacercarial challenge, (b) drainage to reduce the rate of egg hatching and survival of free-living stages of *F hepatica* and to prevent the establishment of adult snail populations, and (c) grazing management strategies to avoid contact between metacercariae and susceptible final hosts. Most successful control programs involve the strategic application of all of these methods, but rely on the use of effective fasciolacidal drugs.

Various anthelmintic drugs are licensed for use against *F hepatica* in sheep. All are effective against adult flukes in the bile ducts, but the drugs differ in their efficacy against immature flukes in the liver parenchyma. The benzimidazole anthelmintic drug triclabendazole is effective against immature flukes from 2 days after infection,[87] whereas albendazole and netobimin are effective only against adult flukes when used at a higher dose (7.5 mg/kg body weight) than that required for parasitic nematodes.

Of the salicylanilide derivatives, nitroxynil and closantel are effective against immature flukes from 6 weeks after infection, whereas oxyclozanide is only effective against adult flukes. The benzenesulfonamide drug, clorsulon, is only effective against adult flukes. Most of these drugs have long meat withdrawal periods. Fasciolacidal drugs are commonly used in combination with other anthelmintic drugs, for example levamisole-triclabendazole combinations in sheep (and triclabendazole-moxidectin, clorsulon-ivermectin, or closantel-ivermectin combinations for cattle). These products are convenient to use, but their use often involves inappropriate timing of one component. It has also been suggested that the effects of the 2 drugs in the combination might be synergistic.

Triclabendazole is the only drug with practical efficacy against immature *F hepatica* larvae less than 5 weeks after infection of the final host and is, therefore, the drug of choice for early winter treatments aimed at the prevention of subacute fasciolosis.[87] Flock health planning involving timely metaphylactic treatments can prove to be simpler and more acceptable to farmers than complex preventive strategies, provided that the cost of medicines is low when compared with the potential losses from disease. The administration of regular triclabendazole treatments to sheep between October and January, with the aim of ensuring adequate productivity, has therefore become common practice on farms following the diagnosis of fasciolosis. Suppression of egg shedding in grazing animals to limit miracidial infection of snails is most efficiently achieved using triclabendazole, closantel, or nitroxynil anthelmintics that kill flukes before they reach maturity, whereas albendazole, netobimin, or oxyclozanide, which are only effective against adult flukes, are most effective when used for suppressive treatments of housed sheep before turnout in the spring. Both metaphylactic and strategic anthelmintic control of fasciolosis in sheep are, therefore, highly dependent on the use of triclabendazole. Dependence on triclabendazole in this manner is potentially unsustainable, given the enormous evolutionary potential of *F hepatica* to adapt to changes in their environment. This evolutionary potential is conferred by a life cycle that involves hermaphroditic self-fertilization and parthenogenic egg production in the final mammalian hosts and clonal, asexual reproduction in intermediate mud snail host. Furthermore, the existence of triploidy in some populations of *F hepatica* confers a 50% higher rate of mutations,[88] for example to detoxify or excrete anthelmintic drugs. Not surprisingly, therefore, triclabendazole resistance has become a problem in many countries,[89–95] occurring where sheep that are kept all year round on rough grazings are repeatedly treated with triclabendazole in an attempt to maintain adequate productivity in heavily fluke-infested areas. Confirmation of the diagnosis of triclabendazole resistance is not straightforward,[96] because the presence of helminth eggs in feces following anthelmintic treatment could arise due to underexposure of helminths to an effective anthelmintic drug concentration, following underdosing, or due to factors influencing drug bioavailability.[97,98]

Where triclabendazole resistance is suspected, both the treatment of subacute fasciolosis in sheep and strategic anthelmintic treatments to suppress egg shedding rely on the frequent use of the salicylanilide drug, closantel. However, the efficacy of closantel against migrating stages of *F hepatica* is poor, because it is dependent on the breakdown of drug-albumin bonds that occurs within the liver parenchyma. Once triclabendazole resistance has been diagnosed, farmers have little choice other than to adopt preventive evasive management strategies combined with strategic fasciolacidal drug treatments to suppress fluke egg output, thereby limiting miracidial infection of snails and consequent pasture metacercarial challenge. The optimal timing of strategic fasciolacidal anthelmintic treatments depends on forecasts of the effects of summer temperature and rainfall on the rate of fluke development, the availability of snail intermediate hosts, and the effects of previous animal grazing management on the number of miracidiae that would have found a snail host.[99–103]

The molecular and genetic basis of triclabendazole resistance is not understood,[104,105] so advice concerning management of the problem is largely pragmatic. Administration of the correct drug dose is important, and the importance of evasive and strategic treatment strategies is intuitive. Quarantine treatments of introduced sheep and cattle using a sequentially administered combination of a benzimidazole and salicylanilide derivative anthelmintics are recommended to reduce the spread of resistant *F hepatica* into new areas.[106] However, this strategy may prove to be inadequate because triclabendazole-resistant *F hepatica* may be spread between farms, with miracidiae, cercariae, or infected intermediate snail hosts after flooding and in the normal passage of watercourses, or with wildlife final hosts.

Pharmaceutical Control of Dicrocoelium Dendriticum and Paramphistomum spp

The action of triclabendazole is *Fasciola* spp specific. Anthelmintic control of *D dendriticum*[107] and *Paramphistomum* spp[108] therefore requires the use of salicylanilide-derivative anthelmintics or administration of high dose rates of albendazole or netobimin (20 mg/kg body weight).

CONTROL OF CESTODE PARASITES

There is little evidence to show any need to control *M expansa*, although many farmers selling store or breeding sheep irrationally prefer to do so because the physical appearance of tapeworm segments in feces is unsightly. Modern benzimidazole anthelmintics are effective against *M expansa*, whereas the imidazothiazole and macrocyclic lactone anthelmintics are not. Praziquantel (usually in combination with levamisole) is effective against adult *M expansa* in sheep.[109]

The cestode parasites that have sheep as their intermediate hosts must be controlled by preventing access to sheep carcasses by dogs, coyotes, or wolves. Prompt disposal of deadstock, proper composting facilities (subject to legal permission in different countries) that limit access to carcasses by canids, and when feeding offal to dogs either thoroughly cooking to 56°C or freezing to −10°C for 10 days, thus assuring death of the larval cysts, will lower the risk of transmission. Although foxes are sometimes implicated in transmission, they are less efficient than canids as definitive hosts. It is also useful to treat farm dogs with a cestocide at 6- to 8-week intervals. Praziquantel is effective against all of the common dog tapeworms, including *E granulosus*,[110] while normal therapeutic doses of nitroscanate are effective against *T ovis* and *T hydatigena*, but not against *E granulosus*.[111] Dogs should be confined for 48 hours after treatment, and any infected feces collected and carefully disposed of. Outbreaks of coenurosis sometimes occur despite the diligent application of preventive measures, including tapeworm treatments of farm dogs. These cases are associated with stray dogs or public access, and highlight the need for a concerted approach to tapeworm control on a district level.

SUMMARY

Helminth parasites are an important cause of production-limiting diseases. Their proper treatment and control requires knowledge of the epidemiology of these parasites in the region where the farm is located, including knowledge of the important species and their pathogenic effects, the role of immunity and resilience of the sheep, survival of L_3 on pasture under different conditions, and farm management practices. Use of anthelmintics must be combined with this knowledge to reduce risk of development of anthelmintic resistance, particularly with the control of gastrointestinal nematode parasites. Nonchemotherapeutic control measures must be used in conjunction or instead of chemotherapies in order to reduce this risk. Proper implementation of these practices on-farm requires working closely with producers to aid in their understanding of these factors, and thus improves compliance.

REFERENCES

1. Stewart TB, Gasbarre LC. The veterinary importance of nodular worms (*Oesophagostomum* spp). Parasitol Today 1989;5:209–13.
2. Greer AW. Trade-offs and benefits: implications of promoting a strong immunity to gastrointestinal parasites in sheep. Parasite Immunol 2008;30:123–32.
3. Fox MT. Pathophysiology of infection with gastrointestinal nematodes in domestic ruminants: recent developments. Vet Parasitol 1977;71:285–308.
4. Greer AW, McAnulty AW, Stankiewicz M, et al. Corticosteroid treatment prevents the reduction in food intake and growth in lambs infected with the abomasal parasite *Teladorsagia circumcincta*. In: Proceedings of the New Zealand Society of Animal Production, vol 65. New Zealand: New Zealand Society of Animal Production; 2005. p. 9–13.
5. Greer AW, Stankiewicz M, Jay NP, et al. The effect of concurrent corticosteroid induced immune suppression and infection with the intestinal parasite *Trichostrongylus colubriformis* on food intake and utilization in both immunologically naïve and competent sheep. Anim Sci 2005;80:89–99.
6. Stear M, Park M, Bishop S. The key components of resistance to *Ostertagia circumcincta* in lambs. Parasitol Today 1996;12:438–41.
7. Bisset SA, Morris CA. Feasibility and implications of breeding sheep for resilience to nematode challenge. Int J Parasitol 1996;26:857–68.
8. Coop RL. Production loss in subclinical helminth infections. Vet Rec 1979;105:89.
9. Coop RL, Field AC. Effect of phosphorus intake on growth rate, food intake and quality of the skeleton of growing lambs infected with the intestinal nematode *Trichostrongylus vitrinus*. Res Vet Sci 1983;35:175–81.
10. Coop RL, Jackson F, Graham RB, et al. Influence of two levels of concurrent infection with *Ostertagia circumcincta* and *Trichostrongylus vitrinus* on the growth performance of lambs. Res Vet Sci 1988;45:275–80.
11. Coop RL, Sykes AR, Angus KW. The effect of three levels of intake of *Ostertagia circumcincta* larvae on growth rate, food intake and body composition of growing lambs. J Agric Sci 1982;98:247–55.
12. Edwards GT. Tapeworm control in sheep. Vet Rec 2005;157:268.
13. Wilson DJ, Sargison ND, Scott PR, et al. Epidemiology of gastrointestinal nematode parasitism in a commercial sheep flock and its implications for control programs. Vet Rec 2008;162:546–50.
14. Gibson TE. Recent advances in the epidemiology and control of parasitic gastroenteritis in sheep. Vet Rec 1973;92:469–73.
15. Barger I. Control by management. Vet Parasitol 1997;72:493–506.
16. Gordon HM. Phenothiazine as an anthelmintic. Aust Vet J 1945;1:90–5.
17. Borgers M, De Nollin S, De Brabander M, et al. Influence of the anthelmintic mebendazole on microtubules and intracellular organelle movement in nematode intestinal cells. Am J Vet Res 1975;36:1153–66.
18. Coles GC, East JM, Jenkins SN. The mechanism of action of the anthelmintic levamisole. Gen Pharmacol 1974;6:309–13.

19. Turner MJ, Schaeffer JM. Mode of action of ivermectin. In: Campbell WE, editor. Ivermectin and abermectin. New York: Springer; 1989. p. 73–88.
20. Kaminsky R, Ducray P, Jung M, et al. A new class of anthelmintics effective against drug-resistant nematodes. Nature 2008;452:176–80.
21. Dash KM. Control of helminthosis in lambs by strategic treatment with closantel and broad spectrum anthelmintics. Aust Vet J 1986;63:4–8.
22. Hennessy DR. The disposition of antiparasitic drugs in relation to the development of resistance by parasites of livestock. Acta Trop 1994;56:125–41.
23. Kenyon F, Sargison ND, Skuce PJ, et al. Sheep helminth parasitic disease in south eastern Scotland arising as a possible consequence of climate change. Vet Parasitol 2009;163:293–7.
24. Sargison ND, Wilson DJ, Bartley DJ, et al. Haemonchosis and teladorsagiosis in a Scottish sheep flock putatively associated with the overwintering of hypobiotic fourth stage larvae. Vet Parasitol 2007;147:326–31.
25. Van Dijk J, Morgan ER. The influence of temperature on the development, hatching and survival of *Nematodirus battus* larvae. Parasitology 2008;135:269–83.
26. Sargison ND, Jackson F, Scott PR. Teladorsagiosis (ostertagiosis) in young lambs and an extended post-parturient susceptibility in moxidectin treated ewes grazing heavily contaminated pastures. Vet Rec 2002;151:353–5.
27. Blake N, Coles GC. Flock cull due to anthelmintic-resistant nematodes. Vet Rec 2007;161:36.
28. Barger I. Control of nematodes in the presence of anthelmintic resistance—Australian experience. In: Proceedings of the Sheep and Beef Cattle Society of the New Zealand Veterinary Association. New Zealand: Foundation for Continuing Education of the N.Z. Veterinary Association; 1995. p. 87–92.
29. Barnes EH, Dobson RJ, Barger IA. Worm control and anthelmintic resistance: adventures with a model. Parasitol Today 1995;11:56–63.
30. Van Wyk JA. Principles for the use of macrocyclic lactones to minimise selection for resistance. Aust Vet J 2002;80:437–8.
31. Prichard RK, Hall CA, Kelly JD, et al. The problem of anthelmintic resistance in nematodes. Aust Vet J 1980;56:239–51.
32. Martin PJ. Development and control of resistance to anthelmintics. Int J Parasitol 1987;17:493–501.
33. West DM, Probert AD. The rapid appearance of anthelmintic resistance on a sheep farm. N Z Vet J 1989;37:126–7.
34. Orpin PG. Anthelmintic resistance. Vet Rec 1991;129:475.
35. Coles GC, Roush RT. Slowing the spread of anthelmintic resistant nematodes of sheep and goats in the United Kingdom. Vet Rec 1992;130:505–10.
36. Sargison ND, Jackson F, Scott PR. Multiple anthelmintic resistance in sheep. Vet Rec 2001;149:778–9.
37. Sargison ND, Jackson F, Gilleard JS, et al. Ivermectin resistance in a terminal sire sheep flock. Vet Rec 2004;155:343.
38. Sargison ND, Jackson F, Bartley DJ, et al. Failure of moxidectin to control benzimidazole, levamisole and ivermectin resistant *Teladorsagia circumcincta* in a sheep flock. Vet Rec 2005;156:106–9.
39. Sargison ND, Jackson F, Wilson DJ, et al. Characterisation of milbemycin, avermectin, imidazothiazole and benzimidazole resistant *Teladorsagia circumcincta* from a sheep flock. Vet Rec 2010;166:681–6.
40. Dobson RJ, Besier RB, Barnes EH, et al. Principles for the use of macrocyclic lactones to minimise selection for resistance. Aust Vet J 2001;79:756–61.

41. Sargison N, Taylor D, Dun K. Regional control of sheep scab in UK flocks. In Pract 2006;28:62–9.
42. Martin PJ. Selection for thiabendazole resistance in *Ostertagia* spp. by low efficacy of anthelmintic treatment. Int J Parasitol 1989;19:317–25.
43. Besier RB, Hopkins DL. Anthelmintic dose selection by farmers. Aust Vet J 1988; 65:193–4.
44. Waller PJ, Echevarria F, Eddi C, et al. The prevalence of anthelmintic resistance in nematode parasites of sheep in southern Latin America: general overview. Vet Parasitol 1996;62:181–7.
45. Sargison N, Scott P. Sheep welfare—supply of trace element supplements and unbranded anthelmintics for sheep. Vet Rec 2009;165:215–6.
46. Hennessy DR, Ali DN, Tremain S. The partition and fate of soluble and digesta-particulate associated oxfendazole and its metabolites in the gastrointestinal tract of sheep. Int J Parasitol 1994;24:327–33.
47. Ali DN, Hennessy DR. The effect of level of feed intake on the pharmacokinetic disposition of oxfendazole in sheep. Int J Parasitol 1995;25:63–70.
48. Hennessy DR. Pharmacokinetic disposition of benzimidazole drugs in the ruminant gastrointestinal tract. Parasitol Today 1993;9:329–33.
49. Sargison ND, Stafford KJ, West DM. The effects of age, weaning, drench volume and yarding on ruminoreticulum bypass in sheep, with reference to the anthelmintic efficacy of benzimidazole drenches. N Z Vet J 1998;46:20–7.
50. Prichard RK, Hennessy DR. Effect of oesophageal groove closure on the pharmacokinetic behaviour and efficacy of oxfendazole in sheep. Res Vet Sci 1981; 30:22–7.
51. Hennessy DR, Martin PJ, Murray S. Influence of drench volume on the disposition of oxfendazole in sheep. Vet Rec 1997;40:429–30.
52. Watson TG. Anthelmintic resistance in the New Zealand animal production industries. In: Proceedings of the New Zealand Society of Animal Production, vol 54. New Zealand: New Zealand Society of Animal Production; 1994. p.1–4.
53. Gopal RM, Pomroy WE, West DM. Resistance of field isolates of *Trichostrongylus colubriformis* and *Ostertagia circumcincta* to ivermectin. Int J Parasitol 1999; 29:781–6.
54. Chartier C, Pors I, Hubert J, et al. Prevalence of anthelmintic resistant nematodes in sheep and goats in western France. Small Rumin Res 1998;29: 33–41.
55. Waller PJ, Dobson RJ, Obendorf DL, et al. Resistance of *Trichostrongylus columbriformis* to levamisole and morantel: differences in relation to selection history. Vet Parasitol 1986;21:255–63.
56. Jackson F, Coop RL, Jackson E, et al. Anthelmintic nematodes in goats. Vet Rec 1991;129:39.
57. Jackson F, Jackson E, Little S, et al. Prevalence of anthelmintic resistant nematodes in fibre producing goats in Scotland. Vet Rec 1992;131:282–5.
58. Michel JF. Strategies for the use of anthelmintics in livestock and their implications for the development of drug resistance. Parasitology 1985;90:621–8.
59. Van Wyk JA. Refugia—overlooked as perhaps the most potent factor concerning the development of anthelmintic resistance. Onderstepoort J Vet Res 2001; 68:55–67.
60. Coles GC. Sustainable use of anthelmintics in grazing animals. Vet Rec 2002; 151:165–9.
61. Taylor MA, Hunt KR. Field observations on the control of ovine parasitic gastroenteritis in south-east England. Vet Rec 1988;123:241–5.

62. Roush RT, McKenzie JA. Ecological genetics of insecticide and acaricide resistance. Annu Rev Entomol 1987;32:361–80.
63. Anderson N. Trichostrongylid infections of sheep in a winter rainfall region. 1. Epizootiological studies in the Western District of Victoria. Aust J Agric Res 1972;23:1113–29.
64. Besier RB. Ivermectin resistant Ostertagia in Western Australia. In: Proceedings of the Sheep and Beef Cattle Society of the New Zealand Veterinary Association. New Zealand: Foundation for Continuing Education of the N.Z. Veterinary Association; 1996. p. 195–207.
65. Palmer DG, Besier RB, Lyon J, et al. Detecting macrocyclic lactone resistance using the faecal egg count reduction test—the Western Australian experience. In: Proceedings of the 5th International Sheep Veterinary Congress. Onderstepoort (South Africa); 2001. p. 186–7.
66. Dobson RJ, Le Jambre LF, Gill JH. Management of anthelmintic resistance: inheritance of resistance and selection with persistent drugs. Int J Parasitol 1996;26:993–1000.
67. Houdijk JCM, Kyriazakis I, Jackson F, et al. The relationship between protein nutrition, reproductive effort and breakdown in immunity to *Teladorsagia circumcincta* in periparturient ewes. Anim Sci 2001;72:595–606.
68. Hoste H, Chartier C, Le Frileux Y. Control of gastrointestinal parasitism with nematodes in dairy goats by treating the host category at risk. Vet Res 2002;33:531–45.
69. Van Wyk JA. Production trials involving use of the FAMACHA copyright system for haemonchosis in sheep: preliminary results. Onderstepoort J Vet Res 2008;75:331–45.
70. Jackson F, Coles G, Cabaret J, et al. Targeted selective treatments an innovative strategy for the control of nematode infection in sheep and goats. In: Claerbout E, Vercruysse J, editors. Proceedings of the 21st International Conference of World Association for the Advancement of Veterinary Parasitology. Ghent (Belgium): World Association for the Advancement of Veterinary Parasitology; 2007. p. 146.
71. Waghorn TS, Leathwick DM, Miller CM, et al. Brave or gullible: testing the concept that leaving susceptible parasites in refugia will slow the development of anthelmintic resistance. N Z Vet J 2008;56:158–63.
72. Leathwick DM, Miller CM, Atkinson DS, et al. Drenching adult ewes: implications of anthelmintic treatment pre- and post-lambing on the development of anthelmintic resistance. N Z Vet J 2006;54:297–304.
73. Pomroy WE. Anthelmintic resistance in New Zealand: a perspective on recent findings and options for the future. N Z Vet J 2006;54:265–70.
74. Leathwick DM, Barlow ND, Vlassoff A. A model for nematodiasis in New Zealand lambs: the effect of drenching regime and grazing management on the development of anthelmintic resistance. Int J Parasitol 1995;25:1479–90.
75. Lawrence KE, Rhodes AP, Jackson R, et al. Farm management practices associated with macrocyclic lactone resistance on sheep farms in New Zealand. N Z Vet J 2006;54:283–8.
76. Vlassoff A, Leathwick DM, Heath AGG. The epidemiology of nematode infections of sheep. N Z Vet J 2001;49:213–21.
77. Sargison N, Roger P, Stubbings L, et al. Sheep scab control can only be achieved through eradication. Vet Rec 2007;160:491–2.
78. Alvinerie M. Comparative pharmacokinetic properties of moxidectin and ivermectin in different animal species. J Vet Pharmacol Ther 1997;20:74.

79. Marriner SE, McKinnon I, Bogan JA. The pharmacokinetics of ivermectin after oral and subcutaneous administration to sheep and horses. J Vet Pharmacol Ther 1987;10:175–9.
80. Alvinerie M, Escudero E, Sutra J, et al. The pharmacokinetics of moxidectin after oral and subcutaneous administration to sheep. Vet Res 1998;29:113–8.
81. Borgsteede FHM. The efficacy and persistent anthelmintic effect of ivermectin in sheep. Vet Parasitol 1993;50:117–24.
82. Gopal RM, West DM, Pomroy WE. The difference in efficacy of ivermectin oral, moxidectin oral and moxidectin injectable formulations against an ivermectin resistant strain of *Trichostrongylus colubriformis* in sheep. N Z Vet J 2001;49: 133–7.
83. Alka RM, Gopal KS, Sandhu KS, et al. Efficacy of abamectin against ivermectin resistant strain of *Trichostrongylus colubriformis* in sheep. Vet Parasitol 2004; 121:277–83.
84. Lespine A, Alvinerie M, Sutra JF, et al. Influence of the route of administration on efficacy and tissue distribution of ivermectin in goat. Vet Parasitol 2005;128: 251–60.
85. Blitz NM, Gibbs HC. Studies on the arrested development of *Haemonchus contortus* in sheep. I. The induction of arrested development. II. Termination of arrested development and the spring rise phenomenon. Int J Parasitol 1972;2: 5–22.
86. Taylor MA, Hunt KR. Anthelmintic drug resistance in UK. Vet Rec 1989;125: 143–7.
87. Boray JC, Crowfoot PD, Strong MB, et al. Treatment of immature and mature *Fasciola hepatica* infections in sheep with triclabendazole. Vet Rec 1983;113: 315–7.
88. Fletcher HL, Hoey EM, Orr N, et al. The occurrence and significance of triploidy in the liver fluke, *Fasciola hepatica*. Parasitology 2004;128:69–72.
89. Mitchell GB, Maris L, Bonniwell MA. Triclabendazole-resistant liver fluke in Scottish sheep. Vet Rec 1998;143:399.
90. Lane G. Anthelmintic resistance. Vet Rec 1998;143:232.
91. Moll L, Gaasenbeek CPH, Vellema P, et al. Resistance of *Fasciola hepatica* against triclabendazole in cattle and sheep in the Netherlands. Vet Rec 2000; 91:153–8.
92. Thomas I, Coles GC, Duffus K. Triclabendazole-resistant *Fasciola hepatica* in southwest Wales. Vet Rec 2000;146:200.
93. Borgsteede FHM, Moll L, Vellema P, et al. Lack of reversion in triclabendazole-resistant *Fasciola hepatica*. Vet Rec 2005;156:350–1.
94. Alvarez-Sánchez MA, Mainar-Jaime RC, Pérez-García J, et al. Resistance of *Fasciola hepatica* to triclabendazole and albendazole in sheep in Spain. Vet Rec 2006;159:424–5.
95. Mooney L, Good B, Hanrahan JP, et al. The comparative efficacy of four anthelmintics against a natural acquired *Fasciola hepatica* infection in hill sheep flock in the west of Ireland. Vet Parasitol 2009;164:201–5.
96. Coles GC, Jackson F, Pomroy WE, et al. The detection of anthelmintic resistance in nematodes of veterinary importance. Vet Parasitol 2006;136:167–85.
97. Hennessy DR, Lacey E, Steel JW, et al. The kinetics of triclabendazole disposition in sheep. J Vet Pharmacol Ther 1987;10:64–72.
98. Halferty L, Brennan GP, Trudgett A, et al. Relative activity of triclabendazole metabolites against the liver fluke, *Fasciola hepatica*. Vet Parasitol 2009;159: 126–38.

99. Kendall SB, McCullough FS. The emergence of the cercariae of *Fasciola hepatica* from the snail *Lymnaea truncatula*. J Helminthol 1951;25:77–92.

100. Ollerenshaw CB, Rowlands WT. A method of forecasting the incidence of fascioliasis in Anglesey. Vet Rec 1959;71:591–8.

101. Armour J, Urquhart GM, Jennings FW, et al. Studies on ovine fasciolosis II. The relationship between the availability of metacercariae of *Fasciola hepatica* on pastures and the development of clinical disease. Vet Rec 1970;86:274–7.

102. Ross JG. A five year study of the epidemiology of fascioliasis in the North, East and West of Scotland. Br Vet J 1977;133:263–72.

103. Whitelaw A, Fawcett AR. A study of a strategic dosing programme against fascioliasis on a hill farm. Vet Rec 1977;100:443–7.

104. Robinson MW, Trudgett A, Hoey EM, et al. Triclabendazole-resistant *Fasciola hepatica*: b-tubulin and response to *in vitro* treatment with triclabendazole. Parasitology 2002;124:325–38.

105. Robinson MW, Lawson J, Trudgett A, et al. The comparative metabolism of triclabendazole sulphoxide by triclabendazole-susceptible and triclabendazole-resistant *Fasciola hepatica*. Parasitol Res 2004;92:205–10.

106. Fairweather I, Boray JP. Fasciolicides: efficacy, actions, resistance and its management. Vet J 1999;158:81–112.

107. Rojo-Vazquez FA, Meana A, Tarazona JM, et al. The efficacy of netobimin, 15 mg/kg, against *Dicrocoelium dendriticum* in sheep. Vet Rec 1989;124:512–3.

108. De Waal T. Paramphistomum—a brief review. Ir Vet J 2010;63:313–5.

109. Bauer C. Comparative efficacy of praziquantel, albendazole, febantel and oxfendazole against *Moniezia expansa*. Vet Rec 1990;127:353–4.

110. Walters TMH. Echinococcosis hydatidosis and the South Powys control scheme. State Veterinary Journal 1986;40:130–40.

111. Boray JC, Strong MB, Allison JR, et al. Nitroscanate: a new broad spectrum anthelmintic against nematodes of cats and dogs. Aust Vet J 1979;55:45–53.

Non-pharmaceutical Control of Endoparasitic Infections in Sheep

Gareth F. Bath, BVSc

KEYWORDS

• Control • Endoparasites • Non-pharmaceutical • Sheep

Before 1960, researchers, advisors and farmers were forced to consider and use several non-pharmaceutical options to control internal parasites, but this changed as a number of highly effective, safe, and relatively cheap anthelmintic drug groups came into use over the next 25 years. Worldwide, this resulted in an almost total reliance on anthelmintics to control sheep worms; initially, this was rewarded by dramatic suppression of worm burdens. Systems such as regular, blanket deworming of the flock with immediate movement to fresh (uncontaminated) pasture after treatment became universally advocated. However, the very success of these drugs carried with them the seeds of their own destruction, since the only worms that could survive this treatment onslaught were those that had genes for anthelmintic resistance (AR), now a major international problem. Unintended selection for AR has to be stopped, since there will nearly always be a need for treatment with highly effective remedies when circumstances dictate. Non-pharmaceutical control is thus not in opposition to conventional drug therapy, but rather an adjunct and ally. The need for sustainable, holistic, and integrated parasite management (SHIPM) is now almost universally recognized.[1–5] Veterinary advisors and their clients should accept this paradigm shift. Admittedly, SHIPM is more difficult to implement and manage than purely pharmaceutical methods, but in every country where it has been tried, these holistic measures have proven to be practical and sustainable.[2,6,7]

REDUCE THE RATE AND AMOUNT OF CONTAMINATION

This applies firstly to the pastures and secondly to the sheep.

- Internal parasites build up in worm hotspots, such as continually wet areas, where sheep are attracted to graze intensively. This causes greater

The author is co-originator and developer of the FAMACHA and FIVE POINT CHECK systems.
Department of Production Animal Studies, Faculty of Veterinary Science, University of Pretoria, Private Bag X04, Onderstepoort 0110, Gauteng, South Africa
E-mail address: gareth.bath@up.ac.za

Vet Clin Food Anim 27 (2011) 157–162
doi:10.1016/j.cvfa.2010.10.002
0749-0720/11/$ – see front matter © 2011 Elsevier Inc. All rights reserved.

vetfood.theclinics.com

contamination of these areas; moisture then ensures a higher larval survival, while intensive grazing means the sheep are eating very short grass, heavily contaminated by larvae. Examples are marshes, around leaking water troughs, or overnight pens. Either eliminate these areas or manage them carefully.[7]

- Short cropped grass contains more concentrated larvae, so do not use such pastures for susceptible sheep.
- The greater the grazing pressure (number of sheep per area per time), the more the contamination of the pasture there will be. Reduce this where possible.
- By resting a pasture for long enough, fewer larvae will survive. The time needed for this varies with the worm species and climate, but generally a rest of 2 to 3 months is helpful in a temperate climate during the hot, summer months.[1]
- Alternating pasture use with grazing species that are not susceptible to sheep worms (this excludes goats) will assist in that the pasture can be grazed more intensively or more often; the other grazers actually clean up the pasture by consuming larvae, but not allowing them to survive.[7,8]
- The type of pasture influences larval survival and ingestion by sheep; thus alfalfa and shrubs may be less dangerous than grass.

IDENTIFY AND PROTECT THE MOST VULNERABLE SHEEP

This usually applies to nursing and weaned lambs, as well as to lactating ewes and ewes in late pregnancy. Old or sick animals also need extra attention.[7] These sheep should be given the safest grazing by allowing them to graze new or well rested pastures first. They will require extra monitoring and probably also more treatment. Sheep on the farm that do not fit these categories will not require the same treatment protocol. To treat all categories similarly is unnecessary and uneconomical and will lead to AR.

REDUCE THE SELECTION PRESSURE FOR AR

If all the sheep in a group are treated and immediately moved to a clean pasture (with very few larvae) the only worms (and thus worm eggs) that survive to contaminate the new pasture are resistant to the anthelmintic drug used.[8] This is a potent but unintended way to hasten the onset of AR, since these refractive parasites quickly become the dominant population on a farm. There are several ways to prevent this:

- First, treat only the animals that are likely to benefit from it. This is known as targeted selective treatment (TST),[2] which can be done on-farm by the use of several techniques that require direct monitoring. By only treating some sheep, it takes much longer for the resistant worms to become dominant.
- Second, the entire flock can be treated, but at times when this is most useful and when there are many worm eggs or larvae in refugia (mainly on the pastures), which escape exposure to the drug and thus escape selection for AR. This is known as targeted treatment (TT).[2]
- Third, if the whole flock is to be treated, the sheep should be kept on the pasture where they have been grazing for a few more days to weeks to allow them to ingest unselected larvae and thus slow AR development. This is termed treat all then stay (TATS).[7] With TATS, the time needed to leave sheep on that pasture is related to the action of the anthelmintic used. Drugs that have a prolonged action require the sheep be left longer, since unselected larvae can only establish themselves in the host after the effective residual drug action ends.
- The fourth option is to move the flock onto fresh pasture and delay treatment for a few weeks to contaminate it with unselected eggs (move first then treat, [MFTT]).

- The final action to be taken to prevent the rapid onset of AR in a flock is to apply strict quarantine on all sheep or goats that enter the property. This prevents the unwitting importation of resistant parasites from other farms. In practice, this requires that no new animals go straight onto pasture. Instead they must be kept in pens without pasture or grass, and subjected to intensive treatment with a range of effective remedies. Before release and after a suitable waiting period, they are checked for surviving worms using a quantitative fecal egg count (FEC) to ensure minimal contamination of pastures with imported AR worm eggs. Then, the new sheep must be put onto pastures contaminated with eggs and larvae present on the farm. These will help dilute out any remaining AR worm population that survive in the new animals.

MONITORING OF WORM INFECTIONS

The era of fixed treatment programs, strategic treatment, and repeated treatment of entire flocks has passed, since although these work well for some time, they are a sure recipe for creating widespread and severe AR.[1,8] Instead, a flock should be monitored and treated according to current circumstances as well as parasite load. There are several practical, economical, simple, and reliable ways to achieve this. The FEC is widely used for monitoring worm species but has several serious limitations. Each species has its own egg laying capacity, *Haemonchus contortus* being very prolific, while *Nematodirus* species are the opposite. Unless this is taken into account by identifying the eggs, the numbers in the FEC can be very misleading. Secondly, the count will not accurately reflect the number of worms in the host, except in lambs. This is because adults can become resistant to worms and suppress egg laying. The sample taken must also be representative of the flock and, at least 10 and up to 20 animals should be sampled. If the same volume of feces is taken from each sheep, then the sample can be pooled to save costs. The FEC is a good indicator of pasture contamination rate and gives a warning of approaching danger, if it is done on a flock basis every 1 to 2 months depending on the season.[7,8] Allied to the FEC is the reduction test (FECRT), which measures the efficacy of the drugs tested and is useful in giving early warnings of AR and identifying which drugs to use (see the article by Neil D. Sargison elsewhere in this issue for further exploration of this topic).[9]

Identifying animals that can benefit from treatment is a good way to reduce the onset of AR and is economically sound. Most of the tests proposed for this are impractical for on-farm use, but clinical anemia caused by hematophagous worms is a well proven exception.[6] This system, known as FAMACHA, only requires the examination of the ocular mucous membrane and comparing the color seen with a standard, five-category illustration. Paler shades are treated, and redder shades are not. This means that only animals compromised by blood-sucking worms (mainly *H contortus*) are exposed to the drug, while the rest retain unselected worms, thus slowing AR. Savings on deworming are considerable, usually in excess of 50%. Very susceptible sheep also can be identified for culling.

A further extension of the principle of TST was announced in 2009, known as the FIVE POINT CHECK.[10] In this system

- The nose is checked for discharge that indicates nasal bots.
- The eyes are checked for anemia, indicating blood-sucking worms
- The jaw is checked for submandibular edema that also accompanies anemia and protein-losing enteropathies caused by parasites such as the conical fluke *Callicophoron* species

- The back for body condition score (BCS) indicating possible infection by internal parasites like *Teladorsagia* and *Trichostrongylus* species.
- Finally, the tail is checked for signs of diarrhea, indicating mainly worms that also cause loss in body condition score.

This quick, easy, and cheap checking system is readily adopted by farmers, since they can do this in the crush and immediately identify which sheep are likely to benefit from treatment. While there are many other causes of these signs, the most important ones include internal parasites; the sheep least likely to benefit from treatment can be passed over, slowing the onset of severe AR. The BCS system does require some practice and expertise in performing body condition scoring accurately and repeatedly; however, this is a skill every stock farmer should have, as it is also useful to monitor nutrition and the correct condition for each phase in the reproductive cycle. The FIVE POINT CHECK needs further testing and refinement to make it useful in various conditions. Apart from the scoring systems, it contains tables of the likely parasites involved as well as which drug groups should be used. The mottos of TST summarize the intentions: "Leave the best, and treat the rest" or "Look before you treat."

Another way to apply TST is by measuring changes in body weight, but this will only work where the farm is geared up for regular (twice monthly) weighing.[2] Animals showing the slowest growth rates can be identified for treatment, but more importantly those with the fastest growth rates can be left untreated. Obviously, this only applies to young weaned sheep, which are most at risk from helminthosis. If tapeworms are seen to be a problem, then lambs with potbellies and poor growth or condition can be identified for treatment.

A test on feces for occult blood has been developed, but it is unsuitable for TST due to the time and expense of individual testing and, like FAMACHA, it is only applicable to hematophagous worms.[11] Its use lies at a group or flock level, since it gives a quick, easy, and cheap warning of a build-up of these parasites and the need for enhanced surveillance and control measures (TTS).[2]

Monitoring the weather and the grazing management applied also can give timely warnings of potential or impending conditions conducive to worm infections so that appropriate measures are taken in good time.

INCREASING RESISTANCE TO WORMS IN SHEEP

In the past, far too much attention was given to making the environment suitable to sheep, rather than the other way around. Deficiencies in the animal were covered up by increasing treatments, and this reliance on drugs has led to widespread AR. However, resistance (the capacity of the animal to prevent infection) and resilience (the capacity of the animal to cope with infection) have not been given the attention they deserve. It has been shown that these traits do not compromise key production or reproduction parameters much, if at all.[12–14] Furthermore, they are heritable at levels (typically around 25% to 30%) that allow practical selection and culling to have a meaningful impact within 5 years.

There are practical and economical ways of identifying and selecting rams that show superior resistance or resilience. By using an index of FECs, those rams with the lowest counts in a group of animals exposed to the same parasite challenge can be selected for resistance with confidence.[13,15] More recently clinical anemia (FAMACHA findings) and hematocrit results also have been shown to be reliable indicators of resistance and resilience to *H contortus*.[16] Since these traits usually apply to other worms too, selection will assist in breeding sheep with a strong ability to withstand internal parasites. The same is true of selection based on changes in body weight, provided in all cases that the animals are subjected to a realistic parasite challenge before selection. Ewes in large flocks may be more difficult to select, but at least the poorest group (usually less than 10%) can be easily identified by the FIVE POINT CHECK and culled from the breeding group. The motto should be "Stop selecting sissy sheep."

Animals can only express inherent resistance and resilience if they are adequately fed. This applies especially to protein, although, in addition, insufficient copper, iron, selenium, vitamin A, and zinc intakes may inhibit the immune response of the animals.[17]

It is often forgotten that sheep will develop effective immunity only if they are exposed to regular low levels of parasite challenge. Aggressive treatment results in negligible larval challenge and thus a loss of immunity. Aim for safe, not worm-free, environments. Unfortunately, although vaccines are a theoretical possibility, no vaccine has thus far proceeded to the commercial implementation stage.

Another factor to consider is that a sick sheep is a susceptible sheep. By controlling other diseases, one enables the animals to mount an effective immune response to worms. Finally, by separating the most susceptible categories of sheep (lambs, lactating and heavily pregnant ewes), one can ensure that animals of approximately equal abilities to mount an immune response are run together and can thus be managed accordingly.

CONTROL MEASURES UNDER DEVELOPMENT OR UNPROVEN

The use of copper oxide wire particles dosed by capsule into the rumen has recently been proven to control *H contortus* for a prolonged period in goats, but also in sheep.[17] In most situations, this extra copper is quite safe, but sheep are peculiarly susceptible to poisoning; hence the level of copper in grazing and supplements needs to be established beforehand. The legume *Sericia lespedeza* has been shown to suppress *H contortus* worm burdens and FECs, probably by virtue of its high levels of condensed tannins.[17] Several other tanniniferous plants also been identified. Collectively, these plants promise to make an important contribution to worm control, although the exact methods of management and implementation remain to be determined.

Several herbal preparations are claimed to be effective, but in nearly all these cases good scientific evidence is either lacking or extremely limited. Extravagant claims may be found on the Internet, but these have to be treated cautiously until they have been properly evaluated. The same is true of natural products like diatomaceous earth, which has good science behind its use against insects in grain silos, but much less to support its use against worms. In all these cases, it must be remembered that a measurable effect on worms does not necessarily mean a meaningful effect in parasite control. An efficacy of 20% is measurable, but not necessarily meaningful. In most countries that would not entitle such a product to be registered for use as an anthelmintic.

The use of nematophagous fungi has been extensively investigated, but although the theory is good, no practical product has emerged. Since it is known that some fungi are able to immobilize and then consume larvae in dung pats or on the pasture, it was hoped that dosing animals with these fungal spores could lead to effective worm control.

SUMMARY

The need for sustainable, holistic, and integrated parasite management against sheep worms is emphasized. Approaches include lowering the rate and amount of contamination of pastures, identifying and protecting the most vulnerable animals, reducing the selection pressure for AR, monitoring of parasite infections, and increasing the resistance and resilience of sheep. Control measures under development are briefly discussed.

REFERENCES

1. Waller PJ. International approaches to the concept of integrated control of nematode parasites of livestock. Int J Parasitol 1999;29:155–64.
2. Kenyon F, Greer AW, Coles GC, et al. The role of targeted and targeted selective treatments in the development of refugia-based approaches to the control of gastrointestinal nematodes of small ruminants. Vet Parasitol 2009;164:3–11.
3. Besier RB, Love SCJ. Anthelmintic resistance in sheep: the need for new approaches. Aust J Exp Agric 2003;43:1383–91.
4. Jackson F, Bartley D, Bartley Y, et al. Worm control in sheep in the future. Small Rumin Res 2009;86:40–5.
5. Papadopoulos E. Anthelmintic resistance in sheep nematodes. Small Rumin Res 2008;76:99–103.
6. Van Wyk JA, Bath GF. The FAMACHA system for managing haemonchosis in sheep and goats by clinically identifying individual animals for treatment. Vet Res 2002;33:509–29.
7. Bath GF. Practical implementation of holistic internal parasite management in sheep. Small Rumin Res 2006;62:13–8.
8. Van Wyk JA. Refugia—overlooked as perhaps the most potent factor concerning the development of anthelmintic resistance. Onderstepoort J Vet Res 2001;68:55–67.
9. Taylor MA. Parasitological examinations in sheep health management. Small Rumin Res 2010;92:120–5.
10. Bath GF, Van Wyk JA. The FIVE POINT CHECK for targeted selective treatment of internal parasites in small ruminants. Small Rumin Res 2009;86:6–13.
11. Colditz IG, Le Jambre LF. Development of a faecal occult blood test to determine the severity of Haemonchus contortus infections in sheep. Vet Parasitol 2008;153:93–9.
12. Larsen JWA, Anderson N, Vizard AL, et al. Diarrhoea in Merino ewes during winter: association with trichostrogylid larvae. Aust Vet J 1994;71:365–72.
13. Bisset SA, Morris CA. Feasibility and implications of breeding sheep for resilience to nematode challenge. Int J Parasitol 1996;26:857–68.
14. Albers GAA, Gray GD, Piper LA, et al. The genetics of resistance and resilience to Haemonchus contortus infection in young merino sheep. Int J Parasitol 1987; 17:1355–63.
15. Karlsson LJE, Greeff JC. Selection response in faecal worm egg counts in the rylington merino parasite-resistant flock. Aust J Exp Agric 2006;46:809–11.
16. Riley DG, Van Wyk JA. Genetic parameters for FAMACHA score and related traits for host resistance/resilience and production at differing severities of worm challenge in a merino flock in South Africa. Vet Parasitol 2009;164:44–52.
17. Terrill T, Southern Consortium for Small Ruminant Parasite Control. Available at: http://www.scsrpc.org. Accessed August, 2010.

Control of Endoparasitic Nematode Infections in Goats

Hervé Hoste, DVM, PhD[a],*, Smaragda Sotiraki, DVM, PhD[b],
Juan Felipe de Jesús Torres-Acosta, DVM, PhD[c]

KEYWORDS

- Alternative method of control • Anthelmintic • Goat
- Grazing management • Nematodes • Treatment

In 2007, the world goat population was estimated at 831 million, compared with 1.09 billion sheep, but the goat population is expanding more rapidly. More than 90% of goats are found in developing countries, with the primary commodity being its meat. The commonly used description of the goat as "the cow of the poorest" underlines its importance for small farmers. However, in the developed world (eg, the European Union and much of North America), the value of goats relates to its select ability to produce high yields of milk and the increased returns associated with the dairy products, particularly artisanal cheeses. Therefore, the current success of goats seems to be related to 2 characteristics: (1) its ability to efficiently convert low-quality forages into high-quality protein sources, that is, milk and meat, in developing countries and (2) its ability to produce commodities for valuable niche markets in developed countries.

GASTROINTESTINAL NEMATODES IN GOATS

Parasitism with gastrointestinal nematodes (GINs) remains a major threat for small ruminant health and production. Both sheep and goats are infected by the same nematode species, although the occurrence of some caprine-adapted strains has

The COST Action FA 0805 project CAPARA (Goat-Parasite Interactions: from knowledge to control) is sincerely thanked for financial support. The authors have nothing to disclose.
[a] UMR 1225, INRA/ENVT, Ecole Nationale Vétérinaire de Toulouse, 23 Chemin des Capelles, 31076 Toulouse Cedex, France
[b] National Agricultural Research Foundation, VRI NAGREF Campus, PO Box 60272, 57001 Thermi Thessaloniki, Greece
[c] Facultad de Medicina Veterinaria y Zootecnia, Universidad Autónoma de Yucatán, Km 15.5 Carretera Mérida-Xmatkuil, Mérida, Yucatán, México
* Corresponding author.
E-mail address: h.hoste@envt.fr

been suggested.[1] In both host species, the parasitic GINs are responsible for major economic costs because of the direct losses (reduced production, lower product quality, mortalities) and the indirect losses (costs associated with treatment and control, such as laboratory diagnostics, drugs, and labor for administration).

These economic losses underline the need for better control measures. The routine use of commercial chemical anthelmintics has been the cornerstone of GIN control programs for more than 5 decades.[2,3] These drugs are applied either curatively, to save animals from death or preserve productivity by avoiding excessive uncontrolled production losses, or preventively, to break the parasite's life cycle before the level of parasitism reaches clinical levels. However, the rapid development and wide distribution of anthelmintic resistance (AR) in nematode populations,[4] a major issue in goats, has renewed interest in promoting more integrated and sustainable approaches of control. Nematode control is done by combining more than one control approach,[2,5] that is, not only by using anthelmintic treatments but also by reducing the contamination of pastures and improving the host immunity against parasites. These 3 principles (ie, treatment, hygienic measures, and immune prophylaxis) are the paradigms of control for most pathogens. For the control of GINs, many solutions have been explored first in sheep[6,7] (see the articles by Gareth F. Bath; and Neil D. Sargison for further exploration of this topic). This article focuses specifically on caprine physiologic, metabolic, and behavioral differences to demonstrate how these various methods can be adapted to goat production.

TARGETING THE WORM POPULATION IN THE HOST: CHEMICAL TREATMENT
Differences Specific to Goats

Goats are different in several important regards compared with sheep and cattle. Goats are described as browsers or intermediate browsers, whereas sheep and cattle are grazers. From an evolutionary perspective, it is thought that this major behavioral difference has led to (1) an increased contact with a wide range of plant secondary metabolites, some of them considered toxic, and (2) a reduced contact with infective nematode larvae (L3).[8] It is hypothesized that the above-mentioned differences might explain, respectively, (1) the goat's remarkable ability to detoxify exogenous chemicals, including anthelmintic drugs, and (2) its decreased ability to develop a fully effective immune response against GINs.[8]

The Adapted Use of Anthelmintics in Goats

For years, anthelmintic drugs from the 3 broad-spectrum families: benzimidazoles and probenzimidazoles, levamisole, and macrocyclic lactones, have been used worldwide to control GINs, their use varying by production type. For example, there is evidence that levamisole should not be used in fiber-producing goats because of toxicity issues.[7] In addition, the oral route of administration should always be preferred, and the intramuscular injectable route should not be used in any goat breed. The subcutaneous injectable route is widely used in goats without any toxic effects in some parts of Latin America. In lactating dairy goats, the national regulations governing withdrawal times and extralabel drug use must be followed to avoid milk residues. In addition, it is widely acknowledged that goats metabolize anthelmintic drugs more rapidly than do sheep. Some key pharmacokinetic parameters (eg, area under the curve, plasmatic half-life) that may influence the drug efficacy against worms highly differ between goats and sheep. This metabolic difference has been shown for various molecules of each family of anthelmintic drugs, that is, benzimidazoles,[8–10] levamisole,[11] and macrocyclic lactones.[12,13]

The existence of such metabolic differences has been ignored for many years. Consequently, the treatment of goats at the recommended sheep dose rates resulted in routine underdosing, leading to reduced efficacy of the drug. This underdosing partly explains the high prevalence of anthelmintic drug resistance in worm populations in goats when compared with other livestock species, including sheep.[4,14,15] This scenario also includes cases of multiresistant nematode strains.[16–19]

These identified differences have led to recommendations to increase the dosage when treating goats to achieve an efficacy that is comparable to that in sheep (**Table 1**).[20,21] These adaptations in doses are usually associated with some general practical recommendations to improve the use of anthelmintics and reduce the risk of AR when treating a herd of goats.[22] Most of these practical recommendations are similar to those for sheep, although some of the recommendations relate to some caprine physiologic differences (eg, reflex of esophageal groove).

Targeted Selective Treatment in Goats

As with sheep, parasitic infections of goats follow a negative binomial distribution, in which most animals have a low fecal egg count (FEC), and only a few have a high FEC, indicating a higher level of infection.[23] This distribution gives the possibility to administer anthelmintic drugs selectively by targeting only the highly infected animals. In dairy goats, schemes for selective treatments have been developed

Table 1 Recommendations for the use of chemical anthelmintics in goats	
Animals	Accurate weighing of animals Correct dosing; no underdosing Calculation of the dosage by reference to the heavier animal in a group
Administration	For oral administration, small volumes should be delivered beyond the tongue to avoid closure of the esophageal groove
Drugs	
General issues	Suitable route of administration
Benzimidazoles: Probenzimidazoles	Repetition of the sheep dose after 12 or 24 h; if not feasible, sheep dose × 2 to be administered[22]
Levamisole	Recommended sheep dose × 1.5[22] Administration of injectable product better to be avoided[7] (if injectable form is the only pharmaceutical form available, it should be administered by the subcutaneous route)
Macrocyclic lactones	Ivermectin: recommended sheep dose × 1.5[22] Eprinomectin: recommended sheep dose × 2,[22] for pour-on application Moxidectin injectable: recommended sheep dose × 1.5[21]
Equipment	Accuracy and calibration of dosing gun should be checked regularly
Withdrawal period for meat and milk	Follow advice by Food Animal Residue Avoidance & Depletion Program or an appropriate national organization for recommended meat and milk withdrawals when using these products in an extralabel manner; all withdrawals should be based on the dosages recommended earlier

based on the differences in resistance and resilience depending on either the age or the level of milk production.[24] Under hot humid conditions, in which *Haemonchus contortus* is the dominant pathogenic species, the FAMACHA method has been applied as a tool for selective treatment both in sheep and goats.[25] A new approach that has produced good results under subhumid tropical conditions has been obtained through fecal sampling of animals with a high FAMACHA value (ie, 3–5 indicating a high level of anemia) and/or low condition score, and then treating only those animals classified higher than a certain FEC level.

ALTERNATIVE TREATMENTS
Copper Supplementation

Supplementation with copper, in the form of either copper oxide wire particles (COWPs) or a sustained-release multitrace element/vitamin ruminal bolus (TEB), provide an anthelmintic effect against *H contortus* in goats, causing a temporary reduction in FEC. Its use should be targeted during the warm humid months when *Haemonchus* infection is abundant. Supplementation with copper sulfate has failed to show any anthelmintic effect in goats.[26] The first evidence of anthelmintic activity of copper against established *H contortus* populations in naturally infected goats was obtained using COWPs.[27] A dose of 2 g of COWPs proved to be effective against adult *H contortus* in kids[28] and a dose of 4 g was effective in adult goats.[29] Moreover, field trials on naturally infected goats showed that COWP doses of 0.5 g in kids and 5 g in adult goats caused a significant reduction of FEC.[29] Similar reductions in FEC were reported for adult goats supplemented with 3.7 g of Cu contained in a TEB.[30] However, no information on worm burdens was included.

COWP administration in gelatin capsules can be difficult, but a recent study confirmed that when administered in feed, COWPs are as effective as those in gelatin capsules in reducing FEC.[31] Thus, COWPs may be administered in farms by using supplementary feeding. However, the animals would need to consume the full dose (2 or 4 g/day) in 1 or 2 rations. Thus, the palatability of the feed and adaptation of the animals are crucial to recommend this approach. Also, investigators warned about possible copper toxicity if some animals eat more of their share of feed with COWPs. Furthermore, the combination of COWPs and supplementary feeding can improve the growth of kids compared with that with each separate solution.[32]

It is difficult to determine if the efficacy of COWPs differs between sheep and goats because of the differences in the doses administered, the nature of COWP commercial products, differences in pasture infectivity, differences in diets (influencing the abomasal pH), and so forth. A recent comparison between lambs and kids, under similar management conditions, showed that COWPs are effective against *H contortus* for up to 6 weeks after weaning.[33] However, 3 possible differences may exist. First, a difference between sheep and goats in the persistent effect of COWPs; although it is considered that COWPs have an extended period of efficacy (preventing incoming larvae to infect the host) in sheep, trials in goats failed to find such a persistency.[27,28] Second, differences related to the absorption and metabolism of copper; although the reasons are unclear, goats supplemented with COWP or copper sulfate gave birth to kids with reduced birth weight, an effect that continued for up to 60 days.[29,31] Third, goats are more tolerant than sheep to copper, and the use of copper in sheep may result in mortality because of copper toxicity in some regions.[27] Because COWPs and TEB were developed to supplement copper to grazing ruminants in copper-deficient areas, goats supplemented with those supplements increase their liver cupric content[28,31]; moreover, COWPs and TEB should not be used in animals receiving other copper supplementation.

Plant Nutraceuticals

The possible use of plants to control helminths in humans or animals is acknowledged by centuries of use in ethnomedical traditions. After 50 years of successful use of chemical anthelmintic drugs in the control of helminths of veterinary importance, the renewed impetus given to plants as a possible sustainable alternative to chemotherapy was initiated by field studies in New Zealand, which indicated positive results when infected sheep received different tannin-containing legume forages.[34] Since then, several studies have shown that the use of nutraceuticals is an option in goats.[35] The negative effects on various key steps and stages of the life cycle of nematodes (ie, a reduced level of host invasion by disturbing the infective process related to L3, and a reduced contamination of pastures by significant decreases in egg output) have been found when goats consumed either legume fodders, such as *Sericea lespedeza*[36] and sainfoin,[37] or other temperate[38] or tropical browses.[39,40]

Because of major differences in feeding behavior between sheep and goats, it is suspected that some adaptive mechanisms might explain the greater ability of goats to neutralize tannins because of either specialized protein-binding ability of the saliva or tannin-resistant ruminal flora.[41] The influence of such mechanisms of detoxification on the efficiency of tannin-rich plants against GINs in goats versus sheep has received little attention. In particular, detoxification mechanisms might modulate the proportion of tannins needed in feed to achieve full efficiency. Only a few studies have compared the effects of the same tannin-rich resources in the 2 hosts under similar experimental conditions.[42,43] The current results suggest a need to increase the dose in goats compared with sheep but this needs further investigation.

Use of Nematophagous Fungi

Because the use of nematophagous fungi represents a multivalent solution against a wide range of parasite species, applicable in many livestock species and complementary to the chemical control of GINs, the effect of the distribution of the fungi spores in altering the dynamics of infection has also been explored in goats. In particular, the administration of *Duddingtonia flagrans* spores as a feed additive on a daily basis has demonstrated its efficacy to reduce the preparasitic stages of different GIN species, for example, by more than 80% for *Teladorsagia circumcincta* and *Trichostrongylus colubriformis* populations in experimental infections[44,45] and from 50% to 80% in a plot study.[46] No main differences in results have been observed in goats when compared with sheep, except that in the former, a higher daily dose may be required, possibly because of their behavioral ability to sort diet at the trough.[44] Recent evidence highlights the importance of the relationship between FEC and the number of chlamydospores reaching the feces.[47] The best efficacy is achieved with animals presenting a ratio of 5 to 10 chlamydospores per egg in feces. Therefore, the proposed difference in dose between sheeps and goats might relate to FECs because goats tend to have higher FECs than sheep after the same parasitic challenges. Thus, goats need higher chlamydospore doses than sheep to achieve the ratio mentioned earlier. A further aspect that should be considered is that goats can consume a higher amount of feed containing plant secondary metabolites. These metabolites can affect nematode egg hatching, reducing the quantity of infective larvae stimulating the formation of trapping structures in the feces.

GRAZING MANAGEMENT

The 3 general principles of grazing management (ie, escaping, evading, and diluting L3) should be applied in goat breeding systems to lower the risk of infections associated with pasture grazing. Some caprine differences are discussed.

Goat Grazing Behavior

The preference of goats to browse compared with sheep leads to 3 possible synergistic positive effects in regard of GIN infections. Goats are at a lower risk of ingesting infective stages because L3 are absent on trees and bushes. This behavior also allows them to better exploit some extensive grazing systems, which may dilute the risk of infection. The species can better exploit the possible anthelmintic properties of various temperate or tropical browse plant species,[48,49] particularly when considering the recent hypothesis regarding the ability of small ruminants to self-medicate when raised in a biodiverse environment.[50,51]

Alternate Species Grazing

Most results obtained on the positive effects associated with mixed or alternate grazing between cattle and small ruminants with regard to GIN infections involved sheep. Only a few studies examining the consequences of mixed grazing on GINs have directly involved goats.[52] Some studies from French West Indies have shown results similar to those obtained from studies with sheep and cattle, that is, whether simultaneous or alternate mode, mixed grazing contributes to reduced levels of infection in goats.[53] In sheep, this decrease in worm populations was particularly prominent with H contortus.[54] This finding remains to be confirmed in goats. On the other hand, mixed grazing usually increased the diversity of the helminthofauna, particularly by increasing the number of abomasal cattle parasites in small ruminants.

STIMULATION OF THE IMMUNE RESPONSES AGAINST GINs
Goat versus Sheep Immune Responses Against GINs and Related Consequences

It is usually assumed that the greater avoidance of nematode L3 by goats because of its browsing behavior is the reason behind the differences between sheep and goat immune responses to GIN species. Many studies have shown that the development of an immune response in goats might be less efficient than that in sheep in several aspects; for example, the reduction of larval establishment and expulsion of adult worms are rarely observed in goats.[6,55] However, genotypic (eg, possible breed differences) and phenotypic (eg, including selection for high levels of milk production) variations should also be considered. These fundamental differences might have an effect on the development and efficacy of alternative methods of control, relying on the host ability to raise an immune response.

Genetic Selection for Resistance to GINs

There is ample evidence to suggest that the negative binomial distribution of nematodes in host populations relates to some host genetic factors. Although caprine programs to study the genetic response to GINs and its possible exploitation to select for resistance are less common than in sheep, some prolonged studies have shown the validity of the concept by demonstrating the existence of genetic variability either between[56] or within breeds.[53,57] The program set up to study fiber-producing Cashmere goats in Scotland[57] has now been discontinued, but several ongoing studies persist in breeds of meat-producing goats under tropical conditions, particularly in the French West Indies.[53,58]

Nutrition-Parasite Interactions

As in sheep, the possibility to manipulate nutrition, primarily by improving dietary protein, particularly rumen nondegradable or bypass proteins, has shown its efficiency in goats and has been the subject of recent reviews.[59,60] A few studies in dairy goats have shown that a higher-protein diet offers the possibility to alleviate the periparturient rise and partly compensate milk losses in high-yielding goats.[61] In growing kids of meat-producing breeds, early attempts to improve resilience through a higher plane of nutrition provided promising responses.[62] However, a pen trial with kids, in which the amount of protein administered alone was increased, failed to show a clear improvement in resilience against *H contortus*, contrary to what has been reported in lambs. Furthermore, kids tended to urinate the excess nitrogen provided in the high-protein diet.[63] This nitrogen excretion could be because of the different ability to mobilize fat reserves to fuel the metabolism of high amounts of protein that is available in kids compared with lambs. Similarly, studies exploring the use of urea as a possible source of nonprotein nitrogen underline the need to associate urea and cotton seed to achieve better results on caprine resilience and resistance.[59,64]

Field trials performed under tropical browsing conditions with naturally infected growing kids showed that dietary supplementation (combining an increase of protein and energy) improved resilience and, to a lesser extent, resistance against GINs in the wet and the dry seasons.[65,66] Considering the high level of protein provided by the browse legume fodders, a series of trials have compared the efficacy of dietary supplementation based on protein plus energy versus energy alone, provided by sorghum meal.[67] The results showed that energy supplementation can cause similar improvement of resilience and a further reduction in FEC compared with protein plus energy supplementation. The overall result supports the idea that, under conditions of high protein availability (from browsing trees), energy supplementation can improve resilience to an economically viable level. Also, some recent trials have examined the effect of protein supplementation on the periparturient egg increase in pregnant West African Dwarf goats.[68,69] Overall, the results showed that an increase in dietary protein was protective against early parasite establishment, body-weight losses, and deterioration in body-condition score during pregnancy and significantly increased kid birth weight and survival. All these findings are similar to those found in adult sheep.

SUMMARY

Because the same nematode species infect the gastrointestinal tract of sheep and goats, it is logical to initially consider that most research findings on the control of GINs acquired in sheep might be applied to goats. However, it is essential to take into account the differences in the caprine species. This difference has been clearly shown with the application of anthelmintic drugs and elaboration of recommendations for adapted doses in goats based on scientific evidence. This example highlights the need for more specific caprine studies in general.

REFERENCES

1. Gasnier N, Cabaret J. Evidence for a sheep and a goat line of *Teladorsagia circumcincta*. Parasitol Res 1996;82:546–50.
2. Waller PJ. Sustainable nematode parasite control strategies for ruminant livestock by grazing management and biological control. Anim Feed Sci Technol 2006;126: 277–89.

3. James CE, Hudson AL, Davey MW. Drug resistance mechanisms in helminths: is it survival of the fittest? Trends Parasitol 2009;25:328–35.

4. Kaplan RM. Drug resistance in nematodes of veterinary importance: a status report. Trends Parasitol 2004;20:477–81.

5. Waller PJ. International approaches to the concept of integrated control of nematode parasites of livestock. Int J Parasitol 1999;29:155–64.

6. Hoste H, Sotiraki S, Landau SY, et al. Goat nematode interactions: think differently. Trends Parasitol 2010;26:376–81.

7. Cawley GD, Shaw IC, Jackson F, et al. Levamisole toxicity in fibre goats. Vet Rec 1993;133:627–8.

8. Hennessy DR. Physiology, pharmacology and parasitology. Int J Parasitol 1997; 27:145–52.

9. Bogan J, Benoit E, Delatour P. Pharmacokinetics of oxfendazole in goats: a comparison with sheep. J Vet Pharmacol Ther 1987;10:305–9.

10. Hennessy DR, Sangster NC, Steel JW, et al. Comparative pharmacokinetic behaviour of albendazole in sheep and goats. Int J Parasitol 1993;23:321–5.

11. Galtier P, Escoula L, Camguilhem R, et al. Comparative availability of levamisole in non lactating ewes and goats. Ann Rech Vet 1981;12:109–15.

12. Dupuy J, Chartier C, Sutra JF, Alvinerie M. Eprinomectin in dairy goats: dose influence on plasma levels and excretion in milk. Parasitol Res 2001;87: 294–8.

13. Alvinerie M, Lacoste E, Sutra JF, et al. Some pharmacokinetic parameters of eprinomectin in goats following pour-on administration. Vet Res Commun 1999; 23:449–55.

14. Jackson F, Coop RL. The development of anthelmintic resistance in sheep nematodes. Parasitology 2000;120:S95–107.

15. Chartier C, Pors I, Hubert J, et al. Prevalence of anthelmintic resistant nematodes in sheep and goats in Western France. Small Rumin Res 1998;29:33–41.

16. Jackson F, Jackson E, Coop RL. Evidence of multiple anthelmintic resistance in a strain of Teladorsagia circumcincta (Ostertagia circumcincta) isolated from goats in Scotland. Multiple anthelmintic resistant nematodes in goats. Res Vet Sci 1992;53:371–4.

17. Zajac AM, Gipson TA. Multiple anthelmintic resistance in a goat herd. Vet Parasitol 2000;87:163–72.

18. Chandrawathani P, Adnan M, Waller PJ. Anthelmintic resistance in sheep and goat farms on Peninsular Malaysia. Vet Parasitol 1999;82:305–10.

19. Paraud C, Kulo A, Pors I, et al. Resistance of goat nematodes to multiple anthelmintics on a farm in France. Vet Rec 2009;164:563–4.

20. Edwards GT, Sian E, Mitchell ESE, et al. Anthelmintic use in goats. Vet Rec 2007; 161:763–4.

21. Mavrogianni VS, Fthenakis GC, Papadopoulos E, et al. Safety and reproductive safety of moxidectin in goats. Small Rumin Res 2004;54:33–41.

22. Chartier C. Parasitisme helminthique des caprins. In: Pathologie caprine: du diagnostic à la prevention. Maisons-Alfort (France): Point Vétérinaire; 2009. p. 159–79.

23. Hoste H, Le Frileux Y, Pommaret A. Distribution and repeatability of fecal egg counts and blood parameters in dairy goats naturally infected with gastrointestinal nematodes. Res Vet Sci 2001;70:57–60.

24. Hoste H, Chartier C, LeFrileux Y. Control of gastrointestinal parasitism with nematodes in dairy goats by treating the host category at risk. Vet Res 2002; 33:531–45.

25. Mahieu M, Arquet R, Kandassamy T, et al. Evaluation of targeted drenching using Famacha method in Creole goat: reduction of anthelmintic use, and effects on kid production and pasture contamination. Vet Parasitol 2007;146:135–47.

26. Burke JM, Miller JE. Dietary copper sulfate for control of gastrointestinal nematodes in goats. Vet Parasitol 2008;154:289–93.

27. Chartier C, Etter E, Hoste H, et al. Efficacy of copper oxide needles for the control of nematode parasites of dairy goats. Vet Res Commun 2000;24:389–99.

28. Vatta AF, Waller PJ, Githiori JB, et al. The potential to control *Haemonchus contortus* in indigenous South African goats with copper oxide wire particles. Vet Parasitol 2009;162:306–13.

29. Burke JM, Terrill TH, Kallu RR, et al. Use of copper oxide wire particles to control gastrointestinal nematodes in goats. J Anim Sci 2007;85:2753–61.

30. Burke JM, Miller JE. Control of *Haemonchus contortus* in goats with a sustained-release multi-trace element/vitamin ruminal bolus containing copper. Vet Parasitol 2006;141:132–7.

31. Burke JM, Soli F, Miller JE, et al. Administration of copper oxide wire particles in a capsule or feed for gastrointestinal nematode control in goats. Vet Parasitol 2010;168:346–50.

32. Martínez-Ortiz-de-Montellano C, Vargas-Magaña JJ, Aguilar-Caballero AJ, et al. Combining the effects of supplementary feeding and copper oxide needles improves the control of gastrointestinal nematodes in browsing goats. Vet Parasitol 2007;146:66–76.

33. Soli F, Terrill TH, Shaik SA, et al. Efficacy of copper oxide wire particles against gastrointestinal nematodes in sheep and goats. Vet Parasitol 2010;168:93–6.

34. Niezen JH, Robertson HA, Waghorn GC, et al. Production, faecal egg counts and worm burdens of ewe lambs which grazed six contrasting forages. Vet Parasitol 1998;80:15–27.

35. Hoste H, Jackson F, Athanasiadou S, et al. The effects of tannin-rich plants on parasitic nematodes in ruminants. Trends Parasitol 2006;32:253–61.

36. Shaik SA, Terrill TH, Miller JE, et al. Effects of feeding *Sericea lespedeza* hay to goats infected with *Haemonchus contortus*. S Afr J Anim Sci 2004;34(Suppl 1): 234–7.

37. Paolini V, De La Farge F, Prevot F, et al. Effects of the repeated distribution of sainfoin hay on the resistance and the resilience of goats naturally infected with gastrointestinal nematodes. Vet Parasitol 2005;127:277–83.

38. Osoro K, Benito-Peña A, Frutos P, et al. The effect of heather supplementation on gastrointestinal nematode infections and performance in Cashmere and local Celtiberic goats on pasture. Small Rumin Res 2007;67:184–91.

39. Brunet S, Martinez-Ortiz De Montellano C, Torres-Acosta JF, et al. Effect of the consumption of *Lysiloma latisilliquum* on the larval establishment of parasitic nematodes in goats. Vet Parasitol 2008;157:81–8.

40. Kabasa JD, Opuda-Asibo J, Ter Meulen U. The effect of oral administration of polyethylene glycol on faecal helminth egg counts in pregnant goats grazed on browse containing condensed tannins. Trop Anim Health Prod 2000;32: 73–86.

41. Alonso Diaz MA, Torres-Acosta JF, Sandoval Castro M, et al. Tannins in tropical tree fodders fed to small ruminants: a friendly foe? Small Rumin Res 2010;89: 164–73.

42. Max RA, Kassuku AA, Kimambo AE, et al. The effect of wattle tannin drenches on gastrointestinal nematodes of tropical sheep and goats during experimental and natural infections. J Agric Sci (Camb) 2009;147:1–8.

43. Max RA. Effect of repeated wattle tannin drenches on worm burdens, faecal egg counts and egg hatchability during naturally acquired nematode infections in sheep and goats. Vet Parasitol 2010;169:138–43.

44. Paraud C, Hoste H, LeFrileux Y, et al. Administration of *Duddingtonia flagrans* chlamydospores to goats to control gastro-intestinal nematodes: dose trials. Vet Res 2005;36:157–66.

45. Paraud C, Chartier C. Biological control of infective larvae of a gastro-intestinal nematode (*Teladorsagia circumcincta*) and a small lungworm (*Muellerius capillaris*) by *Duddingtonia flagrans* in goat faeces. Parasitol Res 2003;89:102–6.

46. Chartier C, Pors I. Effect of the nematophagous fungus, *Duddingtonia flagrans*, on the larval development of goat parasitic nematodes: a plot study. Vet Res 2003;34:1–10.

47. Ojeda-Robertos NF, Torres-Acosta JF, Aguilar-Caballero AJ, et al. Assessing the efficacy of *Duddingtonia flagrans* chlamydospores per gram of faeces to control *Haemonchus contortus* larvae. Vet Parasitol 2008;158:329–35.

48. Alonso-Díaz MA, Torres-Acosta JF, Sandoval-Castro C, et al. In vitro larval migration and kinetics of exsheathment of *Haemonchus contortus* exposed to four tropical taniniferous plants. Vet Parasitol 2008;153:313–9.

49. Manolaraki F, Sotiraki S, Stefanakis A, et al. Anthelmintic activity of some Mediterranean browse plants against parasitic nematodes. Parasitology 2010;137: 685–96.

50. Lisonbee LD, Villalba JJ, Provenza FD, et al. Tannins and self-medication: implications for sustainable parasite control in herbivores. Behav Processes 2009;82: 184–9.

51. Villalba JJ, Provenza FD, Hall JO, et al. Selection of tannins by sheep in response to gastrointestinal nematode infection. J Anim Sci 2010;88:2189–98.

52. Doumenc V. In: *Helminthofaune des caprins en Saone-et-Loire. Influence du pâturage mixte avec les bovins*. Thèse de doctorat vétérinaire. Toulouse, France: Ecole Nationale Vétérinaire de Toulouse; 1975.

53. Alexandre G, González-García E, Lallo CH, et al. Goat management and systems of production: global framework and study cases in the Caribbean. Small Rumin Res 2010;89:193–206.

54. Hoste H, Cabaret J, Grosmond G, et al. [Alternatives aux traitements anthelminthiques en élevage biologique des ruminants]. Productions Animales 2009;22: 245–54 [in French].

55. Hoste H, Torres-Acosta JF, Aguilar-Caballero AJ. Nutrition-parasite interactions in goats: is immunoregulation involved in the control of gastrointestinal nematodes? Parasite Immunol 2008;30:79–88.

56. Pralomkarn W, Pandey VS, Ngampongsai W, et al. Genetic resistance of three genotypes of goats to experimental infection with *Haemonchus contortus*. Vet Parasitol 1997;68:79–90.

57. Vagenas D, Jackson F, Russel AJ, et al. Genetic control of resistance to gastrointestinal parasites in crossbred cashmere-producing goats: responses to selection, genetic parameters and relationships with production traits. Anim Sci 2002; 74:199–208.

58. Mandonnet N, Menendez-Buxadera A, Arquet R, et al. Genetic variability in resistance to gastrointestinal strongyles during early lactation in Creole goats. Anim Sci 2006;82:283–7.

59. Hoste H, Torres Acosta JF, Paolini V, et al. Interactions between nutrition and gastrointestinal infections with parasitic nematodes in goats. Small Rumin Res 2005;60:141–51.

60. Knox MR, Torres Acosta JF, Aguilar Caballero AJ. Exploiting the effects of dietary supplementation of small ruminants on resilience and resistance against gastrointestinal nematodes. Vet Parasitol 2006;139:385–93.

61. Etter E, Hoste H, Chartier C, et al. The effect of two levels of dietary protein on resistance and resilience of dairy goats experimentally infected with *Trichostrongylus colubriformis*: comparison between high and low producers. Vet Res 2000; 31:247–58.

62. Blackburn HD, Rocha JL, Figueiredo EP, et al. Interaction of parasitism and nutrition and their effects on production and clinical parameters in goats. Vet Parasitol 1991;40:99–112.

63. Torres-Acosta JF. In: *Supplementary feeding and the control of gastrointestinal nematodes of goats in Yucatan Mexico* [PhD thesis]. London: The Royal Veterinary College, University of London; 1999.

64. Knox MR, Steel J. Nutritional enhancement of parasite control in small ruminant production systems in developing countries of South East Asia and the Pacific. Int J Parasitol 1996;26:963–70.

65. Torres-Acosta JF, Jacobs D, Aguilar-Caballero AJ, et al. The effect of supplementary feeding on the resilience and resistance of browsing Criollo kids against natural gastrointestinal nematode infections during the rainy season in tropical Mexico. Vet Parasitol 2004;124:217–38.

66. Torres-Acosta JF, Jacobs D, Aguilar-Caballero AJ, et al. Improving resilience against natural gastrointestinal nematode infections in browsing kids during the dry season in tropical Mexico. Vet Parasitol 2006;135:163–73.

67. Gutierrez-Segura SI, Torres-Acosta JF, Aguilar-Caballero AJ, et al. Supplementation can improve resilience and resistance of browsing Criollo kids against nematode infections during wet season. Trop Subtrop Agroecosystems 2003;3: 537–40.

68. Nnadi PA, Kamalu TN, Onah DN. The effect of dietary protein supplementation on the pathophysiology of *Haemonchus contortus* infection in West African Dwarf goats. Vet Parasitol 2007;148:256–61.

69. Nnadi PA, Kamalu TN, Onah DN. Effect of dietary protein supplementation on performance of West Africa Dwarf goats during pregnancy and lactation. Small Rumin Res 2007;71:200–4.

Treatment and Control of Respiratory Disease in Sheep

Philip R. Scott, DVMS, MPhil, FRCVS

KEYWORDS

- Atypical pneumonia • Goat • *Mannheimia haemolytica*
- *Mycoplasma ovipneumoniae* • Pasteurellosis • Prevention
- Sheep • Treatment

Respiratory disease results in poor liveweight gain and mortality, thus causing considerable financial losses for lamb producers.[1,2] The disease is also an important animal welfare concern. Respiratory diseases in sheep and goats often result from adverse weather conditions[3] and physiologic stress combined with viral and bacterial infections.[4] Virus infections alone do not cause acute respiratory disease.[5] Risk factors predisposing lambs to the outbreaks of *Mannheimia haemolytica* pneumonia are listed in **Box 1**.

An etiologic approach to the diagnosis, treatment, and control of ovine respiratory diseases is adopted in most review articles[6] and book chapters.[7] However, such precise classification is unrealistic in most general veterinary practice situations because clinical signs are not pathognomonic for particular causative agents, costs limit laboratory resources to isolate the causal agents, and necropsy findings are easily confused.

The presumptive clinical diagnosis of acute respiratory disease caused by *M haemolytica* or *Bibersteinia trehalosi* (pasteurellosis, reclassified from *Pasteurella trehalosi*) in growing lambs and adult sheep is based on findings of sudden severe illness, inappetence, pyrexia, marked toxemia, and tachypnea consistent with endotoxemia,[7] but many other infectious diseases have a similar clinical presentation. The response of pasteurellosis to treatment by antibiotics or nonsteroidal antiinflammatory drugs (NSAIDs) does not necessarily support the diagnosis because many bacterial infections that present with profound endotoxemia[8,9] may also recover similarly. Therefore, at the farm level, efforts should be directed toward prompt detection of all sick sheep rather than concentrate on identifying respiratory disease.

Publication of auscultated sounds recorded over respiratory tract pathology defined during simultaneous ultrasonographic investigation has questioned the value of

The author has nothing to disclose.

Division of Veterinary Clinical Sciences, R(D)SVS, University of Edinburgh, Easter Bush, Roslin, Midlothian, Scotland, EH25 9RG, UK

E-mail address: philip.r.scott@ed.ac.uk

Vet Clin Food Anim 27 (2011) 175–186

doi:10.1016/j.cvfa.2010.10.016

Box 1
Risk factors predisposing lambs to outbreaks of _M haemolytica_ pneumonia
Concurrent infections involving other respiratory pathogens
Housing conditions (eg, stocking density, humidity, ammonia levels, temperature fluctuations)
Marked changes in weather conditions, such as rain and severe winds
Mixing sheep from multiple sources
Moving lambs from poor pasture to silage aftermath
Stress due to repeated handling and transportation

auscultation of the chest performed as part of the standard veterinary clinical examination.[10,11] It is therefore essential to critically assess clinical diagnostic methods for the common respiratory diseases affecting sheep before embarking on a review of treatment and control measures.

DIAGNOSIS OF RESPIRATORY DISEASE
History

Recent management events that could precipitate respiratory disease include weaning, purchase, source, transport, vaccination, housing, severe weather changes, and diet.

Auscultation Findings

Adventitious lung sounds are noises superimposed on normal lung sounds,[12] with a wide range of descriptors.[13–16] Investigators in more recent papers on ovine respiratory disease[17,18] have not described auscultation findings but have instead referred to their distribution. Recent studies have highlighted the lack of correlation between lungs sounds and distribution of pathologic condition in ovine pulmonary adenocarcinoma.[19] Routine interpretation of auscultated sound did not allow the presence of superficial lung pathology or its distribution to be accurately defined in the respiratory diseases represented in recent publications.[10,11]

Laboratory Tests

Changes in the leukogram and the haptoglobin, fibrinogen, and serum protein concentrations may indicate an inflammatory response to bacterial infection, but these changes are not specific for respiratory disease.

Bronchoalveolar Lavage

The detection of _M haemolytica_, _Mycoplasma ovipneumoniae_, parainfluenza virus 3, and bovine respiratory syncytial virus antigen in transtracheal bronchoalveolar lavage samples is closely correlated with clinical disease. However, this technique is not commonly used in general practice.

Radiographic Examination of the Thorax

The position of the thoracic limbs and associated musculature in the standing animal largely restricts radiographic examinations to the caudodorsal thorax when pathologic changes associated with aerosol infection more commonly involve the cranioventral lung field.

Ultrasonographic Examination of the Thorax

Ultrasonographic examination of the ovine chest provides an accurate assessment of the pleural surfaces and superficial lung parenchyma.[20,21] Examination is inexpensive and noninvasive, and unlike radiography, there are no special health and safety procedures or restrictions with ultrasonographic examination.

TREATMENT AND CONTROL OF PASTEURELLOSIS

Despite different bacterial etiologies, pasteurellosis is the term commonly used by veterinarians and farmers to describe acute respiratory disease in growing lambs or adult sheep. *M haemolytica* is of considerable economic importance to the sheep industry, causing septicemia in young lambs and pneumonia in older sheep. *B trehalosi* causes septicemia in 4- to 9-month-old lambs (systemic pasteurellosis). Recent reports have also described septicemia in young lambs caused by *Pasteurella multocida*.[22]

Disease Caused by M Haemolytica

M haemolytica is the most important bacterial infection of the ovine respiratory system,[7] the infection being an important cause of sudden death in lambs up to 12 weeks old. Affected adult sheep and those lambs found alive are profoundly depressed, pyrexic (rectal temperature often >41°C) with injected mucous membranes, marked tachypnea, and hyperpnea.

Treatment

A good treatment response to antibiotic therapy necessitates rapid detection of sick sheep by shepherds. The isolates of *M haemolytica* are sensitive to penicillin, ampicillin, oxytetracycline, erythromycin, and streptomycin,[23] as well as to amoxicillin-clavulanic acid combination.[24] Oxytetracycline, administered by slow intravenous injection at a dose rate of 10 mg/kg body weight (BW) in the first instance possible, is the antibiotic most commonly selected for pasteurellosis.[7,25] Thereafter, the drug is injected intramuscularly daily for 3 to 4 consecutive days at 10 mg/kg BW or with a single long-acting injection at 20 mg/kg BW. Unlike in cattle, there are few reported oxytetracycline-resistant strains in sheep. An improvement in demeanor and appetite is expected within 24 to 48 hours, with a corresponding fall in rectal temperature to the normal range (from >41.0°C–39.5°C).

Antibiotics that have recently been introduced for the treatment of bovine respiratory disease, including tilmicosin (5–10 mg/kg BW, once only by subcutaneous injection to sheep heavier than 15 kg[14]) and florfenicol (20 mg/kg BW, twice with a 48-hour interval by intramuscular injection), have been tested for treating sheep, but there are few comparative efficacy data and these drugs are considerably more expensive than oxytetracycline (**Boxes 2** and **3**). Some of these antibiotic treatment regimes, especially those in **Box 3**, do not have a regulatory license (off-label use) in many countries of the world. Moreover, in certain countries, tilmicosin has health and safety restrictions concerning its administration. Trials using danofloxacin have also suggested that this drug is effective for treating *Mannheimia* infections,[26,27] although not licensed for use in sheep at present. It should be noted that use of antimicrobials of high importance to human health, such as fluoroquinolones, is discouraged or forbidden in many countries. The veterinary practitioner must be acquainted with national regulations regarding extralabel drug use. There is evidence that antimicrobial drugs licensed for the treatment of bovine respiratory disease (see **Box 3**) can also be effective in the treatment of pneumonia in sheep.

Box 2
Antimicrobial drugs licensed for the treatment of ovine respiratory diseases in many countries worldwide

Amoxicillin trihydrate

Amoxicillin–clavulanic acid combination

Ampicillin trihydrate

Oxytetracycline dihydrate/hydrochloride

Procaine benzylpenicillin

Procaine penicillin–dihydrostreptomycin sulfate combination

Tilmicosin (not for use in lambs weighing <15 kg)

Under experimental conditions, severity of clinical pneumonic pasteurellosis correlated with episodes of endotoxemia, bacteremia, and elevated eicosanoid concentrations[28]; therefore, there is good reason to administer an NSAID preparation at first presentation[29] in conjunction with antibiotic therapy. However, in many countries worldwide, no NSAIDs are licensed for the treatment of ovine respiratory disease (**Box 4**). There is support for NSAID administration in respiratory disease from the results of studies of infections of other organs or systems in small ruminants. For example, flunixin meglumine was shown to confer more rapid improvement in clinical signs in a case-controlled study comparing cefuroxime plus flunixin with cefuroxime alone in sheep[30] or goats[31] predominantly with *Staphylococcus aureus* mastitis.

The basic therapeutic strategy involves the combination of an antibiotic to act against the relevant pathogens and an NSAID to act against the deleterious effects of inflammation.[32] However, in a study performed in cattle, in which 3 NSAIDS, flunixin, ketoprofen, and carprofen, were used in conjunction with ceftiofur in the treatment of spontaneous respiratory disease, no differences were evident among the treatment regimes with respect to clinical signs observed.[33] Studies on the use of NSAIDs in cattle with endotoxemic conditions have produced equivocal results. The single administration of flunixin at a dose rate of 2.2 mg/kg BW, in addition to systemic antibiotic treatment of cows with acute puerperal metritis[34] or acute toxic mastitis,[35] did not result in beneficial effects on clinical cure. Although administration of the drug resulted in the decrease of the rectal temperature of cows with endotoxin-induced mastitis, it has not been established that reduction of fever is beneficial to cows with naturally occurring mastitis.[36]

NSAIDs can also be administered to sheep with acute infections for their analgesic properties, but there is no consensus for such benefit in the published literature.

Box 3
Antimicrobial drugs licensed for the treatment of bovine respiratory diseases in many countries worldwide for potential use in sheep

Florfenicol

Fluoroquinolones (eg, danofloxacin, difloxacin, marbofloxacin)

Tulathromycin

Tylosin

Box 4
NSAIDs licensed for the treatment of bovine respiratory diseases in many countries worldwide
Carprofen
Flunixin meglumine
Ketoprofen
Meloxicam
Tolfenamic acid

Flunixin was considered to be ineffective for the management of acute and chronic pain in sheep.[37,38] In another clinical study, intramuscular xylazine administration provided the best combination of onset, duration, and total analgesic response for the routine management of acute pain.[6]

In cattle, corticosteroids are used successfully in the treatment of peracute infections with bovine respiratory syncytial virus because of the allergic nature of this severe presentation. Similar allergic-type reactions have not been reported in sheep; therefore, NSAIDs seem to be a more rational treatment to combat endotoxemia present. A prescribing dilemma can arise in countries in which corticosteroids are licensed for use in sheep but NSAIDs are not.

Hypertonic saline is routinely used as a supportive therapy for generalized endotoxemia in cattle,[39] but such treatment is rarely used in sheep. Supportive therapy comprising 45 L of intravenous isotonic electrolyte solution and flunixin meglumine (2000 mg) had no significant effect on the survival rate of cows with endotoxemia.[40] In sheep, however, fluids administered by orogastric tube, combined with intravenous flunixin injection, may prove the best compromise.

Control

Because many risk factors cannot be avoided, prevention is best attempted using vaccines incorporating iron-regulated proteins produced by the causative organisms.[7] Because these proteins are antigenically similar, they confer cross-protection against all isolates of M haemolytica and B trehalosi. Breeding ewes require a primary course of 2 injections 4 to 6 weeks apart, followed by an annual booster 4 to 6 weeks before lambing. However, this vaccination regimen only provides passive immunity to the lambs for up to 5 weeks after birth. Lambs can be protected by 2 doses of vaccine, administered 4 to 6 weeks apart from the age of 3 weeks; at that age, colostral antibodies do not interfere with the development of active immunity. However, not all field studies have found a benefit from vaccination. For example, in New Zealand, vaccinated lambs had a lower mean daily weight gain between first vaccination and 11 weeks and there were no significant differences between the frequency of isolation of M haemolytica and B trehalosi or the histopathologic classification of disease lesions between pneumonic lung samples from the placebo-treated and vaccinated lambs.[41]

Good husbandry practices (**Box 5**) should help to reduce respiratory disease in sheep following housing. Shelter from adverse climatic conditions in exposed grazing areas, eg, woodlands, should be provided during the winter months.[3] The possibility of trace element deficiency states, particularly of cobalt or selenium, should be investigated in geographic areas with known soil types or where there is a high incidence of disease; these should be corrected with appropriate means.

Box 5
Husbandry practices to reduce the incidence of respiratory disease in housed sheep

Ensure appropriate ventilation

Avoid housing in drafty or poorly ventilated barns

Reduce number of sheep in the same airspace

Divide animals in groups according to age, BW, and origin

Do not house young sheep with adult animals

Disease Caused by B Trehalosi

Systemic pasteurellosis caused by *B trehalosi* is the most common cause of sudden death in 4- to 9-month-old lambs after weaning in the United Kingdom.

Oxytetracycline is the antibiotic of choice for systemic pasteurellosis, but the prognosis should be guarded because of the advanced state of the disease when animals are presented for treatment. Intravenous injection of NSAIDs, such as flunixin meglumine or ketoprofen, helps counter the endotoxemia.

For control of the disease, it is important to limit potential predisposing factors after weaning, which may trigger clinical disease; these factors include handling stresses, long periods held in markets without food, mixing with other stock, repeated journeys to markets, and sudden dietary changes. Lambs can also be protected by 2 doses of vaccines containing iron-regulated proteins, given 4 weeks apart, with the second injection 2 weeks before weaning or sale.[42]

Antibiotic metaphylaxis with a single long-acting injection of oxytetracycline at 20 mg/kg BW in the face of mounting deaths has produced equivocal results in split-flock trials in the United Kingdom with a favorable benefit:cost ratio found in only 1 of 10 test flocks.[43] Injection with long-acting oxytetracycline or tilmicosin is often delayed until losses exceed 1%, whereas total losses are unlikely to exceed 2%. Medication of the drinking water with sulfonamides (200 mg/kg BW on the first day, followed by 66 mg/kg BW/d for further 4 days) is restricted to housed or feedlot situations. In this case, there is of course concern that sick animals may not drink adequate amount of water and thus not receive adequate amount of the drug.

TREATMENT AND CONTROL OF *MYCOPLASMA* PNEUMONIA

Mycoplasma pneumonia (atypical pneumonia, enzootic pneumonia) is a nonprogressive chronic pneumonia of housed sheep, younger than 1 year, and caused by *M ovipneumoniae* and possibly other organisms.[44,45] Typical pathologic findings of sharply demarcated, dark red/brown anteroventral consolidation of the lungs are common in lambs at slaughter plants, without apparent adverse effects on growth rate. Abscessation of the lungs and pleurisy are uncommon.

Treatment is generally not necessary because clinical signs are mild.[46] Oxytetracycline (single intramuscular injection of a long-acting preparation at a dose rate of 20 mg/kg BW) should be given to inappetant sick lambs. Mycoplasmas are also sensitive to macrolide and fluoroquinolone antibiotics, but such treatment is rarely needed.

Control can be attempted by improving the building's ventilation and by reducing stocking density. The airspace should not be shared with older sheep, carriers of the causative agents. Purchased lambs should be housed separately from homebred stock.

CONTROL OF PARAINFLUENZA VIRUS 3

The single serotype of ovine parainfluenza virus 3 infection causes a mild undifferentiated interstitial pneumonia without clinical signs. The bovine parainfluenza virus 3 used in an attenuated cattle intranasal vaccine is antigenically related to the ovine strain[5] and has been used off-license for vaccinating sheep in experimental studies.[47] In one study, the vaccine was given intranasally to ewes on one farm, resulting in seroconversion of many sheep and negligible outbreaks of pneumonia around the subsequent lambing time; protection of the flock appeared to last for one season. Subsequently, ewes and lambs on other farms were vaccinated, and on these farms, there were fewer deaths than expected as a result of pasteurellosis.[48] However, in more recent studies,[49] vaccination against this virus did not seem to reduce the incidence of pneumonia. Care must be taken using unapproved vaccines for sheep containing modified live virus for which no safety data exist.

CONTROL OF OVINE PULMONARY ADENOCARCINOMA

Ovine pulmonary adenocarcinoma (jaagsiekte, pulmonary carcinoma) is a contagious tumor of the lungs of sheep, with a worldwide distribution caused by infection with a β-retrovirus known as jaagsiekte sheep retrovirus.[50]

There is no treatment of the disease. Affected sheep must be culled as soon as clinical suspicions are confirmed, either by clinical detection of the copious clear nasal discharge or by ultrasonographic examination of the chest.[20]

A disease-free closed flock is the only reliable means of controlling pulmonary adenocarcinoma. The disease is introduced into flocks with purchased infected sheep, which shed the virus before illness becomes apparent. The main route of infection is by respiratory aerosol, with housing increasing the rate of spread of infection.

Regular flock inspection with prompt isolation and culling of lean and/or dyspneic sheep may identify early clinical cases and slow the spread of infection. Maintaining sheep in single age groups during housing has been shown to be the most important management factor in reducing clinical disease. Most sheep flocks are grouped during housing on their late gestation nutritional requirements based on fetal number; therefore age-grouping may prove problematic. The offspring of affected sheep frequently develop pulmonary adenocarcinoma by the age of 2 years and must not be kept as replacement breeding stock.

CONTROL OF ENZOOTIC NASAL ADENOCARCINOMA

Enzootic nasal adenocarcinoma (also called enzootic nasal adenomatosis) is caused by a β-retrovirus, enzootic nasal tumor virus 1 and occurs throughout North America and Europe.[50,51] Infection cannot be detected by a serologic test because the virus stimulates no immune response. Signs of the disease occur in adult sheep and may present as severe upper respiratory stertor and noise of days to months duration or sudden death due to occlusion of both nares. The tumors are unilateral, causing decreased to absent breaths from one nostril. Affected sheep are distressed and show weight loss. The virus is contagious, but other factors may play a role in its ability to cause clinical disease. Flock mortality rates vary annually from low sporadic to 10%. The breed or line of the animal may play a role, but little is currently understood about the epidemiology of this disease. Sheep with suspected infection should be culled as quickly as possible and nursing lambs marketed as appropriate.

CONTROL OF OVINE ADENOVIRUS AND RESPIRATORY SYNCYTIAL VIRUS INFECTIONS

The significance of these 2 viruses as causes of naturally occurring pneumonia in sheep remains unknown.

CONTROL OF MAEDI-VISNA

Respiratory disease (maedi, ovine progressive pneumonia), nervous disease (visna), mastitis, and arthritis are caused by infections with small ruminant lentivirus. There is no effective treatment of this disease.

Prevention of infection is best achieved by maintaining a disease-free closed flock with stringent biosecurity measures and, when absolutely necessary, purchase of adult animals from a reputable source, confirmed to be free from infection. Control can be attempted in an infected closed flock by regular 3- to 6-month serologic testing with culling of seropositive sheep and their offspring, but this is a costly and protracted protocol over several years and requires biosecurity of new introductions. The sensitivity of available tests is low and sheep may seroconvert up to 2 years after acquiring infection. Alternatively, removal of lambs from their dams immediately after birth, before they ingest colostrum, breaks the lactogenic route of transmission. Artificial rearing systems using automated machines have greatly improved the rearing of young lambs in such a way that this method is now a realistic option.

TREATMENT AND CONTROL OF CHRONIC SUPPURATIVE PNEUMONIA/LUNG ABSCESSES

Lung abscesses are common in adult sheep, especially rams, but are difficult to diagnose by clinical examination alone.[52] Affected sheep are presented with chronic weight loss over several weeks to months and are often dull although appetite may appear normal. The rectal temperature is only slightly elevated (up to 40°C). At rest, affected sheep are tachypneic and cough occasionally, and there may be a scant mucopurulent nasal discharge. *Arcanobacterium pyogenes* is a common isolate from lung abscesses.[53]

Penicillin is the antibiotic of choice for chronic respiratory disease because of the frequent isolation of *A pyogenes*. A 4- to 6-week duration of daily penicillin injection, necessary because of the severity of chronicity of infection and time-dependent action of this antibiotic, has produced encouraging results in sheep with pleural and superficial lung abscesses identified during ultrasonographic examination.[20,52,54] Other potentially effective antibiotics include ceftiofur, amoxicillin, and amoxicillin/clavulanic acid combination but are considerably more expensive.

Prolonged housing and respiratory viral infections are considered to be risk factors for the disease (see **Box 5**).

TREATMENT AND CONTROL OF PARASITIC PNEUMONIA

Dictyocaulus filaria may cause mild coughing, especially after exercise, in growing lambs during autumn and winter, although large infestations can be encountered in sheep with paratuberculosis and other immunosuppressive conditions. Evidence of *Protostrongylus rufescens* and *Muellerius capillaris* may be found at necropsy without premonitory signs.

Nematodes of the respiratory tract are responsive to benzimidazoles[55] and macrocyclic lactones[56,57] and are usually controlled by most flock health anthelmintic strategies for parasitic gastroenteritis.

TREATMENT AND CONTROL OF LARYNGEAL CHONDRITIS

Laryngeal chondritis is an obstructive upper respiratory tract disease characterized by severe dyspnea, most commonly encountered in 18- to 24-month-old meat breed rams, during the late summer and autumn months. There is acute onset severe respiratory distress, with marked inspiratory effort and stertor, caused by edema of the arytenoid cartilages of the larynx, resulting in narrowing of the lumen. Delayed identification and/or inadequate duration of antibiotic therapy may result in abscess formation within the arytenoid cartilages.

Treatment involves intravenous or intramuscular administration of dexamethasone once only at presentation, with the aim to reduce edema. This treatment should be followed by a course of intramuscular administration of a broad-spectrum antibiotic for at least 7 to 10 consecutive days.

The sporadic occurrence of laryngeal chondritis means that little constructive advice can be given to breeders regarding prevention. Reducing the level of supplementary feeding may reduce the prevalence of this problem, but farmers are most reluctant to not have rams in top condition for the sales. Reducing dust in the environment is considered an important preventive measure but may be difficult, if not impossible, to achieve in commercial farms.

TREATMENT AND CONTROL OF *OESTRUS OVIS* INFESTATION

Oestrus ovis larvae (nasal bots) are obligatory parasites of the nasal and sinus cavities of sheep and goats. Infestation is prevalent in hot and dry regions, such as Mediterranean countries. Affected sheep have a nasal discharge, sneeze frequently, and rub their heads against objects. The activity of adult flies before larval deposition in the nasal passages can disrupt grazing, leading to weight loss if severe. Treatment is only necessary with heavy infestations; closantel, nitroxynil, and the group III anthelmintics, such as ivermectin or moxidectin, are effective.

SUMMARY

Early detection of sick sheep with acute respiratory disease caused by *M haemolytica* and *B trehalosi* (pasteurellosis) is essential to achieve a successful outcome. Treatment associated with these infections comprises intravenous antibiotic and NSAID therapy. Control measures include good husbandry practices and iron-regulated protein vaccines. Chronic bacterial infection of the respiratory tract is altogether different, and affected sheep usually present with weight loss over several weeks or months. Auscultation fails to identify and define specific lesions, but diagnosis is readily achieved using ultrasonography. *A pyogenes* is the most common bacterial isolate and such chronic infections are treated with a 4- to 6-week course of procaine penicillin with reasonable success. Specific control measures apply to certain chronic slow viral diseases of the respiratory tract.

REFERENCES

1. Jones GE, Field AC, Gilmour JS, et al. Effects of experimental chronic pneumonia on bodyweight, feed intake and carcase composition of lambs. Vet Rec 1982; 110:168–73.
2. Goodwin-Ray KA, Jackson R, Brown C, et al. Pneumonic lesions in lambs in New Zealand: patterns of prevalence and effects on production. N Z Vet J 2004;52: 175–9.

3. McIlroy SG, Goodall EA, McCracken RM, et al. Rain and windchill as factors in the occurrence of pneumonia in sheep. Vet Rec 1989;125:79–82.

4. Brogden KA, Lehmkuhl HD, Cutlip RC. Pasteurella haemolytica complicated respiratory infections in sheep and goats. Vet Res 1998;29:233–54.

5. Sharp JM, Nettleton PF. Acute respiratory viral infections. In: Aitken ID, editor. Diseases of sheep. 4th edition. Oxford(UK): Blackwell Publishing; 2007. p. 207–11.

6. Bell S. Respiratory disease in sheep 1. Differential diagnosis and epidemiology. In Pract 2008;30:200–7.

7. Donachie W. Pasteurellosis. In: Aitken ID, editor. Diseases of sheep. 4th edition. Oxford(UK): Blackwell Publishing; 2007. p. 224–35.

8. Tzora A, Leontides LS, Amiridis GS, et al. Bacteriological and epidemiological findings during examination of the uterine content of ewes with retention of fetal membranes. Theriogenology 2002;57:1809–17.

9. Jiménez A, Sánchez J, Andrés S, et al. Evaluation of endotoxaemia in the prognosis and treatment of scouring Merino lambs. J Vet Med A Physiol Pathol Clin Med 2007;54:103–6.

10. Scott PR. Lung auscultation recordings from normal sheep and from sheep with well-defined respiratory tract pathology. Small Rumin Res 2010;92:104–7.

11. Scott P, Collie D, McGorum B, et al. Relationship between thoracic auscultation and lung pathology detected by ultrasonography in sheep. Vet J 2010;186:53–7.

12. Cugell DW. Lung sound nomenclature. Am Rev Respir Dis 1987;136:1016.

13. Braun U, Flukiger M, Sicher D, et al. Suppurative pleuropneumonia and a pulmonary abscess in a ram: ultrasonographic and radiographic findings. Schweiz Arch Tierheilkd 1995;137:272–8.

14. Naccari F, Giofrè F, Pellegrino M, et al. Effectiveness and kinetic behaviour of tilmicosin in the treatment of respiratory infections in sheep. Vet Rec 2001;148:773–6.

15. Jackson PGG, Cockcroft PD. Clinical examination of farm animals. Oxford (UK): Blackwell Publishing; 2002.

16. McGorum BC, Dixon PM. Clinical examination of the respiratory tract. In: McGorum BC, Dixon PM, Robinson NE, et al, editors. Equine respiratory medicine and surgery. London: Saunders; 2007. p. 103–19.

17. Mavrogianni VS, Fthenakis GC. Efficacy of difloxacin against respiratory infections of lambs. J Vet Pharmacol Ther 2005;28:325–8.

18. Skoufos J, Christodoulopoulos G, Fragkou IA, et al. Efficacy of marbofloxacin against respiratory infections of lambs. Small Rumin Res 2007;71:304–9.

19. Cousens C, Graham M, Sales J, et al. Evaluation of the efficacy of clinical diagnosis of ovine pulmonary adenocarcinoma. Vet Rec 2008;162:88–90.

20. Scott PR, Gessert ME. Ultrasonographic examination of the ovine thorax. Vet J 1998;155:305–10.

21. Scott PR, Sargison ND. Ultrasonography as an adjunct to clinical examination in sheep. Small Rumin Res 2010;92:108–19.

22. Watson PJ, Davies RL. Outbreak of Pasteurella multocida septicaemia in neonatal lambs. Vet Rec 2002;154:420–2.

23. Diker KS, Akan M, Haziroglu R. Antimicrobial susceptibility of Pasteurella haemolytica and Pasteurella multocida isolated from pneumonic ovine lungs. Vet Rec 1994;134:597–8.

24. Gilmour NJL, Gilmour JS, Quirie M, et al. Treatment of experimental pasteurellosis in lambs with clavulanic acid and amoxicillin. Vet Rec 1990;126:311.

25. Sargison ND, Scott PR. Evaluation of antibiotic treatment of respiratory disease including suspected septicaemic pasteurellosis in 5 week-old lambs. Agri Pract 1995;16:25–8.

26. McKellar QA, Gibson FI, McCormack ZR. Pharmacokinetics and tissue disposition of danofloxacin in sheep. Biopharm Drug Dispos 1998;19:123–9.

27. Aliabadi FS, Landoni MF, Lees P. Pharmacokinetics (PK), pharmacodynamics (PD) and PK–PD integration of danofloxacin in sheep biological fluids. Antimicrob Agents Chemother 2003;47:626–35.

28. Hodgson JC, Moon GM, Quirie M, et al. Association of LPS chemotype of *Mannheimia (Pasteurella) haemolytica* A1 with disease virulence in a model of ovine pneumonic pasteurellosis. J Endotoxin Res 2003;9:25–32.

29. MacKay RJ. Endotoxemia. In: Smith BP, editor. Large animal internal medicine. 3rd edition. St Louis(MO): Mosby; 2002. p. 633–41.

30. Fthenakis GC. Field evaluation of flunixin meglumine in the supportive treatment of ovine mastitis. J Vet Pharmacol Ther 2000;28:405–7.

31. Mavrogianni VS, Alexopoulos C, Fthenakis GC. Field evaluation of flunixin meglumine in the supportive treatment of caprine mastitis. J Vet Pharmacol Ther 2004; 27:373–5.

32. Lekeux P. A therapeutic strategy for treatment of the bovine respiratory disease complex: the rationale for the combination of a nonsteroidal anti-inflammatory drug with an antibiotic. Cattle Pract 2007;15:115–9.

33. Lockwood PW, Johnson JC, Katz TL. Clinical efficacy of flunixin, carprofen and ketoprofen as adjuncts to the antibacterial treatment of bovine respiratory disease. Vet Rec 2003;152:392–4.

34. Drillich M, Voigt D, Forderung D, et al. Treatment of acute puerperal metritis with flunixin meglumine in addition to antibiotic treatment. J Dairy Sci 2007;90: 3758–63.

35. Dascanio JJ, Mechor GD, Grohn YT, et al. Effect of phenylbutazone and flunixin meglumine on acute toxic mastitis in dairy cows. Am J Vet Res 1995;56:1213–8.

36. Wagner SA, Apley MD. Effects of two anti-inflammatory drugs on physiologic variables and milk production in cows with endotoxin-induced mastitis. Am J Vet Res 2004;65:64–8.

37. Welsh EM, Nolan AM. Effect of flunixin meglumine on the thresholds to mechanical stimulation in healthy and lame sheep. Res Vet Sci 1995;58:61–6.

38. Grant C, Upton RN, Kuchel TR. Efficacy of intra-muscular analgesics for acute pain in sheep. Aust Vet J 1996;73:129–32.

39. Sargison N, Scott P. Supportive therapy of generalised endotoxaemia in cattle using hypertonic saline. In Pract 1996;18:18–9.

40. Green MJ, Green LE, Cripps PJ. Comparison of fluid and flunixin meglumine therapy in combination and individually in the treatment of toxic mastitis. Vet Rec 1997;140:149–52.

41. Goodwin-Ray KA, Stevenson MA, Heuer C. Effect of vaccinating lambs against pneumonic pasteurellosis under New Zealand field conditions on their s gain and pneumonic lung lesions at slaughter. Vet Rec 2008;162:9–11.

42. Suarez-Guemes F, Collins MT, Whiteman CE. Experimental reproduction of septicaemic pasteurellosis in feedlot lambs: bacteriological and pathological examinations. Am J Vet Res 1985;46:185–92.

43. Gilmour NJL, Quirie M, Jones GE, et al. Metaphylactic use of long-acting oxytetracycline in pasteurellosis in lambs. Vet Rec 1988;123:443–4.

44. Alley MR, Ionas G, Clarke JK. Chronic non-progressive pneumonia of sheep in New Zealand—a review of the role of *Mycoplasma ovipneumoniae*. N Z Vet J 1999;47:155–60.

45. Sheehan M, Cassidy JP, Brady J, et al. An aetiopathological study of chronic bronchopneumonia in lambs in Ireland. Vet J 2007;173:630–7.

46. Malone FE, McCullough SJ, McLoughlin MF, et al. Infectious agents in respiratory disease of housed, fattening lambs in Northern Ireland. Vet Rec 1988;122:203–7.

47. Davies DH, McCarthy AR, Penwarden RA. The effect of vaccination of lambs with live parainfluenza virus type 3 on pneumonia produced by parainfluenza virus type 3 and *Pasteurella haemolytica*. N Z Vet J 1980;28:201–2.

48. Rodger JL. Parainfluenza-3 vaccination of sheep. Vet Rec 1989;125:453–6.

49. Thonney ML, Smith MC, Mateescu RG, et al. Vaccination of ewes and lambs against parainfluenza 3 to prevent lamb pneumonia. Small Rumin Res 2008;74: 30–6.

50. Sharp JM, De Las Heras M. Contagious respiratory tumours. In: Aitken ID, editor. Diseases of sheep. 4th edition. Oxford(UK): Blackwell Publishing; 2007. p. 211–7.

51. Walsh SR, Linnerth-Petrik NM, Laporte AN, et al. Full-length genome sequence analysis of enzootic nasal tumor virus reveals an unusually high degree of genetic stability. Virus Res 2010;151:74–87.

52. Scott PR. Sheep medicine. London: Manson Publishing; 2007.

53. Barbour EK, Nabbut NH, Hamadeh SK, et al. Bacterial identity and characteristics in healthy and unhealthy respiratory tracts of sheep and calves. Vet Res Commun 1997;21:421–30.

54. Scott P. The role of ultrasonography as an adjunct to clinical examination in sheep practice. Ir Vet J 2008;61:474–80.

55. Banos PD, Pelayo PM, Gonzalez EBC, et al. Assessment of albendazole treatment against ovine lungworms in north-west Spain. Rev Vet Mex 1995;26:117–21.

56. Rehbein S, Visser M. Efficacy of ivermectin delivered via a controlled-release capsule against small lungworms (Protostrongylidae) in sheep. J Vet Med B Infect Dis Vet Public Health 2002;49:313–6.

57. Papadopoulos E, Sotiraki S, Himonas C, et al. Treatment of small lungworm infestation in sheep by using moxidectin. Vet Parasitol 2004;121:329–36.

Treatment and Control of Hoof Disorders in Sheep and Goats

Agnes C. Winter, BVSc, PhD, DSHP, MRCVS, FRAgs[a,b,*]

KEYWORDS

- Contagious ovine digital dermatitis • Footrot • Goats
- Interdigital dermatitis • Lameness • Sheep

Foot lameness in sheep and goats is a worldwide problem, leading to compromised welfare, loss of production, and consequent financial loss. The diseases that are mainly considered in this article are those caused by infections that can affect a considerable proportion of the flock or herd. These diseases are interdigital dermatitis (ID), footrot (FR), and contagious ovine digital dermatitis (CODD). Other more sporadic problems, such as white line disease and deep sepsis of the pedal joint, are also addressed briefly. In general, sheep and goats are susceptible to the same foot diseases, although CODD, a problem only seen in sheep in the United Kingdom, has not been reported in goats. Details of differential diagnosis have already been described.[1,2] The management of FR has also been reviewed[3,4] and, more recently, the effect of treating individual sheep with ID and FR on reducing overall flock prevalence has been reported.[5] Current knowledge of *Dichelobacter nodosus*, the causal agent of FR, and its implications for control and elimination strategies have also been assessed.[6]

Pain relief as part of treatment of lameness has received little attention until recently. In any case of significant lameness, administration of agents for pain relief should be considered, such as flunixin meglumine or meloxicam.

AVAILABLE METHODS AND THEIR EFFICACY IN THE TREATMENT AND CONTROL OF INTERDIGITAL DERMATITIS, FOOTROT, AND CONTAGIOUS OVINE DIGITAL DERMATITIS
Foot Trimming

Often, foot trimming is done harshly and can cause damage. Although careful minimal trimming of obviously loose horn or very overgrown or distorted feet, or to aid in diagnosis, is acceptable and often necessary, it does not prevent any of these diseases.

The author has nothing to disclose.
[a] 2Fossbridge House, Walmgate York, North Yorkshire, YO1 9SY, UK
[b] School of Veterinary Science, University of Liverpool, UK
* 2Fossbridge House, Walmgate York, North Yorkshire, YO1 9SY, UK.
E-mail address: a.winter@liverpool.ac.uk

Indeed, gathering sheep into poorly maintained or dirty handling pens may facilitate spread of the causative agents. A recent report has shown that recovery from FR took longer in sheep whose feet were trimmed in addition to being given other treatments.[7]

Vaccination

Currently, vaccination is only available to control FR, with the additional benefit that its use often causes an improvement in already infected animals. The commonly used vaccine contains 10 strains of *D nodosus*, because many sheep flocks have infections with multiple strains of this bacterium. The vaccine has also been used in goats. Local reactions to the vaccine may develop in both sheep and goats. Concerns exist about antigenic competition, and therefore monovalent vaccines have been used in countries or individual flocks in which single-strain infections have been identified.[8] After sequencing of the *D nodosus* genome, current research is aimed at improving the vaccine through identifying candidate antigens, which could protect against all strains.[9,10] Vaccination programs must be tailored to individual flocks based on high-risk periods for transmission, such as in warm wet weather or during housing. No vaccines are available to control ID or CODD, although recent work on subspecies of *Fusobacterium necrophorum* may lead to advances in control of diseases involving this organism in the future.[11]

Use of Antibiotics

Treatment of dairy goats or sheep with antibiotics usually results in periods of milk withdrawal. Because some periods can be long, this creates problems in parenteral treatment of these animals. Withdrawal periods in meat-producing animals also apply.

Injection of antibiotic, such as long-acting oxytetracycline (200 mg/mL) at 1 mL per 10 kg of body weight once, is now the preferred method of treatment of FR. A combination of procaine penicillin (200 mg/mL) and dihydrostreptomycin (250 mg/mL) given at twice the recommended dose, where licensed, has also been used successfully. Animals that fail to respond to two successive treatments are likely to remain chronically infected and should preferably be culled. Injectable antibiotics should not be used to treat ID, which is a superficial infection of the interdigital skin. The response of animals with CODD to injection of these antibiotics has been mixed. Treatment of CODD cases with tilmicosin injection (300 mg/mL) at 1 mL per 30 kg of body weight once has been successful.

Topical application of antibiotic, such as oxytetracycline as a spray, is usually successful in treating ID, provided it is not immediately washed off by wet underfoot conditions. Antibiotic spray is a useful adjunct to parenteral treatment for FR, but is not sufficient alone for established cases. Early cases of CODD have been treated successfully with repeated spray application of combined lincomycin and spectinomycin soluble powder or tylosin soluble powder made up at 1 g per 2 L in water. These products also have been used successfully as footbaths, but are expensive to use in quantity and raise the issue of safe disposal. Neither of these products is licensed for use in these ways.

Footbathing

Footbathing is a common method of treatment that has been used for many years. Footbaths and their surroundings, including a dry area for standing after treatment, must be well maintained and regularly cleaned to be effective. Dirty or poorly maintained facilities may actually damage feet, facilitating disease spread, and returning sheep to wet pasture or along muddy tracks will negate any beneficial effect.

Products commonly used for footbathing are formalin, zinc sulfate, and copper sulfate. Various proprietary products consisting of different combinations of chemicals are also available. For any particular product, the instructions for use should be followed carefully.

Formalin has been used for many years, and still is in some countries; however, it is unpleasant, an irritant for both animals and people, and is a known carcinogen. Its advantages are the low cost and the fact that animals only need to be walked through rather than stood in it; therefore, many animals can be treated rapidly and with a small cost. It should be used only at a concentration of 2% to 3%, because strong solutions can harden the horn to the point of causing cracking of the hooves if used repeatedly. Weak formalin, if available for use, may be the most practical way of treating a large number of cases of ID, but its use for treating FR or CODD must be seriously questioned on welfare grounds, because it is extremely painful when applied to open wounds.

Zinc sulfate is probably the preferred chemical to be used in footbaths for treating ID and FR. It is nonirritant but is relatively expensive and has the disadvantage that animals are required to stand in it for a time (2–20 minutes, depending on the formulation and on the severity of the cases being treated). The usual concentration is 10%, but stronger solutions can be used if desired. Stand-in time can be reduced through addition of a surfactant (detergent). In most FR control programs, footbathing once weekly for at least 3 weeks is recommended, although it may be used more frequently to achieve a faster result if desired. Anecdotal evidence suggests that variable results have been obtained from footbathing animals with CODD in zinc sulfate; it has apparently had some success in some cases, but little benefit in others.

Copper sulfate (5% solution) is effective in treating FR, but because of the susceptibility of sheep to copper toxicity, particularly European continental breeds such as the Texel, it should be used with caution.

Antibiotic footbaths are effective in treating CODD, although chronic cases may not respond to any treatment. These footbaths are also effective in treating ID and FR, but should not be used because other licensed products are available.

Culling Chronically Infected Animals

ID is an acute infection that will usually resolve in time, even if untreated, if FR is not present in the flock. For successful control of FR within a flock, culling chronically infected animals is crucial, because these act as an ongoing source of infection for other animals during transmission periods. Breeders of pedigree animals are often unwilling to cull because of the perceived value of some breeding stock, but this is counterproductive for two reasons: first, the sheep present a constant source of FR infection, and second, they are probably more genetically susceptible to infection.

In neglected cases of CODD, permanent damage to the foot may occur, with little prospect of recovery of normal form and function.[12]

Farm Biosecurity

Because ID is caused by the common environmental bacterium *F necrophorum*, quarantining incoming animals is irrelevant in preventing this condition. However, because both FR and CODD can be introduced into previously uninfected flocks/herds with extremely serious consequences, and to guard against many other infectious diseases, incoming animals should be quarantined for at least 4 weeks, carefully examined, and preferably footbathed before being mixed with resident animals. For self-contained flocks/herds, maintenance of perimeter fences is extremely important to prevent access of straying animals. Where common grazing occurs, the diseases are much more difficult to control because this requires good cooperation among all owners.

Genetic Improvement

Nothing is known about possible genetic susceptibility or resistance to CODD, and no well-documented evidence on natural resistance to ID seems to be available. However, although because ID is the precursor to infection with FR, animals that are less susceptible to FR also may be less susceptible to ID. Differences in susceptibility to FR between and within sheep breeds have been known for some time.[13] A gene test was developed in New Zealand,[14] but whether it will be effective in other countries with different breeds is unknown. More widely applicable genetic tests likely will be developed in future and will form a component of estimated breeding values for buyers of purebred stock. Whether these techniques will be applicable to goats seems to be unknown.

CONTROL OR ERADICATION?

ID cannot be eradicated because of the ubiquitous presence of the causal organism in the environment, particularly in mud and feces. Therefore, it can only be controlled by improving the environment, where possible, to reduce damage to the interdigital skin, or through providing prompt treatment for affected animals. Virtually nothing is known about the epidemiology of CODD, apart from the likely involvement of treponemes, and therefore affected animals must be treated promptly to keep the disease under control.

FR has been successfully eradicated in New South Wales, Australia[15] through a state-run program involving a combination of vaccine use, treatment, strict culling, and quarantine. This program has required huge commitment and cooperation of all sides of the industry. The existence of predictable nontransmission periods has played a large part in the success of the scheme. In the United Kingdom and other temperate countries, eradication on a country or area basis poses much greater problems, although eradication has been successful in some individual flocks. Possible ways have been proposed in which long-term control or eradication could be managed in situations such as in the United Kingdom.[6]

Clearly, there are far too many chronically lame sheep in the United Kingdom and elsewhere in the world. Making a concerted effort to reduce this number to an acceptable level will require a large commitment in terms of labor, time, and financial resources, followed by constant vigilance to prevent reversion to the current situation.

TREATMENT AND CONTROL OF OTHER IMPORTANT HOOF DISORDERS
White Line Lesions (Toe Abscess, White Line Abscess, Shelly Hoof)

White line lesions are extremely common in sheep[16] and goats, and vary from small discrete areas of discoloration of the horn of the white line to separation along much of the lateral wall of the hoof (shelly hoof). Virtually nothing is known about the possible causes, and therefore no method of prevention has been established. Although minor separations are often only of cosmetic significance, a proportion of affected animals develop acute lameness from mud or debris becoming impacted in the defect or under the loosened horn, with accompanying infection development and pus formation. After a few days, pus bursts out at the coronary band and recovery gradually occurs. In the acute stage, careful trimming along the white line in the area of the defect may release pus, or poulticing may encourage pus release. In cases uncomplicated by pus formation, careful trimming of loose horn on a regular basis is all that can be done.

Deep Sepsis of the Pedal Joint (Pedal Joint Abscess, Septic Pedal Arthritis)

Deep sepsis of the pedal joint is a sporadic but serious problem that causes great pain and, unless recognized and treated aggressively in the very early stages, leads to swelling and deformity of the affected claw, and consequently to chronic lameness. If diagnosed early, flushing of the pedal joint with sterile water or saline twice daily, together with administration of a broad-spectrum antibiotic and pain relief, can be successful. Access to the pedal joint can be gained by inserting a cannula either through a discharging sinus or by drilling into the joint from the lateral hoof wall. This technique should be performed under intravenous regional anesthesia. Cases with a longer duration have irreversible changes to the pedal bone and joint, with amputation of the affected digit the only solution.

Apart from trying to provide underfoot conditions that do not damage the interdigital space, there is no method of preventing this condition.

Toe Granuloma

Toe granuloma is the development of a strawberry-like piece of granulation tissue, usually at the toe, but occasionally in the sole of the hoof. Most are the result of unskilled overtrimming of the hoof, causing bleeding, but some follow accidental penetration of the sole with a sharp object or may be found in chronic FR cases. Treatment consists of removing the granulation tissue with a sharp knife followed by pressure bandaging or cauterization, or encouraging gradual cornification through careful application of a drying agent such as copper sulfate crystals.

The most important aspect of treatment is to prevent disease formation through controlling footrot and educating people who trim feet to do this much more sparingly.

SUMMARY

Lame sheep experience pain and should be treated as soon as reasonably practical. Treatment and control should be based on a firm diagnosis, and farmers should be encouraged to seek veterinary attention for animals that do not respond quickly to administered treatment. Overall flock lameness should be minimized through implementing appropriate control measures for the common types of foot lameness caused by infectious agents, including vaccination, antibiotic treatment, footbathing, biosecurity, and culling.

REFERENCES

1. Winter A. Lameness in sheep: 1 diagnosis. In Pract 2004;26:58–63.
2. Hodgkinson O. The importance of feet examination in sheep health management. Small Rumin Res 2010;92:67–71.
3. Abbott KA, Lewis CJ. Current approaches to the management of ovine footrot. Vet J 2005;169:28–41.
4. Winter AC. Footrot control and eradication (elimination) strategies. Small Rumin Res 2009;85:90–3.
5. Green LE, Wassink GJ, Grogono-Thomas R, et al. Looking after the individual to reduce disease in the flock: a binomial mixed effects model investigating the impact of individual sheep management of footrot and interdigital dermatitis in a prospective longitudinal study on one farm. Prev Vet Med 2007;78:172–8.
6. Green LE, George TR. Assessment of current knowledge of footrot in sheep with particular reference to Dichelobacter nodosus and implications for elimination or control strategies for sheep in Great Britain. Vet J 2008;175:173–80.
7. Kaler J, Daniels SL, Wright JL, et al. Randomised clinical trial of long-acting oxytetracycline, foot trimming and flunixin meglumine on time to recovery of sheep with footrot. J Vet Intern Med 2010;24:420–5.

8. Egerton JR, Ghimire SC, Dhungyel OP, et al. Eradication of virulent footrot from sheep and goats in an endemic area of Nepal and an evaluation of specific vaccination. Vet Rec 2002;151:290–5.

9. Myers GS, Parker D, Al-Hasani K, et al. Genome sequence and identification of candidate vaccine antigens from the animal pathogen Dichelobacter nodosus. Nat Biotechnol 2007;25:569–75.

10. Ennen S, Hamann H, Distl O, et al. A field trial to control ovine footrot via vaccination and genetic markers. Small Rumin Res 2009;86:22–5.

11. Zhou H, Bennett G, Hickford JG. Variation in Fusobacterium necrophorum strains present on the hooves of footrot infected sheep, goats and cattle. Vet Microbiol 2009;135:363–7.

12. Scott P. Chronic contagious ovine digital dermatitis-like lesions in a Scottish flock. Livestock 2010;15:32–5.

13. Emery DL, Stewart DJ, Clark BL. The comparative susceptibility of five breeds of sheep to footrot. Aust Vet J 1984;61:85–8.

14. Bishop SC, Morris CA. Genetics of disease resistance in sheep and goats. Small Rumin Res 2007;70:48–59.

15. Egerton JR, Seaman JT, Walker RI. Eradication of footrot from New South Wales. In: Proceedings of 13th international symposium and 5th conference on lameness in Ruminants. Maribor (Slovenia); 2004.

16. Winter AC, Arsenos G. Diagnosis of white line lesions sheep. In Pract 2009;31:17–21.

Control of Caseous Lymphadenitis

Peter A. Windsor, DVSc, PhD, GradCertEdStud

KEYWORDS

- Caseous lymphadenitis • Cheesy gland • Chronic abscess
- Goat • Sheep • CLA • Vaccination

Corynebacterium pseudotuberculosis may infect numerous mammalian species, the most significant being farmed small ruminants, which develop chronic caseous lymphadenitis (CLA). CLA was first identified in 1888. It is characterized by abscess formation in the lymph nodes, lungs, and other visceral organs[1] and occurs in most sheep farming countries, presumably spread globally by sheep exported by the eighteenth-century colonialists.[2] Merino sheep from Spain exported first to South America and then Australia and North America, with more recent export from Australia to countries in the Middle East, are possibly the most responsible for this spread.[3] CLA emerged recently in the United Kingdom and is becoming endemic because it is regulated only in Northern Ireland.[2]

The prevalence of CLA is considered high in many countries, but detailed research on prevalence rates, farm practices, and abattoir findings is limited to Australian wool sheep; surveys in 1995 identified that cheesy gland was extremely widespread and present on 97% of farms in New South Wales (NSW), 91% in Victoria, and 88% in Western Australia (WA).[4] However, the average prevalence of CLA in the adult sheep population has been declining and was found in WA to be 58% in 1973 and 53% in 1984, after the introduction of a CLA vaccine in 1983. In 1995, abattoir and postal surveys of farmers estimated the average prevalence of CLA in adult sheep at 26%, varying from 20% in WA to 29% in NSW.[4] Routine abattoir surveillance was introduced in 2006 to monitor the prevalence of ovine paratuberculosis (OPTB) and has also provided current insights into CLA prevalence, with 17% of 3608 consignments of sheep to NSW abattoirs in that year having sheep with CLA and 1.3% of all sheep found with CLA lesions. Because consignments can include sheep from different farms, this rate does not translate directly to the prevalence of the properties affected.

Significant economic losses to the Australian sheep industry because of CLA have been recognized through long-term ill thrift, costs of carcass inspection and condemnations, and reduced wool yields and have been estimated in 1991–1992 at A$30

The author has nothing to disclose.
Farm Animal and Veterinary Public Health Group, Faculty of Veterinary Science, University of Sydney, 425 Werombi Road, Camden, New South Wales 2570, Australia
E-mail address: peter.windsor@sydney.edu.au

million to A$40 million (US $29,630–$39,500). In addition, the presence of CLA lesions in exported live sheep and nil tolerance for sheep carcasses affected with CLA lesions exported from Australia are of concern to the reputation of Australian sheep meat products.

Control of CLA depends on vaccination in most countries, with the notable exception of the United Kingdom. However, the disease has persisted even after prolonged vaccination, indicating the suppressive nature of CLA vaccination. A 1990 study in Australia concluded that with only 10% to 15% of sheep producers using the recommended CLA vaccination program, persistence of the infection is not surprising.[5–7] Because these data are now 15 years old and the current abattoir data suggest further decline in CLA prevalence, it is appropriate to revisit the current vaccination practices on-farm. Furthermore, the emergence of OPTB in Australia has led to a renewed interest in CLA control. The owners of many OPTB-infected flocks suffering significant mortalities observed that Gudair vaccination for OPTB rapidly resolved the losses, leading to efforts to use other best practice animal health strategies. Most owners also observed that the injection lesions in a substantial number of sheep after Gudair vaccination for OPTB closely resemble CLA lesions.[8] Furthermore, the recent occurrence of false-positive reactors to OPTB on serologic tests in a consignment of goats for export was attributed to a serologic cross-reaction to CLA vaccination, confirming the importance of the knowledge of CLA control procedures when preparing animals for export. For these reasons, it is timely that research on CLA prevalence and vaccine usage would recommence and that the current control options for management of CLA would be reviewed.

LESIONS AND TRANSMISSION

The lymph nodes of CLA-affected animals are enlarged, frequently between 5 and 15 cm in diameter. In Australia, the prefemoral, prescapular, mediastinal, and bronchial nodes are mostly affected (**Fig. 1**). In North America, external abscesses are most commonly found in the parotid and submandibular regions of the head[6]; this infection may spread because of transmission by feeders in the confinement housing. The infectious organism can survive for several weeks in feces and on fomites, as well as at least 2 hours in sheep dips (dips contaminated by open skin or bronchial abscesses are

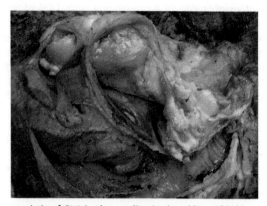

Fig. 1. Lesions characteristic of CLA in the mediastinal and bronchial lymph nodes of a sheep at necropsy; erosion of the capsule of the lesion allowing pus into the bronchioles is considered a major source of transmission.

a potential source of infection). Sheep with lung lesions (see **Fig. 1**) are considered the main source of new infections because, when infected sheep with no externally discharging CLA abscesses are penned together with recently shorn uninfected sheep, infection is readily transmitted.[7] Lung abscesses examined at necropsy frequently have fistulae, and infectious organisms have been isolated from the tracheas of the infected sheep. When *C pseudotuberculosis* is applied to skin wounds or to intact, recently shorn, or nonwool skin, CLA lesions develop in the skin and spread through the lymphatic drainage or bloodstream, causing lesions in the peripheral lymph nodes, lungs, and other viscera, followed by elimination or containment of infection.[8]

The prevalence of CLA infection is very low in sheep up to 1 year of age but increases dramatically after shearing, presumably because of close contact between susceptible fleece-free sheep and sheep with lung lesions excreting organisms. Because the prevalence of CLA in adult sheep varies between flocks from approximately 0% to more than 90%, the risk factors for a high incidence of CLA include[8] a high seroprevalence among animals, indicating high challenge; a high prevalence of lesions in aged ewes, also indicating high challenge; the use of a dip (shower dipping significantly increased the risk of having a high CLA incidence); and time under cover after shearing. When sheep were held together for more than 1 hour after shearing, there was a 3-fold increase in the risk of being in the high-incidence group compared with when sheep were held for less than 1 hour. The number of shearing cuts was not a risk factor, possibly because even the lowest frequency of shearing cuts did not limit the incidence of infection.

After entry into the host through the skin, *C pseudotuberculosis* migrates within the phagocytes to the local lymph node,[1] where there is a short period of inflammation.[2] Microabscesses develop within the cortical region of the node within 24 hours of inoculation; after approximately 6 days, they coalesce and enlarge to form more significant lesions, containing clumps of bacteria, cellular debris, and a high proportion of eosinophils (turning the purulent material green). Lesions expand progressively through repeated cycles of necrosis and encapsulation (depending on the location of the node, because subcutaneous nodes may rupture and discharge the contents). Abscess content is initially soft and becomes increasingly solid as inspissation progresses; then, mineralization commences, and concentric capsular layers are formed (the so-called onion ring lesion).

PATHOGENESIS

The pathogenicity of *C pseudotuberculosis* involves the exotoxin phospholipase D (PLD) and a mycolic acid surface lipid, although other virulence factors have been proposed.[2] PLD causes dermal necrosis with inflammation, necrosis, and increased vascular permeability, promoting invasiveness of the organism and transport to the regional lymph nodes through phagocytes, which they ultimately destroy. The surface lipid may provide the organism with resistance to antibacterial activity of the phagocytes. The inflammatory response may prevent infection from progressing beyond the cutaneous lesion, but in most challenged sheep, local lymphadenitis occurs followed by suppuration and destruction of the lymph node; resolution from this stage is unusual. Extension from mediastinal and bronchial lymphadenitis may lead to lung abscesses or multifocal to locally extensive caseopurulent bronchopneumonia and pleuritis with adhesions. Lung infection presumably originates from the hematogenous spread of the organisms and local extension rather than by inhalation, because most early lung lesions have no obvious connection to the air passages and 15% to 20% of the affected sheep have lesions only in the lungs.

CLA of the inguinal and scrotal lymph nodes of rams can be a frequent finding on palpation of rams for breeding soundness.[9] However, these lesions are not connected to the testes or epididymis and usually occur in the tunica adjacent to the spermatic cord in the dorsal scrotum; thus, the semen quality is normal, and the organism is not excreted in the semen. However, if the abscess is large, the heat of inflammation can reduce the semen quality, which improves after the abscess is lanced and has healed.

DIAGNOSIS AND CLA CONTROL BY TEST AND CULL

CLA is usually diagnosed clinically only if infection of the cutaneous lymph nodes progresses to fistulation or, more rarely, visceral organ involvement leads to emaciation (the so-called thin ewe syndrome). Although CLA lesions are characteristic (see **Fig. 1**), the differential diagnosis of clinical cases includes infections by *Actinobacillus*, *Arcanobacterium*, and staphylococcal species as well as OPTB vaccine injection abscesses; hence, bacterial culture to identify *C pseudotuberculosis* from the lesions confirms a diagnosis.[2,10] In Australia and New Zealand, the widespread use of Gudair vaccination for OPTB since 2002 has resulted in sheep presenting clinically and at slaughter (in 0.5% of 3608 consignments to abattoirs) with lesions resembling CLA, but these lesions are really attributable to oil granulomata induced by the oil adjuvant in this vaccine.[8] Palpation of the contents to identify the oil in these lesions assists the diagnosis (**Fig. 2**).

In countries where CLA vaccination is not available (eg, the United Kingdom), control of the disease may require identification of the infected animals to prevent their contact with the uninfected ones, which usually means that serologic testing is required to detect humoral responses to PLD exotoxin, enabling the culling of sero-positive animals.[2] Serologic tests developed for CLA include antihemolysin inhibition,[2] tube agglutination,[11] indirect hemagglutination,[12] double immunodiffusion,[13] and enzyme-linked immunosorbent assays (ELISAs).[14] Initially, CLA-diagnostic ELISAs consisted of crude *C pseudotuberculosis* cell wall preparations or supernate-derived exotoxin as antigen[2] with high sensitivity but poor specificity. More recently, ELISAs based on PLD exotoxin purified from the supernate of *C pseudotuberculosis* culture and polyclonal rabbit anti-PLD serum used as a capture antibody have been reported to have a specificity of 99% $\pm$ 1% and a sensitivity of 79% $\pm$ 5% in sheep. Although

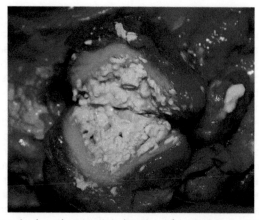

Fig. 2. Oil granuloma in the atlantooccipital region after Gudair vaccination for OPTB.

false-negative results remain an issue for ELISAs, perhaps partly because of samples obtained from animals that have been exposed but subsequently have eliminated the infection, this procedure has contributed to the successful eradication of the disease in several flocks.[15,16] Detection of cell-mediated immunity in CLA by whole blood interferon-γ (IFN-γ) enzyme immunoassay (Bovigam; Pfizer, Parkville, Victoria, Australia) was validated in Canada, and with a sensitivity of 91% and specificity of 98%, it was considered a promising tool for the correct diagnosis of CLA.[17] Moreover, a polymerase chain reaction (PCR) assay using a pair of primers specific to C pseudo-tuberculosis has been used to confirm the phenotypic identification of CLA isolates from sheep and goats at slaughter.[18] With a PCR-positive product on 93 of the 96 suspicious isolates from which DNA was extracted, the specificity and speed of this assay may provide a useful alternative to serologic examination.

CONTROL AND MANAGEMENT BY VACCINATION

The history of the considerable research in South Africa and Australia in the past 75 years exploring the potential of vaccination to prevent CLA and leading to the introduction of commercially available toxoid vaccines has been reviewed later, as have the other approaches used for vaccine development.[2] A brief summary is provided.

Available Vaccines

Bacterin vaccines
A vaccine consisting of formalin-killed whole cells of C pseudotuberculosis was shown to protect sheep against the lethal effects of a subacute infection but not against the formation of the lesions of a chronic infection.[19] A field trial of a formalin-killed whole-cell vaccine in sheep and goats was shown to significantly decrease the incidence of CLA in the sheep, with the suggestion of a similar effect in goats.[6] More recently, a study investigating the immunization of sheep with a formalin-killed virulent C pseudotuberculosis isolate and aluminum hydroxide adjuvant resulted in a statistically significant protection against the homologous challenge, preventing the spread of infection beyond the site of inoculation.[6]

Toxoid vaccines
After the observation that an undefined protoplasmic toxin of C pseudotuberculosis played a role in the induction of protective immunity, administration of the toxoid followed by toxin reduced the extent of experimental CLA in sheep.[20] It was later demonstrated that PLD exotoxin could be used as a protective antigen.[21] An effective toxoid vaccine was provided to the Commonwealth Serum Laboratories (Australia) in 1978, and an optimal antigen dose and combination with clostridial components led to the release of Glanvac[22–24] in 1984. The capacity of a highly purified recombinant derivative of PLD to protect sheep against the homologous challenge with C pseudotuberculosis isolate was also examined, with protection similar to that produced by a bacterin vaccine[6] and leading to the introduction of Glanvac-3; this vaccine protects against the challenge, with decreased numbers of infected loci, suggesting superiority in preventing the spread of infection beyond the site of inoculation and into the superficial lymph nodes compared with Glanvac vaccine.[2]

Combined vaccines
The ability of an alhydrogel-adjuvant vaccine composed of formalin-killed whole C pseudotuberculosis cells enriched with formalin-treated PLD-rich culture supernate to completely protect against experimental C pseudotuberculosis infection suggested that full protection requires the presence of both components.[25] However, during the

development of Glanvac, it was claimed that supplementation of cell-free toxoid vaccine with *C pseudotuberculosis* cells made no difference to the observed protection.[24] Regardless, the commercial CLA vaccine Caseous D-T, containing clostridial toxoids and a combination of *C pseudotuberculosis* bacterin and toxoid, was developed. The product was shown to protect sheep against experimental infection, with reduced incidence of external and internal CLA lesions.[26]

Live vaccines

Because sheep infected experimentally with *C pseudotuberculosis* were found to be protected against further challenge, despite being unable to cure the original infection, possibilities of live attenuated vaccines were proposed.[27] Investigations of sheep immunized with live recombinant vaccine with inactivated *pld* gene (the so-called Toxminus PLD-deficient *C pseudotuberculosis* mutant) and challenged with the wild-type *C pseudotuberculosis* demonstrated protection and strong humoral and cellular immune responses.[28] Concerns that the Toxminus mutant was flawed as one of the major immunodominant antigens (PLD) that have been dispersed led to the oral challenge experiments with the Toxminus mutant carrying inactivated *pld*, demonstrating a rapid amnestic response to PLD but failure to stimulate a significant helper T cell 1 immune response by this route.[20,22,25] Other attempts to create live vaccine vectors against CLA have been less successful, with attenuated strains of the organism showing potential in mice but unsuccessful in the protection of sheep, presumably because of the failure to stimulate specific IFN-γ–secreting lymphocytes and induction of low concentrations of anti–*C pseudotuberculosis* immunoglobulin G.[29]

DNA vaccines

DNA vaccines have been less successful in the immunization of livestock than conventional vaccines against CLA, with weak and short-lived immune responses after challenge and antibody concentrations not significantly higher than those in nonvaccinated animals.[30,31]

Vaccination Strategies and Use in Australia

Glanvac is now available exclusively or in combination with clostridial antigens in Australia (marketed as "6 in 1" with 5 clostridial antigens), but field trials have shown that protection varies from 25% to 90%. Vaccinating a previously unvaccinated, but infected, flock with high challenge means that many sheep become infected, but a reduced number of sheep develop lung abscesses. As older sheep are culled, the challenge of infection decreases over time, fewer sheep have lung abscesses, and continuation of vaccination means that few sheep will be infected. However, it is important that the vaccination program consists of 2 administrations (at least 1 month apart) of the vaccine initially; an annual booster several weeks before lambing or shearing should be administered thereafter. Maternal antibody does interfere with the immune response of lambs; hence, in flocks with a high prevalence of CLA, vaccinating lambs younger than 10 weeks may not produce a strong protection as afforded by later vaccination. However, in commercial flocks, it is practical to administer the initial vaccine 6 to 8 weeks after start of the lambing season, with the second dose administered 4 to 5 weeks later. Protection of lambs younger than 10 weeks is probably satisfactory, if the lambs are not at high risk of exposure to CLA and receive the second dose as indicated.

The use of a vaccine and the prevalence of the disease in sheep flocks were studied in the 1990s[4,29] and were found to vary greatly, with the vaccine efficacy dependent on the vaccination program used. This work led to the development of vaccination extension programs for the sheep industry in 1996 (**Tables 1** and **2**). Only vaccination programs that followed the manufacturer's recommendations of 2 administrations in lambs followed by annual booster vaccinations led to an average prevalence of CLA of 3% compared with 29% in flocks not given any CLA vaccination.[4,5] Use of the non-recommended vaccination program, for example, with sheep given only 1 dose as lambs followed by annual booster vaccinations, led to an average CLA prevalence of 33%. This study also investigated producer's knowledge and beliefs about why producers do not use CLA vaccines and the information that sheep producers consider most likely to persuade them to adopt effective CLA vaccination (see **Table 2**). The effectiveness of this extension program is unknown, with research now commenced to determine whether these attitudes remain or whether sheep producers have become more diligent in their use of vaccination for sheep.

ENVIRONMENTAL CONTROL

Proper vaccination reduces disease and thus the pathogen load in the environment of ruptured abscesses. There are also other means to reduce this pathogen load, although they may not be practical for all farms. For producers with smaller flocks and suitable handling facilities, sheep with abscesses can be identified by routine palpation of the superficial lymph nodes and then quarantined. When ripe, the abscesses should be lanced and cleaned with a strong iodine solution or aqueous chlorhexidine. These sheep should remain in quarantine until the abscess has healed. The quarantine facilities used for sheep with active abscesses should not share feeders or watering places with unaffected animals. The facility should not be used for other sheep at other times, unless thoroughly cleaned and disinfected. Sheep that have repeated abscesses should be culled.

Feeders may be an important source of fomite transmission of *C pseudotuberculosis* because the bacteria can survive for weeks to months on some surfaces. Feeders designed in such a way that sheep do not put their heads through to eat are preferred as of lower risk, because the abscess material is less likely to contaminate the feeder or feed. Shearing equipment and supplies should be routinely cleaned and disinfected before use, particularly if used previously on a flock with CLA. These supplies may include fresh clothing, wool bags, and footwear, if the shearer has worked at other farms without proper biosecurity precautions. If owners of the flocks cured of the disease do not have their own shearing equipment, it is advised that they

| Table 1 | |
| Average prevalence of CLA in flocks using different vaccination programs | |
Vaccination Program Applied	Average Prevalence of CLA (%)
Sheep not vaccinated at all	29
Sheep given only 1 dose as lambs, without annual boosters	31
Sheep given 2 doses as lambs, without annual boosters	22
Sheep given only 1 dose as lambs, with annual boosters	33
Complete scheme: sheep given 2 doses as lambs, with annual boosters	3

Data from Paton MW, Walker SB, Rose IR, et al. Prevalence of caseous lymphadenitis and usage of caseous lymphadenitis vaccines in sheep flocks. Aust Vet J 2003;81:91–5; and Walker B. Cheesy gland caseous lymphadenitis in sheep. Sydney (Australia): NSW Department of Primary Industries; 1996. AgFact A3.9.21.

Table 2	
Reasons why Australian farmers do not vaccinate sheep against CLA	
Reason Provided	**Proportion of Farmers Claiming the Reason for Not Vaccinating (%)**
Never seen the disease in this class of sheep	17
Seen the disease, but do not believe that it causes significant loss	13
Extra cost of CLA component in the vaccine	9
Already using a vaccine for cattle	5
Prevalence of the disease is known to be small from abattoir data	1

Data from Paton MW, Walker SB, Rose IR, et al. Prevalence of caseous lymphadenitis and usage of caseous lymphadenitis vaccines in sheep flocks. Aust Vet J 2003;81:91–5; and Walker B. Cheesy gland caseous lymphadenitis in sheep. Sydney (Australia): NSW Department of Primary Industries; 1996. AgFact A3.9.21.

purchase their own equipment to protect the status of the flock. The goal of all these measures is to reduce environmental sources of infection with the bacteria.

SUMMARY

CLA is a significant cause of economic loss to the global sheep industries. It is difficult to control, particularly in countries where the disease has emerged recently and registered vaccines are unavailable. In Australia, Glanvac vaccination for CLA, mainly in combination with clostridial antigens, has been available for more than 25 years. With studies in the mid-1990s identifying up to 90% of producers failing to comply with the manufacturer's recommendations for vaccine use, extension programs to improve vaccination practices were developed. Management practices addressing the risk factors for transmission, including isolating young recently shorn sheep from older animals, shearing of young sheep first, reducing the time during which sheep are held together under cover off-shears, and minimizing the use of dips for ectoparasites, were also advised, because, although untested, these practices seemed likely to contribute to a decrease in the risk of CLA's causal agent transmission. There seems to be a significant decline in CLA prevalence since the introduction of vaccination, with recent abattoir surveillance identifying 1.3% of sheep and 17% of consignments positive for CLA at slaughter in NSW in 2006. However, many flocks probably remain infected, and current information on vaccination practices is needed to assess the effectiveness of CLA extension programs. Although enhanced diagnostics and new approaches to vaccination have been studied, whether these offer truly superior CLA preventive management options is debatable. The current problem with CLA control may be the inefficient application of a useful but imperfect vaccine rather than the deficiencies in the toxoid vaccine. Addressing CLA as a global economic and welfare problem for sheep producers and their industries requires evolution of best practice extension programs that ensure more efficient application of the available vaccines.

ACKNOWLEDGMENTS

Contributions from R. Barnett, R. Bush, B. Walker, A. Morton, L. Citer, and I. Links are gratefully acknowledged.

REFERENCES

1. Fontaine MC, Baird GJ. Caseous lymphadenitis. Small Rumin Res 2008;76:42–8.
2. Baird GJ, Fontaine MC. *Corynebacterium pseudotuberculosis* and its role in ovine caseous lymphadenitis. J Comp Pathol 2007;137:179–210.
3. Robins R. Focus on caseous lymphadenitis. State Vet J 1991;1:7–10.
4. Paton MW, Walker SB, Rose IR, et al. Prevalence of caseous lymphadenitis and usage of caseous lymphadenitis vaccines in sheep flocks. Aust Vet J 2003;81:91–5.
5. Walker B. Cheesy gland caseous lymphadenitis in sheep. Sydney (Australia): NSW Department of Primary Industries; 1996. AgFact A3.9.21.
6. Menzies PI, Muckle CA, Brogden KA, et al. A field trial to evaluate a whole cell vaccine for the prevention of caseous lymphadenitis in sheep and goat flocks. Can J Vet Res 1991;55:362–6.
7. Walker B. Vaccination programs for sheep. Sydney (Australia): NSW Department of Primary Industries; 1995. AgFact A3.9.47.
8. Windsor PA, Eppleston J. Lesions in sheep following administration of a vaccine of a Freund's complete adjuvant nature used in the control of ovine paratuberculosis. N Z Vet J 2006;54:237–41.
9. Gouletsou PG, Fthenakis GC. Clinical evaluation of reproductive ability of rams. Small Rumin Res 2010;92:45–51.
10. Malone F. Current and emerging flock health concerns. In: Proceedings of Meetings of the British Society of Animal Science. Antrim (Northern Ireland): Greenmount College, Co; 2005. Available at: http://www.afbini.gov.uk/adds-sheeppasteure llosisdec05.pdf. Accessed October 29, 2010.
11. Cameron C, Minnaar JL, Engelbrecht MM, et al. Immune response of merino sheep to inactivated *Corynebacterium pseudotuberculosis* vaccine. Onderstepoort J Vet Res 1972;39:11–24.
12. Shigidi M. An indirect haemagglutination test for the sero-diagnosis of *Corynebacterium ovis* infection in sheep. Res Vet Sci 1978;24:57–60.
13. Burrell D. A simplified double immunodiffusion technique for detection of *Corynebacterium ovis* antitoxin. Res Vet Sci 1980;28:234–7.
14. Schreuder B, Ter Laak E, Dercksen D. Eradication of caseous lymphadenitis in sheep with the help of a newly developed ELISA technique. Vet Rec 1994;135:174–6.
15. Dercksen DP, Brinkhof JMA, Dekker-Nooren T, et al. A comparison of four serological tests for the diagnosis of caseous lymphadenitis in sheep and goats. Vet Microbiol 2000;75:167–75.
16. Baird GJ. Current perspectives on caseous lymphadenitis. In Pract 2003;25: 62–8.
17. Sunil V, Menzies PI, Shewen PE, et al. Performance of a whole blood interferon-gamma assay for detection and eradication of caseous lymphadenitis in sheep. Vet Microbiol 2008;128:288–97.
18. Cetinkaya B, Karahan M, Atil E, et al. Identification of *Corynebacterium pseudotuberculosis* isolated from sheep and goats by PCR. Vet Microbiol 2002;88: 75–83.
19. Cameron CM. Immunity to *Corynebacterium pseudotuberculosis*. J S Afr Vet Assoc 1972;43:343–9.
20. Fontaine MC, Baird G, Connor KM, et al. Vaccination confers significant protection of sheep against infection with a virulent United Kingdom strain of *Corynebacterium pseudotuberculosis*. Vaccine 2006;24:5986–96.
21. Jolly RD. The pathogenic action of exotoxin of *Corynebacterium ovis*. J Comp Pathol 1965;75:417–31.

22. Cameron C, Smit M. Relationship of *Corynebacterium pseudotuberculosis* protoplasmic toxins to the exotoxin. Onderstepoort J Vet Res 1970;37:97–103.
23. Eggleton DW, Doidge CV, Middleton HD, et al. Immunisation against ovine caseous lymphadenitis: efficacy of the monocomponent *Corynebacterium pseudotuberculosis* toxoid vaccine and combined clostridial-corynebacterial vaccines. Aust Vet J 1991;68:320–1.
24. Eggleton DW, Middleton HD, Doidge CV, et al. Immunisation against ovine caseous lymphadenitis: comparison of *Corynebacterium pseudotuberculosis* vaccines with and without bacterial cells. Aust Vet J 1991;68:317–9.
25. Eggleton DW, Haynes JA, Middleton HD, et al. Immunisation against ovine caseous lymphadenitis: correlation between *Corynebacterium pseudotuberculosis* toxoid content and protective efficacy in combined clostridial-corynebacterial vaccines. Aust Vet J 1991;68:322–5.
26. Burrell D. Caseous lymphadenitis vaccine. N S W Vet Proc 1983;19:53–7.
27. Piontkowski MD, Shivvers DW. Evaluation of a commercially available vaccine against *Corynebacterium pseudotuberculosis* for use in sheep. J Am Vet Med Assoc 1998;212:1765–8.
28. Pepin M, Pardon P, Marly J, et al. Acquired immunity after primary caseous lymphadenitis in sheep. Am J Vet Res 1993;54:873–7.
29. Hodgson AL, Tachedjian M, Corner LA, et al. Protection of sheep against caseous lymphadenitis by use of a single oral dose of live recombinant *Corynebacterium pseudotuberculosis*. Infect Immun 1994;62:5275–80.
30. Simmons CP, Dunstan SJ, Tachedjian M, et al. Vaccine potential of attenuated mutants of *Corynebacterium pseudotuberculosis* in sheep. Infect Immun 1998; 66:474–9.
31. De Rose R, Tennent J, McWaters P, et al. Efficacy of DNA vaccination by different routes of immunisation in sheep. Vet Immunol Immunopathol 2002;90:55–63.

Treatment and Control of Ectoparasites in Sheep

John W. Plant, BVSc[a],*, Christopher J. Lewis, BVetMed, DSHP, MRCVS[b]

KEYWORDS

- Blowfly • Control • Ectoparasites • Lice • Scab
- Sheep • Treatment

Ectoparasites are a major concern in sheep flocks, wherever sheep are kept. Techniques to control and eradicate lice, ked, or scab have been available since the beginning of the 20th century, but the parasites still exist. Sheep scab (*Psoroptes ovis*) was eradicated from Australia in the late 1800s, before many of the more effective chemicals were available, and sheep ked is believed to also have been eradicated. Sheep scab has also been eradicated from North America.

In Australia, annual dipping has failed to eradicate sheep lice from many flocks. Similarly, in Britain, annual or biannual dipping has failed to eradicate sheep scab. Surveys in Australia have shown that these failures are from either incorrect application of insecticides or use of ineffective chemicals because of insecticide resistance.[1,2] In some flocks, management factors were incriminated with failure to ensure complete musters or inadequate biosecurity with poor fences, or introduction of infestations.

In most countries, the major cost of ectoparasitic treatments is the cost of chemicals and their application to treat or control infestations. Infested flocks also have significant production losses in meat, wool, or milk production, plus an adverse effect on wool quality, and on fertility and lamb growth rates. A survey of sheep producers estimated that the total costs to sheep producers in New South Wales, because of external parasitic diseases in 1990 and 1991, was approximately AUD 220 million.[1] This cost included the direct losses through mortalities and the loss of production, the costs involved in preventive and strategic treatments, and the effect on product price in the markets.

Because of environmental concerns and insecticide resistance, fewer chemicals are currently available to control or eradicate these parasites. Increasing restrictions are

The authors have nothing to disclose.
[a] 1/54-56 Barclay Road, North Rocks, New South Wales 2151, Australia
[b] Sheep Veterinary Services, Fields Farm, Green Lane, Audlem, Cheshire, CW3 0ES, UK
* Corresponding author.
E-mail address: sheep.vet@bigpond.com

also being placed on the timing and treatments available. The sheep industry is also being put on notice to pay more attention to the welfare and environmental issues associated with ectoparasite treatments used for control and eradication.

THE MAJOR SHEEP ECTOPARASITIC INFESTATIONS
Sheep Blowfly Infestation

In Australia and New Zealand, *Lucilia cuprina* and *L sericata* are the major sheep blow-flies, responsible for more than 90% of the flystrike affecting the body and breech regions. Other flies include *Calliphora* spp and *Chrysomya rufifacies*. *L sericata* also causes problems in the United Kingdom, United States, and Canada. Estimates of annual mortality from flystrike range from 0.1% to 1% of sheep. These low mortalities are a result of the control measures that are applied to flocks in normal seasons.

The major predisposing cause of body strike is the odor and moisture associated with bacterial skin infections, caused by either *Pseudomonas* spp (fleece rot) or *Dermatophilus congolensis* (lumpy wool). Breech strike results from urine staining of the wool or from scouring, usually caused by internal parasites. Poll strike in rams is often associated with the exudates from wounds associated with fighting.

Head Fly (Hydrotea irritans) Infestation

Head fly infestations occur mainly in sheep in the United Kingdom. These cause lesions at the skin–horn junction in young sheep and in wounds associated with fighting in rams.

Sheep Ked (Melophagus ovis) Infestation

Sheep keds spend their entire life cycle on the sheep, although the adult keds can survive for a few days off the animals. The female keds attach pupae to the wool some distance from the skin. These hatch 20 to 22 days later, often when chemical residues remaining after dipping were too low to kill the emerging larvae. They were a problem in many flocks until the advent of the organochlorine and organophosphate insecticides. With these insecticides, sufficient chemical remained in the wool to kill the larvae when they emerged, or adult ked that had been in the environment. Ked infestations have not been seen in sheep in Australia for some years, and therefore the disease may have been eradicated. However, in countries with limited access to persistent chemicals (eg, United States and Canada), keds continue to be a problem, causing pruritus, wool loss and damage to hides. In the United Kingdom, particularly in Wales, keds are making a comeback as the use of organophosphates decreases.

Sheep Lice (Bovicola ovis) Infestation

In Australian flocks, the loss in production from lice-infested sheep varies according to the value of the infested fleece. Sheep that are showing signs of rubbing and biting experience a reduction in fleece value of approximately 40%, which includes lower clean fleece weight and lower yield and discounts at sale, because of cotting and color. Lice usually can only live off the sheep for 1 to 2 days. Despite this and the fact that, in many countries, sheep flocks are subjected to annual or biannual dipping and other insecticide applications, lice are still a problem in many flocks throughout the world. Owners blame neighbors or new sheep as the main reason for lice infestations in their flocks. However, investigations in Australia have shown that the main reason for infestations is the failure to eradicate the resident lice populations in the flock[2] because of the ineffective application of proper chemicals to the skin of the sheep. Not all lice are killed during treatment, and once the chemicals in the wool break down, the lice numbers increase.

Foot Lice (Linognathus pedalis) Infestation

Foot lice are found on the hairy areas of the legs. Affected sheep usually do not show clinical signs. This lice population has appeared in some flocks when the backline applications replaced wet dipping and the insecticide did not reach the affected areas.

Face Lice (Linognathus ovillus) Infestation

Face lice occur at the skin–wool junction on the face and surrounding wool areas. They also appeared in some flocks in which wet dipping was no longer practiced.

Psoroptic Mange ("Sheep Scab")

Psoroptic mange is essentially an acute or chronic allergic skin dermatitis caused by the nonburrowing mite P ovis. The mite is only just visible to the naked eye, with females measuring approximately 1 mm in length. In most cases, transmission occurs among sheep through contact. However, because the mite can remain viable off the sheep for up to 16 days, infestation can be acquired from rubbing on infested posts, fences, and contaminated transporters.[3] Despite compulsory annual and biannual dipping for many years, the disease has not been eradicated from flocks in the United Kingdom.

Itch Mite (Psorergates ovis) Infestation

The itch mite lives in or on the stratum corneum of the skin. Surveys have shown that it was widespread in Australian sheep flocks. This parasite did not cause fleece derangement in many sheep in the flock, unless the sheep were under nutritional stress. P ovis is not considered to be a problem in most flocks. Synthetic pyrethroids are not effective against the parasite, but macrocyclic lactones are, and their widespread use for helminth control might have resulted in the control of the parasite. As distinct from lice infestations, in which sheep usually rub the fleece, the fleece derangement is usually associated with biting and pulled wool in the areas that the sheep can reach to bite. Mites are detected using skin scrapings from affected areas.

Chorioptic Mange

The disorder, caused by sheep-adapted Chorioptes bovis, is more common in rams, in which the hind limbs and scrotum are usually affected. Infestations cause an exudative dermatitis and can affect ram fertility. The number of mites in lesions may be small and hard to find in skin scrapings.

Sarcoptic Mange

Sarcoptic mange, caused by the burrowing mite Sarcoptes scabiei, is a contagious skin parasitic disease, prevalent mainly in Southern European countries. The mite burrows tunnels in the epidermis of sheep, yet is able to live away from animals for a maximum of 18 to 20 days. It is usually transmitted through direct contact between animals or, alternatively, through contact of animals with infested objects in their environment (mainly woods).

Usually the disease starts with focal lesions localized on the nose, with minimal skin damage. The developing lesions are described as crusts, focal alopecia, and hyperkeratosis. The lesions may then spread to various areas of the face, especially around the nostrils and the eyes, and on the pinnae of the ears. In these cases, the skin damage is more severe, but pruritus may not be present in some cases. If the disease remains untreated, extensive lesions on the face with severe blood-stained crusts, skin damage from pruritus, and fissures, and possibly with suppurative bacterial contamination, can develop. In the final stage, the clinical features are extensive pruritus and contaminated lesions on the face and ears. Moreover, lesions can also develop in other parts of the body, mainly on the legs, brisket, and abdominal skin. In rams, the scrotum seems also to be a predilection site for mite localization.[4]

METHODS OF CHEMICAL APPLICATION FOR ECTOPARASITES CONTROL IN SHEEP

For many years, treatment and control of ectoparasites in sheep relied on the application of chemicals to the fleece. With lice, scab, ked, and itch mite, effective treatment relied on the effective wetting of the fleece down to skin level. More recently, systemic insecticides have become available that are effective against parasites that feed on the skin (eg, scab mites), live in the epidermal layers of the skin (eg, itch mite), or suck blood (eg, sheep ked).

For scab, lice, itch mite, and ked, chemical application should have eradication of the parasite from the flock as the ultimate goal. These parasites complete their life-cycle on the sheep and will only survive for a short time off the host. These parasites have been eradicated in many flocks in which effective treatments have been applied in association with good management and biosecurity methods.

Sheep blowflies spend only part of their lifecycle off the sheep, and eradication is not possible. Chemicals have been used to control them for many years, but the flies have developed resistance to most. Hence, other methods of control must be used to reduce reliance on the limited number of chemical groups that are still effective.

The commonly used methods of chemical application include wet dipping, jetting along the backline, backline applications, dusting, injection of macrocyclic lactones, and local applications to affected areas.

Dipping

Shower and plunge dips have been used for many years in an attempt to control or eradicate lice, ked, and scab. However, they have not always been effective because all sheep have not been wet to the skin or resistance to the insecticide has developed.

Experience in Australia has shown that plunge dips should have a swim length of 9 m and the sheep should be dunked twice.[5] The length of the swim is more important in wetting the sheep than the time in the dip. Shower dips are only effective if they are properly maintained, the pump is operating at the correct pressure, and the sheep are left in until they are wet to the skin.[5] Rectangular shower dips are not effective, because these sheep are not wetted to the skin in the neck region. Wetting to the skin level can be checked through using vegetable dyes in the dip wash for some sheep or using special pencils that will only mark in wet areas. For example, for Merino sheep with more than 6 weeks of wool growth, thorough wetting to the skin is hard to achieve.

Jetting

Jetting involves the application of insecticide to the skin of the sheep, through using either specially designed hand pieces or automatic jetting races. Jetting is not effective in eradicating lice from flocks, because the sheep is not wet all over and lice will survive in the wool on untreated areas. Hand jetting, by using an appropriate insecticide, is the most effective method of controlling body strike, applying 0.5 L of jetting fluid per month of wool growth. Poor results usually occur from poor application of insecticide.

Automatic jetting races will treat a lot of sheep quickly. However, they are not as effective in getting the insecticide down to the skin as hand jetting and thus do not provide the same length of protection as obtained with hand jetting.[6]

Back-Line Applications

Back-line formulations are now available for the newer insecticides, including the synthetic pyrethroids (deltamethrin, cypermethrin, alphacypermethrin), insect growth regulators for lice (triflumuron, diflubenzuron), insect growth regulators for flies (cyromazine, dicyclanil), organophosphates (diazinon), extinosad, and, more recently, imidacloprid for lice.

The early application techniques involved applying a single stripe of a small volume of the insecticide formulation along the backline of the sheep within 24 hours of shearing. Later research showed that this technique did not always guarantee that effective concentrations of insecticide reached all woolled areas of the skin. The newer application devices have multiple nozzles and apply a larger volume over a wider area over the back of the sheep.

Formulations are now available for long wool applications to control flystrike and lice infestations. However, they will not eradicate lice in sheep with long wool.

Dusting

Dusting has been used in some countries but is not considered effective because the chemical does not get to the skin in all of the woolly areas. The technique should not be relied on to eradicate lice, ked, or scab. It may also be dangerous to the operator because of the risk of inhalation.

Tip Spraying

Tip spraying involves the application of high concentrations of an organophosphate, usually diazinon, to the fleece of the sheep. The technique was not always effective and also is no longer used because of occupational health and safety risk to the operators.

Local Dressings

Dressings are used largely to treat blowfly strikes in sheep. The main benefit of dressings used to treat struck sheep is in preventing restrike.[7] Many of the treatments would not kill the maggots on the sheep. When treating flystruck sheep, the struck wool and a 5-cm barrier of clean wool around the strike should be shorn close to the skin to remove maggots and allow the skin to heal. A flystrike dressing should then be applied to the shorn area to prevent restrike.

Oral or Injectable Treatments

Macrocyclic lactones, either as a drench, in a capsule, or as an injectable formulation, are effective to control psoroptic mange, itch mite, chorioptic mange, and sarcoptic mange. Some of these drugs have a long persistent efficacy, and thus can prevent reinfection of the animals from the environment.

ERADICATION OF SHEEP LICE INFESTATIONS

Lice can be eradicated from sheep flocks, provided attention is given to management practices in the flock, selection and use of effective chemicals, and correct application of these at the appropriate time. With some of the treatments, poor application techniques result in the need for retreatment of the flock at regular intervals.[2] Some treatment failures have been associated with insecticide resistance.[8]

Control and eradication programs for sheep lice, ked, and scab involve the following four steps:

1. Diagnosing the reason for the infestation. If lice are present in all groups in the flock, then it is more likely to be a treatment failure from poor application or insecticide resistance. Surveys in New South Wales showed that more than 40% of flocks affected with lice for 1 year were still affected the next year, despite one or more treatments after shearing.[2] If lice are present in only one or two groups of sheep, then it may be from the introduction of lice, on either introduced sheep or stray sheep from adjoining properties.
2. Treating the sheep to control the infestation and reduce wool damage until the next shearing. Long wool backline treatments or hand jetting can be used to control the infestation until shearing, but they would not eradicate lice.
3. Treating the flock after shearing to eradicate the parasites. Wet dipping and backline applications using effective chemicals are the only treatments that will eradicate lice under Australian conditions. When using chemicals that strip from the dip wash (eg, diazinon), care must be taken to ensure an effective concentration of insecticide is maintained in the dip wash.[9] For eradication to be achieved, careful attention must be given to management, ensuring clean musters, so that all sheep are treated at one time. Changing shearing times should be considered, so that no young lambs are in the flock at dipping time. Some chemicals take longer to kill adult lice, and the young lambs may provide a reservoir of infection.
4. Taking steps to prevent the reintroduction of lice into the flock with more attention to biosecurity measures. This measure would involve attention to fences and quarantining introduced sheep.

Resistance to Lousicides

Synthetic pyrethroid chemicals are no longer recommended in Australia because of widespread resistance.[8] Resistance has occurred to the insect growth regulators, triflumuron and diflubenzuron; field breakdown, after use of these chemicals, is becoming more common.

Diazinon is still effective, despite having been used and abused for more than 40 years. Unfortunately, it has been withdrawn from use for wet dipping in Australia, because of occupational health and safety concerns to the operators. A backline application formulation is still available, but its use is currently under review.

Effective lousicides currently available in Australia include temephos (an organophosphate), imidacloprid, diazinon as a backline application formulation, magnesium fluosilicate dip, and ectinosad. These lousicides will eradicate lice from sheep flocks if they are applied to all sheep in the flock at the same time. When using wet dipping, it should be performed within 2 to 4 weeks after shearing to allow all sheep to be thoroughly wet to the skin.

ERADICATION OF PSOROPTIC MANGE (SHEEP SCAB)

Eradication and prevention programs against psoroptic mange vary among the various management systems. In closed systems, both eradication and prevention are comparatively easy. In extensive free-range systems, with intermingling of flocks of different owners, eradicating the disease is very difficult. Psoroptic mange was eliminated from England and Scotland by 1948 and from Wales in 1951. Thereafter, Great Britain remained free for a further 20 years. Also, worldwide the disease was reduced to manageable proportions. In 1973, sheep infested with psoroptic mange were imported into Great Britain, specifically into an area of common grazing.

Thereafter, increased movement of sheep led to the rapid spread of infestations throughout the country.

Two alternatives for eradication are available: plunge dipping or the use of macrocyclic lactones. Plunge dipping was the only method of treatment from the late 19th century until the mid-1990s. Various compounds were used with less than 100% efficacy. The organochlorines, introduced in the mid-1940s, resulted in the first really effective acaricide. Nevertheless, they were withdrawn in 1984 and superseded by the organophosphates. Despite strict regulations as to compulsory dipping, psoroptic mange remained. Then, in 1988, only 16 cases were recorded. This incidence coincided with the relaxing of dipping regulations and the opportunity of eliminating scab might have been lost forever.

In 1992, the synthetic pyrethroids were first licensed. However, they seemed to be less effective and also presented major environmental hazards.

Toward the end of the century, the macrocyclic lactones were found to be particularly effective. Of these, moxidectin offers longer residual protection than some others. Irrespective of which specific lactone is used, it must be used correctly as part of a planned program aiming for eradication. Although no resistance has been recorded to these drugs, their widespread use to treat scab mites results in exposure to the chemical of any internal parasites the sheep may be carrying. Extensive use will help select for resistant internal parasites, and therefore may contribute to increased risk for development of anthelmintic resistance.

Eradication of sheep scab from a flock requires the development of a program that ensures that every sheep in the flock is treated correctly. Steps should also be taken to prevent reinfection of the flock. When flocks are closed, quarantine treatment of all incoming sheep can be effective in preventing the resident flock from becoming infected.

Acaricide Resistance as a Limiting Factor in Control of Psoroptic Mange

Acaricide resistance developed initially (1962) to the organochlorines and then (1965) to diazinon in South America. In the United Kingdom, *Psoroptes* mites quickly developed resistance to all of the synthetic pyrethroids.[10] In addition, mites have been shown to be resistant to propetamphos, but without side-resistance to diazinon.[11]

CHEMICAL CONTROL OF BLOWFLY STRIKE

In the past, blowfly strike control and prevention has relied on the use of insecticides. Because of insecticide resistance and increasing concern in wool markets with chemical residues, greater emphasis will have to be given to nonchemical methods of fly control.

Insecticides have been used for local application, either to treat existing strikes or to prevent strikes in various areas (eg, poll, prepuce, body, or breech region) or to the whole body, through hand jetting, automatic jetting races, shower dipping, or using specially formulated spray-on treatments.

The development of resistance by *Lucilia* spp to insecticides was recently reviewed.[12] Resistance to organophosphates is widespread, protection being reduced from 16 weeks to 2 to 4 weeks. Diflubenzuron, a benzoylphenyl urea insecticide, has a cross-resistance with diazinon. Resistance can occur within 2 to 3 years of its release.[13]

Cyromazine, a triazine pesticide first used in 1979, still provides long-term (14 weeks) protection and no resistance has been reported. It can be applied either through jetting or as a backline spray-on formulation. Dicyclanil was introduced in 1998 as a spray-on formulation and provides up to 26 weeks protection against flystrike.

Jetting, dusting, backline application, plunge and shower dipping, and spray races have all been used to control flystrike. Plunge and shower dipping are not recommended because of the health risks associated with dipping sheep in long wool and the high chemical residues that occur in the wool of treated sheep. Hand jetting provides longer protection against body strike than the automatic jetting races.[6]

Nonchemical Methods for Control of Flystrike

Control of scouring
Daggy sheep are more susceptible to flystrike in the breech region.[14] The cause of the scouring (eg, gastrointestinal parasites, coccidiosis) should be determined and steps taken to eliminate the cause or causes. Crutching (removal of wool from the perineal area) also reduces the risk of flystrike in daggy sheep.

Genetic selection
The major predisposing causes of body strike in sheep are fleece-rot and dermatophilosis. Merino sheep can be selected against susceptibility to fleece-rot and body strike, even in high rainfall areas.[15,16] Other flocks have used direct selection, culling any struck sheep from the breeding flock. Studies in the 1940s[17] showed that selection for plainer-bodied animals resulted in less flystrike.

Flock management
Timing of shearing, crutching, and lambing all affect the prevalence of flystrike. Worm control programs to reduce scouring and management to control dermatophilosis can also be helpful.

Tail docking
Trials in the 1940s[17] highlighted the importance of docking the tail at the correct length to reduce urine and fecal staining in the breech area. Weaner sheep with short tails are more prone to flystrike, especially when scouring occurs. Tails should be docked level with the tip of the vulva and be a similar length in male lambs.

Mulesing
Mulesing involves the surgical removal of strips of skin from the breech region. This method is very effective at providing permanent control of breech strike in sheep in Australia. However, it is being phased out in many flocks as better management and selective breeding lead to sheep less susceptible to breech strike, and perceived community concerns for the welfare of sheep during surgery are on the increase.

Vaccination against the blowfly and its larvae or against fleece rot
Several vaccination strategies have been tested. These strategies have been directed against the fly or infection with *P aeruginosa*.[18] In the short term, nothing is offering promise for effective control.

Release of sterile male flies
The release of sterile male flies has been tried with *L cuprina* but, because of the widespread distribution of *Lucilia* in the environment, was not successful.

Use of fly traps
Fly traps may reduce fly numbers in local areas, but their main role may be in indicating when flies are active in the environment. Bait bins, using offal or a sheep carcass as the lure, trap flies indiscriminately. Also, they lose their attractiveness to the primary sheep blowflies as the bait putrefies.

TREATMENT OF SARCOPTIC MANGE

For treating sarcoptic mange, injectable macrocyclic lactones are the preferred drugs. However, several issues should be taken into account during treatment.[19,20] All animals in the flock (even ones with no clinical signs of the disease) should be injected twice, 10 to 11 days apart. Alternatively, spraying with organophosphates can be performed; two treatments of all animals in the flock are advisable. In housed animals (even for part of the day), disinfection of the animal's environment to kill residual mites, is paramount; a strong miticide should be used for this task. Full clinical recovery after treatment, with complete healing and regrowth of the hair, requires at least 3 months.

TREATMENT OF ECTOPARASITES IN NORTH AMERICA

In both the United States and Canada, few pesticides are approved for use in controlling ectoparasites in sheep. Additionally, legislation states that extra-label use of pesticides is not allowed. However, macrocyclic lactones are not included because they are considered a pharmaceutical drug. Veterinarians must check the label of any product approved as a treatment for livestock before using it on sheep.

CONTROL OF SHEEP ECTOPARASITES IN THE FUTURE

With the increasing consumer demands for a clean green (environmentally friendly) product, sheep producers and their advisers will have to change old management systems to meet the new demands. With increasing public concern about the health and welfare of sheep, sound ectoparasite control and eradication programs are necessary.[21] Veterinarians can no longer rely solely on chemicals to control ectoparasites, although their use will still be required for blowfly control. Techniques are currently available that will eradicate lice, ked, itch mite, and scab from flocks, and therefore infestations are unnecessary.

SUMMARY

This article provides an overview of the common ectoparasites of sheep, effective products to control these parasites, and management factors that affect the success of these treatments.

REFERENCES

1. McLeod RS. Costs of major parasites to the Australian livestock industries. Int J Parasitol 1995;25:1363–7.
2. Plant JW. A survey of chemical application techniques for fly and lice control. In: Proceedings of the Australian Sheep Veterinary Society Annual Conference. Keith (Australia): Australian Sheep Veterinary Society; 1993. p. 107–15.
3. O'Brien DJ, Gray JS, O'Reilly PF. Survival and retention of infectivity of the mite Psoroptes ovis off the host. Vet Res Commun 1994;18:27–36.
4. Doukas D, Tontis D, Fthenakis GC. Ovine sarcoptic mange: clinical features and economic impact. In: Wilson D, editor. Proceedings of meetings of the Sheep Veterinary Society. Midlothian (Scotland): Sheep Veterinary Society, Moredun Research Institute; 2007. p. 95–7.
5. Lund RD, Johnson PW, Gould NS, et al. Improved design and use of shower and plunge dipping equipment for the eradication of sheep body lice (Bovicola ovis). In: Watts T, editor. Proceedings of the Australian Sheep Veterinary Society Annual

Conference. Sydney (Australia): Australian Sheep Veterinary Society; 1998. p. 65–72.

6. Lund RD, Kelly PJ, Gould NS. Improve performance characteristics of automatic jetting races for the effective protection of sheep from flystrike. Australian Wool Research and Promotion Organisation. Final Report Project DAN86; 1994. p. 1–33.

7. Levot GW, Sales N, Barchia I. In vitro larvicidal efficacy of flystrike dressings against the Australian sheep blowfly. Aust J Exp Agric 1999;39:541–7.

8. Levot GW, Johnson PW, Hughes PB, et al. Pyrethroid resistance in Australian field populations of the sheep body louse, Bovicola (Damalinia) ovis. Med Vet Entomol 1995;9:59–65.

9. Levot GW, Lund RD. Alternative replenishment regimens to maintain diazinon concentration during shower, plunge and immersion cage dipping of merino sheep. Aust J Exp Agric 2007;47:1326–32.

10. Bates PG. Acaricide resistance in the sheep scab mite. In: Clarkson M, editor. Proceedings of meetings of the Sheep Veterinary Society. Midlothian (Scotland): Sheep Veterinary Society, Moredun Research Institute; 1997. p. 117–22.

11. Synge BA, Bates PG, Clark AM, et al. Apparent resistance of P. ovis to flumethrin. Vet Rec 1995;137:51.

12. Levot G. External parasites of sheep. In: Sheep medicine — Proceedings 355 Post Graduate Foundation in Veterinary Science. Sydney (Australia): Post Graduate Foundation in Veterinary Science, University of Sydney; 2004. p. 101–14.

13. Levot G, Sales N. Resistance to benzoylphenyl urea insecticides in Australian populations of the sheep body louse. Med Vet Entomol 2008;22:331–4.

14. Watts JE, Murray MD, Graham NPH. The blowfly strike problem of sheep in New South Wales. Aust Vet J 1979;55:325–34.

15. Raadsma HW. Fleece rot and body strike in Merino sheep. 5. Heritability of liability to body strike in weaner sheep under flywave conditions. Aust J Agric Res 1991;42:279–93.

16. Raadsma HW. The susceptibility to body strike under high rainfall conditions of flocks selected for and against fleece rot 1991. Aust J Exp Agric 1991;31:757–9.

17. Joint Blowfly Committee. Recent advances in the prevention and treatment of blowfly strike in sheep. Supplement to report No. 2, CSIR Bulletin No 174. Australia: Council for Scientific and Industrial Research, Commonwealth of Australia; 1943. p. 1–20.

18. Sandeman RM. Prospects for the control of sheep blowfly strike by vaccination. Int J Parasitol 1990;20:537–41.

19. Papadopoulos E, Fthenakis GC. Administration of moxidectin for treatment of sarcoptic mange in a flock of sheep. Small Rumin Res 1999;31:165–8.

20. Fthenakis GC, Papadopoulos E, Himonas C, et al. Efficacy of moxidectin against sarcoptic mange and effects on milk yield of ewes and growth of lambs. Vet Parasitol 2000;87:207–16.

21. Plant JW. Sheep ectoparasite control and animal welfare. Small Rumin Res 2006; 62:109–12.

Treatment and Control of Chlamydial and Rickettsial Infections in Sheep and Goats

Snorre Stuen, DVM, PhD, DrPhilos[a],*, David Longbottom, PhD[b]

KEYWORDS

- *Chlamydia* • Control of infection • Diagnosis • *Rickettsia*
- Treatment

Small ruminants are susceptible to several chlamydial and rickettsial infections. Some of them, such as *Ehrlichia ruminantium*, have a great impact on the sheep and goat industry while others, such as *Coxiella burnetii*, are important zoonotic agents. In this review the authors focus on measures of treatment and control for the following organisms: *Chlamydophila abortus* (formerly *Chlamydia psittaci* immunotype 1), *Coxiella burnetii*, *Anaplasma ovis*, *Anaplasma phagocytophilum*, and *Ehrlichia ruminantium*.

ENZOOTIC ABORTION
Etiological Agent

Ovine enzootic abortion (OEA) or enzootic abortion of ewes (EAE) is caused by the obligate intracellular gram-negative organism *Chlamydophila abortus*. The organism belongs to the bacterial family Chlamydiaceae, which undergo a biphasic developmental cycle comprising 2 distinct developmental forms, the small (0.3 μm diameter) extracellular infectious elementary body (EB) and the larger (0.5–1.6 μm) intracellular noninfectious, metabolically active reticulate body (RB).[1] The organism is zoonotic, infecting humans and animals.

Distribution

C abortus is recognized as a major cause of reproductive loss in sheep and goats worldwide, although the disease does not appear to occur in Australia or

---

The authors have nothing to disclose.

[a] Department of Production Animal Clinical Sciences, Norwegian School of Veterinary Science, Kyrkjevegen 332/334, N-4325 Sandnes, Norway

[b] Pentlands Science Park, Moredun Research Institute, International Research Centre, Bush Loan, Penicuik, Midlothian, Scotland, EH26 0PZ, UK

* Corresponding author.

E-mail address: snorre.stuen@nvh.no

New Zealand.[2] In countries of Northern Europe, OEA is the most common infectious cause of abortion in lowland flocks that are intensively managed during the lambing period. In the United Kingdom, OEA accounts for approximately 44% of all diagnosed infectious cases of abortion. The organism can also infect cattle, pigs, horses, and deer, although such infections are thought to be less common.

Clinical Expression

Infection in animals is asymptomatic, displaying no specific premonitory signs of the impending abortion, although some behavioral changes or a vaginal discharge may be observed in some animals up to a couple of days before.[1,2] Usually the first sign of a problem is the discovery of dead lambs 2 to 3 weeks before the expected lambing. Lambs aborted at this late stage of pregnancy appear well developed and normal, but some may show a degree of edema giving rise to a "pot-bellied" appearance. The fleece may be discolored or covered with a pinkish-brown material originating from the placental exudate. The placental membranes can present with a variable degree of necrotic damage, although commonly the majority of the placenta have thickened red intercotyledonary membranes and dark red cotyledons with a creamy-yellow colored exudate on the surface.[1,2] An infectious vaginal discharge may be observed for several days following abortion, but otherwise the ewes are clinically normal and are considered immune to further disease. Occasionally the placenta can be retained, although this appears to occur more frequently in goats than sheep.[3,4] Such retention can lead to the development of an associated metritis, which can result in a loss of condition and death due to secondary bacterial infections. As well as abortion, ewes may deliver stillborn or weakly lambs that fail to survive beyond 2 days of age. Also, it is not uncommon for infected ewes to deliver healthy lambs, with little necrotic damage evident in the placental membranes, as well as delivering one dead and one weakly or healthy lamb.

Although rare, the greatest threat of human infection is to pregnant women, for whom the outcome of infection in the first trimester of pregnancy is likely spontaneous abortion; later, infection causes stillbirths or preterm labor.[5] Several cases of abortion, puerperal sepsis and shock, including renal failure, hepatic dysfunction, and disseminated intravascular coagulation, as well as death have been reported.[6,7] Most cases are associated with direct exposure to infected sheep or goats.[8]

Diagnostics

The choice of tests used to confirm diagnosis is often dictated by the sample received (blood, placental membranes, fetal tissues, swabs), organism viability, the presumptive diagnosis and clinical history.[9] A presumptive diagnosis of infection can be made based on the abortion occurring in the last 2 to 3 weeks of gestation and following examination of the placenta for gross pathology affecting both the intercotyledonary membranes and the cotyledons. The diagnosis is usually confirmed by the identification of large numbers of EBs in smears prepared from the diseased placental membranes and cotyledons, following staining using a modified Ziehl-Neelsen, Giemsa, Gimenez, or Machiavello procedure.[9,10] Other methods of antigen detection include immunohistochemical staining of tissue sections using specific monoclonal antibodies to dominant chlamydial surface antigens, such as the major outer membrane protein (MOMP) and lipopolysaccharide (LPS), immunoassays, DNA amplification methods, microarray, and isolation in cell culture or embryonated hens' eggs.[9,10] Although isolation in cell culture is still considered the gold standard, it is time consuming and expensive, and is restricted to specialist laboratories with the relevant expertise. Instead, several specific polymerase chain reaction (PCR) and real-time PCR protocols, as well as an ArrayTube microarray test that detects and differentiates between *Chlamydiaceae* spp, have been recommended to be used as an alternative gold standard for the detection of chlamydiae in clinical samples.[9]

Serologic testing is generally performed by the complement fixation test[11] on paired blood samples taken at the time of abortion and then at least 3 weeks later, to detect a rising antibody titer.[10] It should be noted that the test also cross-reacts with another common chlamydial species that infects sheep and goats, *Chlamydophila pecorum*.[1] A variety of other serologic tests have been developed, including the microimmuno-fluorescence test, tests based on peptides or recombinant chlamydial antigens, such as LPS, MOMP, and the polymorphic outer membrane proteins (POMPs), and tests based on monoclonal antibodies to MOMP, which vary considerably in their sensitivity and specificity.[9] Recent comparisons of commercial assays with "in-house" developed tests have suggested that tests based on the POMP antigens are more sensitive and specific, with those based on recombinant POMP90 antigen providing the best specificity in terms of lack of cross-reaction with antibodies to *C pecorum*.[12,13]

None of the current serologic tests have been proved to be suitable for detecting infection prior to abortion occurring, and are not able to differentiate vaccinated animals from those infected with wild-type strains. Regarding the latter point, recently molecular tools based on PCR-restriction fragment length polymorphism and sequence analysis of single-nucleotide polymorphisms in the 1B live-attenuated vaccine strain, compared with its parent wild-type strain, have been developed and have been shown to distinguish vaccinal from wild-type infections.[14,15]

Treatment

If OEA is suspected to be present in a flock/herd, the administration of a long-acting oxytetracycline preparation (20 mg/kg body weight [BW] intramuscularly) will reduce the severity of infection and losses resulting from abortion.[1,2] It is important that treatment is given soon after the 95th to 100th day of gestation, the point at which pathologic changes start to occur. Further doses can be subsequently given at 2-week intervals until the time of lambing. Although such treatment reduces losses and limits the shedding of infectious organisms, it does not eliminate the infection nor reverse any pathologic damage already done to the placenta, thus abortions or the delivery of stillborn or weakly lambs can still occur, and the shed organisms are a source of infection for other naïve animals.

In humans, early therapeutic intervention is important. Severely ill patients require supportive therapy, including fluids, oxygen, and measures to combat toxic shock. Tetracyclines, erythromycin, and clarithromycin are administered orally or parenterally, depending on clinical severity.[1,16]

Control

During an OEA outbreak the primary aim is to limit the spread of infection to other naïve animals.[1,2] The major sources of infection are the placental membranes, dead fetuses, coats of live lambs/kids born to infected mothers, and vaginal discharges. Thus, affected animals should be identified and isolated as quickly as possible, and all dead fetuses, placental membranes, and bedding should be carefully disposed of; lambing pens must be cleaned and disinfected.[1] Pregnant women and immunocompromised individuals are advised not to work with sheep, particularly during the lambing period, and should avoid all contact with possible sources of infection, including work clothing.[1,8] Basic hygiene procedures, including thorough washing of hands and the use of disposable gloves, are essential when handling potentially infected materials.

Ewes that have aborted are considered immune to further disease, although this immunity is not sterile. Ewes may become persistently infected carriers and might continue to excrete infectious organisms at next estrus,[17,18] thus providing an opportunity for venereal transmission of infection via the ram, although more recent evidence using quantitative real-time PCR suggests that the risks of this are low.[19]

Although antibiotic treatment (see above) can be used in exceptional circumstances to reduce abortion losses, it should not be used routinely to control infection. Instead it is better to use a combination of flock/herd management and vaccination.[1] Flock/herd management aims to keep animals "clean" by keeping the flock/herd "closed," through breeding own replacement animals or by buying them in from OEA-free accredited sources, such as those that participate in the various United Kingdom Premium Health Schemes.[1,20] If there is any doubt regarding the status of replacements or for animals bought from nonaccredited sources, these should be vaccinated before entering them into the flock/herd.

In most of Europe, there is currently available an attenuated ("live") vaccine based on a temperature-sensitive mutant strain (C abortus strain 1B)[21] that is available from 2 commercial companies. The vaccines must be administered at least 4 weeks before mating and cannot be used in combination with antibiotic treatment. Inactivated vaccines can also be prepared from organisms grown in hens' eggs or cell culture.[22–25] These vaccines are safe for administration during pregnancy.

Both types of vaccines confer good protection from abortion, but do not completely eradicate the shedding of infectious organisms at parturition, and some vaccinated animals still abort as a result of wild-type infections. Recently the live vaccine has been detected in the placentas of vaccinated animals that have aborted as a result of OEA, suggesting a role for the vaccine in causing disease in some animals.[15] However, this requires further investigations to determine the proportion of animals affected in an outbreak. Despite these findings, the importance of continuing the vaccinations is stressed, as this is still the most effective way to protect from disease.[15]

Vaccine development research to produce the next-generation OEA vaccine continues to progress. This treatment is likely to be a subunit vaccine, based on protective recombinant antigens identified through comparative genomic and proteomic approaches, and which is capable of eliciting the required mucosal and systemic cellular and humoral responses.[26]

Q FEVER
Etiological Agent

Q fever is caused by the aerobic intracellular organism Coxiella burnetii. Although Coxiella was historically considered to be a Rickettsia, gene-sequence analysis now classifies the genus Coxiella in the order Legionellales, family Coxiellaceae, with Rickettsiella and Aquicella.[27]

The organism exists in 2 different antigenic phases. In nature, C burnetii exists in phase I form, which is virulent. However, when cultivated in nonimmunocompetent cell cultures or hens' eggs, the organism mutates irreversibly to the phase II form, which is less virulent.[28] C burnetii has 2 different morphologic forms, a large and a small form. In addition, an endospore-like structure is observed in the large form,[29] which is highly resistant to environmental degradation, such as high temperatures, ultraviolet light, and osmotic shock.[30] In the mammalian host, monocyte-macrophages are the only known target cells of the bacteria.[31]

Distribution

Q fever is a worldwide zoonosis that occurs in all geographic and climatic zones, with the exception of Antarctica and possibly New Zealand.[32] However, in many countries Q fever is not a reportable disease, so it is difficult to know exactly where it occurs.

Clinical Expression

In animals, *C burnetii* infections are generally asymptomatic. Except for abortion, still-birth, and the delivery of weak offspring, clinical signs in ruminants are rare. However, *C burnetii* may induce pneumonia, conjunctivitis, and hepatitis.[33] The abortion rate can range from 3% to 80% of pregnant females.[34–36] High abortion rates are rarely observed, although abortion storms in some herds have been described.[34,37] Stress, resulting from overcrowding or poor nutrition, may play an important role in an infected goat aborting.[38] In the majority of cases, abortion or stillbirth occurs at the end of the gestation period, without specific clinical signs, only when placental damage has been severe. Aborted fetuses appear normal, but infected placentas exhibit intercotyledo-nary fibrous thickening and discolored exudates that may be mineralized.[37,39]

In humans, acute Q fever may not be promptly diagnosed, because of nonspecific initial clinical signs such as fever, pneumonia, headache, and weakness, and the time between onset of clinical signs and therapy may be greater than 2 months. Chronic infection may result in severe granulomatous hepatitis, osteomyelitis, and valvular endocarditis with high case fatality rates.[40]

Diagnostics

Current alternatives to diagnose *C burnetii* infection in ruminants include serologic analysis, organism isolation by cell culture (eg, shell vial culture) or live animal inocu-lation, and immunohistochemical and PCR-based detection.[41] For instance, a single touchdown PCR could be used to detect *C burnetii* from genital swabs, milk, and fecal samples.[42] In the acute phase of the infection, *C burnetii* can be detected in lungs, spleen, liver, and blood.[31]

Placental smear or impression of placentas could be stained, for instance using a modified Ziehl-Nielsen procedure. *Coxiella* is stained as acid-fast rod-like organ-isms, observed extra- and intracellularly.[30] Because *C burnetii* can be shed heavily at the time of normal lambing/kidding, isolation of the organisms as a sole procedure is not considered enough to confirm the diagnosis as the cause of abortion.[43,44]

Several serologic tests are available, such as complement fixation test, enzyme-linked immunosorbent assay (ELISA), and a fluorescent antibody test.[45] However, carrier animals may also have an antibody titer increase in late pregnancy.[46] In addi-tion, laboratory animal inoculation and isolation in embryonated eggs are other possible diagnostic techniques. For Q fever diagnostics, it has recently been recom-mended to use PCR and immunofluorescence tests of *Coxiella* on parturition products and vaginal secretions at abortion.[42,47]

Treatment

If Q fever is suspected, aborting animals and other animals in late pregnancy should be treated with tetracycline. The regime consists in 2 injections of oxytetracycline (20 mg/kg BW) during the last month of gestation, although this treatment does not totally suppress abortions and shedding of *C burnetii* at lambing.[48]

Antibiotic treatment is mainly used to minimize shedding of the organisms in the placenta and birth fluids rather than to eliminate it, but its efficacy has not been evaluated.[49] Placentas and aborted fetuses should be destroyed properly, and aborted animals should be isolated. In addition, materials such as bedding and straw contaminated with birth fluids and other secretions from affected animals should be destroyed.

Control

C burnetii is widely spread and is able to infect many animal species, including mammals, birds, and several arthropods. Practically all hematophagous arthropods, such as fleas, bugs, lice, and mites, may serve as a mechanical vector. However, ticks are the principal vector and reservoir of *C burnetii*, because they transmit the agent horizontally and vertically, as well as excreting it in their feces. Every tick species parasitizing a susceptible host in a known area of epidemics can be expected to harbor and spread *C burnetii*.[49] In addition, amoebae have also been found to be infected with *C burnetii* for several weeks. However, cattle, sheep, and goats are the primary animal reservoirs.[31,35,44]

The spread of *C burnetii* infection in domestic animals depends on many factors, such as population density of animals, the system of rearing, and management at parturition.[49] Q-fever abortion is usually prevented by providing good nutrition and management. Because the environment can remain infected for a long time and many species can be carriers, test and cull strategies are not appropriate for infected flocks/herds.[46] However, during the recent outbreak of Q fever in humans in the Netherlands, the Dutch Government ordered the culling of more than 50,000 pregnant goats to halt the worst outbreak of Q fever reported to date, where more than 3000 human cases were recorded from 2007 to 2009. The reason for this strategy is that parturient dairy goats are believed to be the main source of human infection.[50,51]

Serologic tests are not useful for determining which animals represent a current risk for the transmission of *C burnetii*, because some animals shed the bacteria and pose a risk of infection before they develop antibodies, and some infected animals never seroconvert.[36,52] The last situation has an important consequence for animal and public health. However, these shedders may be identified by PCR. A combination of PCR and ELISA seems to be the optimum for diagnosis and tracking the shedding of the organisms.[53]

The uterus and mammary gland of females are sites for persistent *C burnetii* infection.[54] Reactivation of the bacterium in females during pregnancy results in shedding of a great amount of infectious agent into the environment during abortion or via birth fluids, placenta, and fetal membranes.[55] More than 10^9 bacteria per gram of placenta may be released at the time of delivery.[54] In addition, infected animals may excrete the bacteria in the feces, vaginal discharge, and milk for several days or months following parturition.[56] Studies indicate that ewes shed the bacterium mostly in feces and vaginal mucus, with a much lower level in milk.[57] In goats, shedding in milk seems to be the most frequent route.[43,58] In addition, both goats and ewes can shed bacteria at subsequent pregnancies.[59,60]

Contaminated aerosols generated from desiccation of infected placentas, body fluids, or dust from contaminated manure are the main sources of both animal and human infection, and the control of fecal excretion and placental bacterial discharge is essential.[33,61,62] Grazing of contaminated pasture and tick bites are other modes of transmission. The organism is highly contagious, with an infective dose as low as 1 to 10 bacteria.[63] Because *C burnetii* is extremely resistant to desiccation and to physical and chemical agents, it survives in the environment for long periods.[49,54] The small endospore-like form survives in dust for 120 days, in tick feces for 568 days, and in wool for 12 to 16 months at temperatures of 4°C to 6°C.[30]

During a Q-fever outbreak, the contamination of animals and the environment can be prevented or reduced by destroying placentas and fetuses to prevent their ingestion by domestic and wild carnivores, which could disseminate the infection. If possible, births should be confined to a specific location that is disinfected without inducing aerosols.[58] *C burnetii* is resistant to standard disinfectants, but will, for instance, be inactivated within 30 minutes in suspensions of 70% ethyl alcohol or 5% chloroform.[64] Manure should be treated with lime or 0.6% calcium cyanamide before spreading on fields; however, their efficacy has so far been tested only for the treatment of slurry.[58] Manure should not be spread in windy conditions, as the wind may propagate the bacteria over large distances.[48,65,66] To prevent environmental contamination of *C burnetii* during the recent outbreak in the Netherlands, stringent hygiene protocols were implemented on sheep and goat farms. For instance, the farmers were not allowed to take out the manure from their stables for at least 1 month after the lambing/kidding season, they were obliged to cover the manure during storage and transport, and had to plough it under immediately or after it had been composted for at least 3 months.[50]

Vaccine development is progressing. In animals, the most effective vaccines are those composed of inactivated whole phase I bacteria. Bacterial shedding in placentas and milk was strongly reduced in experimental infection or in natural Q-fever infection in ewes vaccinated by phase I vaccines.[48,67–69]

In one study, a commercial vaccine using inactivated phase I *Coxiella* protected against abortion and excretion in milk, feces, and vaginal discharges, whereas an inactivated phase II vaccine did not.[56,70] Because phase I vaccines are dangerous to produce, a subunit vaccine is being investigated.[33]

Vaccination does not eradicate *C burnetii* in animals naturally infected prior to vaccination, and *C burnetii* shedding persisted unchanged after vaccination.[71] In the Netherlands, a compulsory vaccination campaign in the infected area with a phase I inactivated vaccine in dairy sheep and goat flocks has been implemented.[50]

To prevent possible human infection, drinking raw milk or consumption of raw milk products should be restricted. For inactivation, pasteurization of milk at 62.8°C for 30 minutes or at 71.7°C for 15 seconds is required.[49] Q fever often occurs as an occupational disease. People may be infected by handling contaminated wool, manure, or clothes, or indirectly via transport of animals, for instance through a valley.[72] Persons at particular risk are livestock handlers, processors of animal products, abattoir workers, those in contact with dairy products, veterinarians, and laboratory personnel working with *C burnetii*–infected animals.[31] In addition, it is necessary to inform vulnerable persons, such as immunodeficient patients or those suffering from cardiac valvulopathy and pregnant women, that they must avoid contact with animals during lambing/kidding.[33]

ANAPLASMOSIS
Etiological Agent

Anaplasmosis in sheep and goats is caused by *Anaplasma ovis*, belonging to the genus *Anaplasma* (**Box 1**).[73] In addition, a similar pathogen, *A mesaeterum*, may also cause anaplasmosis in small ruminants. Both are obligate pathogens of erythrocytes.[74]

Distribution

Anaplasmosis, caused by *A ovis*, is distributed particularly in tropical Africa, but has also been reported in Europe (mainly in the Mediterranean area), Asia, Russia, and

> **Box 1**
> **New classification of genuses *Anaplasma*, *Ehrlichia*, and *Neorickettsia*, in the family Anaplasmataceae**
>
> Genus
>
> *Anaplasma*
>
>   *A marginale*
>
>   *A bovis*
>
>   *A ovis*
>
>   *A phogocytophilum*
>
>   *A platys*
>
> *Ehrlichia*
>
>   *E canis*
>
>   *E chaffeensis*
>
>   *E ewingii*
>
>   *E muris*
>
>   *E ruminantium*
>
> *Neorickettsia*
>
>   *N risticii*
>
>   *N sennetsu*
>
> *Data from* Dumler JS, Barbet AF, Bekker CPJ, et al. Reorganization of genera in the families *Rickettsiaceae* and *Anaplasmataceae* in the order *Rickettsiales*; unification of some species of *Ehrlichia* with *Anaplasma*, *Cowdria* with *Ehrlichia* and *Ehrlichia* with *Neorickettsia*, descriptions of 6 new species combinations and designation of *Ehrlichia equi* and "HGE agent" as subjective synonyms of *Ehrlichia phagocytophila*. Int J Syst Evol Microbiol 2001;51:2145–65.

the United States. *A ovis* has a wide host range including several deer species. The infection is spread by a variety of ticks, particularly *Rhipicephalus* and *Dermacentor* species.[75]

Clinical Expression

A ovis is commonly reported as causing hemolytic anemia in sheep and goats. Anaplasmosis in sheep is normally subclinical. Outbreaks of severe illness in sheep are rare and seem to occur only under extreme conditions.[75] However, *A ovis* appears to be more pathogenic for goats than for sheep. After an incubation period of 1 to 3 months, infected animals may become depressed and develop fatigue, incoordination, pallor, and icterus, without hemoglobinuria.[76,77] Mortality is low. The bacterium may cause a persistent infection, and clinical cases are mostly identified during periods of nutritional stress.[78,79] In utero transmission of *A ovis* has been recorded in both sheep and goats.[80]

Diagnostics

The organisms can be detected on erythrocytes by microscopy of stained blood smears early in clinical disease.[73] Detection of *A ovis* may also be done by PCR and gene sequencing.[79] In addition, several serologic tests are available, such as the capillary tube agglutination and ELISA.[81,82] Necropsy of infected animals may show watery blood, pallor, icteric tissues, and increased fluid in the body cavities. In addition, the liver may be enlarged.[46]

Treatment

Treatment is most efficient during the bacteremic phase of the infection and is directed at reducing the rate of erythrocyte infection, although treatment during the prepatent period does not prevent bacteremia. Stress should be avoided during handling and treatment. Oxytetracycline or tetracycline hydrochloride has been used successfully to treat clinically affected goats (10 mg/kg BW, once daily for up to 2 days). However, even a 5-day treatment course would not eliminate the carrier state.[46]

Control

Efforts should be focused on controlling tick infestation through regular dipping, spraying, or pour-on treatment. No specific vaccine for *A ovis* is currently available. In the case of an outbreak, prophylactic antibiotic administration might be used to prevent spread of the infection.[46]

TICK-BORNE FEVER
Etiological Agent

Tick-borne fever (TBF) is caused by *Anaplasma phagocytophilum* (formerly *Ehrlichia phagocytophila*), an obligate intracellular microbe in the genus *Anaplasma* (see **Box 1**) that primarily infects phagocytes.[73] Several genetic variants of the bacterium have been found with a variable degree of cross-protective immunity.[83,84]

Distribution

The bacterium is widespread in the northern hemisphere, especially in Europe.[85] *A phagocytophilum* has been detected in several animal species. The infection in humans was first diagnosed in the United States.[86]

Clinical Expression

The most characteristic symptoms of TBF in domestic ruminants is high fever (up to 42°C). Sheep exposed to infected ticks develop clinical signs within 14 days. The fever may last for 1 to 2 weeks.[87] However, the fever reaction may vary according to the age of the animals, the variant of *A phagocytophilum* involved, the host species, and the immunologic status of the host animal.[88]

Other clinical signs are often absent or mild. TBF is seldom fatal, unless complicated by other infections. However, TBF causes immunosuppression and makes the sheep vulnerable to secondary infections, such as tick pyemia caused by *Staphylococcus* spp infections[87] or septicemia caused by *Mannheimia haemolytica*.[89,90] Complications also include abortion,[91] impaired spermatogenesis in rams,[92] reduced weight gain in lambs, and a reduced milk yield in dairy animals.[88,93]

In humans, clinical manifestations range from a mild self-limiting febrile illness to a life-threatening and fatal infection. On average, patients develop a nonspecific influenza-like illness with fever, headache, myalgia, and malaise.[94]

Diagnosis

The clinical diagnosis is based on a sudden onset of very high fever associated with hematological changes and the presence of typical cytoplasmic inclusions in phagocytes, especially in neutrophils. Microscopy of blood smears taken during the fever period is normally sufficient to confirm the diagnosis. Stained with May-Grünwald Giemsa, the organisms appear as blue inclusions.[87] Inoculation of infected blood into susceptible animals was previously used to confirm the diagnosis.[87] A PCR method is now commonly used to identify *A phagocytophilum* infection in blood and tissue samples.[95] Cultivation of *A phagocytophilum* in tissue cultures has also been described.[96]

The presence of specific antibodies may support the diagnosis, the indirect immunofluorescent antibody (IFA) test being commonly used. However, it may be difficult to use the IFA test to diagnose an acute infection in lambs, because the IFA titers persist for months after the primary *A phagocytophilum* infection.[97]

At postmortem examination, an enlarged (up to 4–5 times the normal size) spleen can be regarded as indicative of TBF in sheep.[89,98] No other typical pathologic changes have been described.[99]

Treatment

The safest way to prevent TBF is to avoid areas where ticks are abundant, such as temperate deciduous woodland or mixed forests. However, this is often not feasible. In endemic areas, regular dipping or pour-on treatment with pyrethroids may be necessary against ticks.[100]

In treatment, the drug of choice is tetracycline.[94,101] However, a 5-day long treatment with oxytetracycline (10 mg/kg BW, daily) was not found adequate to clear *A phagocytophilum* from experimentally infected lambs.[102] Data suggest that fluoroquinolone antibiotics and rifampin may be alternative drugs for animals, where allowed, and in patients with intolerance to tetracycline.[103]

Control

In the United Kingdom, it has been estimated that more than 300,000 lambs develop tick pyemia each year[100]; up to 30% of TBF-infected lambs may develop crippling lameness and paralysis following secondary infections. Most of these die or become of reduced economic value.[104] TBF is also one of the main scourges in the sheep industry in Norway, and it has been estimated that more than 300,000 lambs are infected annually.[105]

The main disease problems associated with TBF in sheep are seen in lambs during the first grazing season and in sheep purchased from tick-free areas and placed on tick-infested pastures for the first time.[106] Problems caused by TBF may differ significantly between neighboring pastures, as several variants exist with differing degrees of virulence, and protective immunity is not necessarily transferred between these variants.[107] In one study, 24 msp4 gene variants were found in one sheep flock.[84]

The infection causes persistence in sheep, and variants may therefore be carried between geographic areas by purchasing infected animals. Ticks on the new pastures may become infected from these carriers and later transfer these variants to susceptible animals.

Current control strategies are based on the reduction of tick infestation by application of chemical acaricides at turnout onto a tick-infested pasture, mostly done by dipping or pour-on applications of pyrethroids.[88,101] This treatment has to be repeated several times during the tick season. In the United Kingdom, long-acting oxytetracycline is also used as a prophylactic measure, given before animals are moved from a tick-free environment onto a tick-infested pasture.[104,108] However, there is a growing concern about the environmental safety and human health because of antimicrobial resistance, increasing cost of chemical control, and the increasing resistance of ticks to pesticides.[109]

Another strategy to reduce the losses caused by TBF is to infect the lambs as early as possible. One study indicates that very young lambs (younger than 2 weeks of age)

show milder symptoms than older lambs when experimentally infected with
A phagocytophilum.[110] However, this practice is only feasible if the lambs are infected
immediately after birth, because 3- to 6-week-old lambs are very susceptible to the
infection.[88] Another obstacle to this strategy is that the infection prevalence and
A phagocytophilum variants in ticks may vary during the grazing season and from
year to year.[84]

Pasture management and habitat modification may reduce the density of ticks and
therefore the occurrence of TBF. These changes may destroy the ticks' microhabitat
or at least make the ticks vulnerable to macroclimatic conditions. The methods include
drainage of marshy lands, controlled burning or herbicidal treatment of vegetation,
mechanical clearing of bushes, removal of leaf litter and, in some cases, partial
removal of the forest canopy, all of which require substantial modification of the environment with possible chemical contamination.[111] Alteration of the habitat may also
change the ticks' host availability. However, the tick abundance can only be reduced
by these procedures for a short period, and several of these procedures have to be
repeated periodically and are labor intensive. In addition, sufficient habitat modification is not always feasible and farm animals are always at risk from ticks brought in
from the surrounding areas, especially if other large animal species use the same
pastures. The bacterium is widespread in the environment and may infect several
hosts.[85] However, a recent investigation indicates that there may be natural enzootic
cycles among different strains of *A phagocytophilum*.[112]

Biologic tick control is becoming an attractive approach to tick management. Biologic control of tick infestations has been difficult, because ticks have few natural
enemies. Most predators of ticks are generalists with a limited potential for tick
management. To date, studies have concentrated on examining the potential of
bacteria, entomopathogenic fungi, and nematodes to offer control.[109] However, the
main challenge is to create a sustainable biologic control of ticks in the natural habitat.

A vaccine against *A phagocytophilum* is not yet available. Immunization of susceptible sheep with infected blood from carrier animals should no longer be recommended
or performed, due to a lack of infection control and possible spread of other infectious
agents. The challenge to producing an effective vaccine is to choose antigens that are
conserved among all variants of *A phagocytophilum*. Identification of epitopes involved
in protective immunity combined with the discovery of cytokines involved in pathogenesis is encouraging for future vaccine development.[113] The whole genome of
a human variant of *A phagocytophilum* has recently been sequenced. However, other
strains of the bacterium have to be sequenced to conduct comparative genomics and
develop proper recombinant vaccine antigens for future cross-infection studies.[114]

Vaccines against ticks may be an option. So far, however, only a vaccine against the
one-host cattle tick *Rhipicephalus* (*Boophilus*) *microplus* has been developed.[115]
Control of ticks by vaccination has the advantage of cost-effectiveness, reduced environmental contamination, and prevention of selecting for drug-resistant ticks that may
result from repeated acaricide applications. The identification of tick-protective antigens remains the limiting factor in the development of an effective tick vaccine. Characterization of the ticks' genomes will therefore have a great impact on the discovery
of new protective antigens. Development of vaccines against multiple tick species
may be possible using highly conserved tick-protective antigens or by antigens
showing immune cross-reaction in different tick species.[116] An interesting concept
is the development of transmission-blocking vaccines by using tick immunomodulatory molecules.[117]

The development of vaccines that target both ticks and pathogen transmission may
provide a means of controlling tick-borne infections through immunization of the

human and animal population at risk or by immunization of the mammalian reservoir to reduce pathogen transmission.[116]

In the future, integrated tick control strategies should be implemented. These strategies must be based on host resistance to ticks and to the infections they transmit, strategic tick control on the actual pastures, cost/benefit analyses of the acaricidal applications, and the availability of vaccines against ticks and tick-borne diseases.[118]

HEARTWATER
Etiological Agent

Heartwater is caused by the rickettsia *Ehrlichia ruminantium* (formerly *Cowdria ruminantium*) in the genus *Ehrlichia* (see **Box 1**), which is transmitted by ticks of the genus *Amblyomma*.[73] Various strains of *E ruminantium* exist, but only a variable degree of cross-protective immunity occurs between the different strains.[119–121] The bacteria multiply in neutrophils, monocytes, and vascular endothelial cells.[122]

Distribution

Heartwater is an endemic disease in domestic and some wild ruminants throughout sub-Saharan Africa, including islands in the near-eastern Africa but also in the Caribbean following the introduction of *Amblyomma variegatum* ticks, probably in the 18th century.[123] It has been estimated that more than 150 million animals are at risk in the sub-Saharan area.[124]

Clinical Expression

The incubation period after natural tick-transmitted infection is usually from about 2 to 4 weeks. There are 4 clinical forms of heartwater: peracute, acute, subacute, and subclinical; the most common is the acute form.[46] The clinical symptoms depend on host susceptibility, virulence of the infective strains, and previous exposure. The disease is characterized by sudden onset of high fever (up to 42°C), nervous signs, and rapid and abdominal breathing. Auscultation may detect evidence of pulmonary edema and hydropericardium. Recumbency, convulsions, and death may follow within 24 hours. *E ruminantium* may cause high mortality in sheep, goats, and cattle, largely influenced by breed, age, animal species, and bacterial strains.[125] Small ruminants are very susceptible hosts and greater than 90% and 50% mortality have been observed in nonindigenous goats and sheep, respectively.[122] Subclinical and mild cases are common in young animals and in local indigenous breeds.

An age-related resistance to disease occurs in young domestic ruminants, independent of maternal transferred immunity. The period of resistance in lambs gradually wanes after approximately the first 3 weeks of life. The respective protective period in kids is not well studied, but may be shorter.[46]

Diagnostics

Presumptive diagnosis is based on clinical history and the presence of *Amblyomma* ticks in the region. At postmortem examination, massive transudates into the body cavities, especially hydropericardium, hydrothorax, and edema of the lungs and brain, are recorded. In addition, splenomegaly and enlargement of the lymph nodes are seen. Histologically, heartwater is characterized by the presence of clusters of the organisms in the vascular endothelium of virtually all tissues examined, especially the brain cortex. For rapid field diagnosis, *E ruminantium* can be detected in the vascular endothelial cells by squash preparations of the cerebrum.[46] Confirmation of diagnosis was previously made by the intravenous inoculation of 5 to 10 mL of whole blood from suspected cases into susceptible sheep or goats, but is now done using molecular methods such as PCR.[126] Diagnosis of heartwater based on direct detection of the agent is recommended. Positive PCR should be accompanied by isolation of the organisms in endothelial cell cultures, and corroborated by the presence of infected *Amblyomma* ticks.[125]

Several serologic tests are available for detecting antibodies against *E ruminantium*, such as indirect fluorescent antibody test, Western blot assay, ELISA, and competitive ELISA. Because a large proportion of infected animals die following a primary infection, antibody detection is not often an option. The duration of the antibody response is also questionable. In addition, serology is constrained by cross-reactions with other ehrlichial agents. Serologic methods that have high enough sensitivity and specificity to diagnose heartwater during early infection or after recovery are still lacking.[125]

Treatment

Successful therapy depends on early antibiotic treatment. Animals treated during the febrile stage of acute heartwater respond favorably to oxytetracycline at a dose rate of 5 to 10 mg/kg BW, given intravenously or intramuscularly at the first sign of fever and repeated once more 1 to 2 days later. The use of one dose of long-acting oxytetracycline at a dose rate of 20 mg/kg BW is also effective. Therapy initiated after the onset of neurologic signs is almost always inefficient.[127] Therefore, treatment should not be delayed until laboratory confirmation is established. Recovered animals can be carriers of the infection.[122]

Control

Although heartwater has been known for more than a century, it is still considered as a major obstacle against expansion and development of the livestock industry in Africa.[128] Imported breeds in particular are very susceptible, and severe infection with high mortality rates may occur.[122] There is a considerable concern about the possible spread of heartwater and its vector to tropical and subtropical regions of North, South, and Central America, where other suitable tick vectors exist.[46] *E ruminantium* can be transmitted by at least 13 species of *Amblyomma* ticks, with *A variegatum* (in West, East, and Central Africa) and *A hebraeum* (in South Africa) being the 2 major vectors.[129]

The hosts for *E ruminantium* appear to be restricted to members of the family Bovidae, including both domestic and wild ruminants. The animals most at risk are those introduced to endemic areas from heartwater-free areas. Prolonged survival of *E ruminantium* in ticks maintains the disease, as does the carrier state in ruminants.[130]

The current methods for heartwater control include the use of acaricides to control the tick vector, antibiotic prophylaxis, immunization by infection and treatment, farming with animal breeds resistant to the disease, and establishment of endemic stability.[131–134] All of these methods have serious drawbacks. For instance, acaricides are expensive, environmentally unfriendly, and may induce resistance in ticks. In addition, treatment has to be repeated several times during the tick season. Another drawback of using acaricides is that it hinders creation of endemic stability, as treated animals remain fully susceptible to infection.[125] Other strategies against tick infestation may be applied and have been discussed in the section on control of TBF. Attempts to control heartwater by controlling tick infestation have only partly been successful. Eradication of the disease by vector control therefore seems unlikely.[124]

The best long-term cost-effective control method against heartwater is vaccination.[124] At present, however, there is no safe, user-friendly, and reliable vaccine commercially available. Different vaccines with various efficacies have been produced against *E ruminantium*, including live organisms followed by antibiotic ("infection and treatment method"), live-attenuated vaccines, whole-organism inactivated vaccines, and recombinant protein and DNA vaccines.[135–140] Although many of the vaccines have conferred at least partial protection, a continuing problem is breakdown infection on challenge with organisms heterologous to those included in the vaccines.[114]

There are some barriers to developing an effective vaccine. Attenuation of virulent organisms is imprecise and there is little cross-protection between strains. Moreover, duration of immunity is variable; for example, in some goat breeds it may be as short as 2 months.[46] Vaccination should be timed to precede periods of peak tick feeding activity in wet seasons.[132]

At the moment the only commercially available immunization method is the "infection and treatment method," using an attenuated strain of E ruminantium. At the first signs of fever, vaccinated animals are treated with oxytetracycline to diminish the signs of disease. Successful vaccination depends on the proper timing of treatment. The disadvantages of such a procedure include: the need for chemotherapeutics after immunization; potential difficulties of distributing a deep-frozen vaccine, as the vaccine rapidly loses its infectivity and immunogenicity when thawed; and the requirement for the vaccine to be administered by intravenous injection. However, a recent study indicates that an attenuated vaccine based on the Welgevonden strain, when administrated intramuscularly, seemed to provide good cross-protection in Merino sheep and Angora goats.[141] In addition, attenuated ("live") vaccines induce persistent infection and hence provide a source of infection for ticks. These vaccines should not be used in regions where the disease is absent and where potential vectors exist, such as the United States and Central and South America. An inactivated vaccine may be used in these regions. However, a recombinant vaccine or a marker vaccine should be preferred to differentiate vaccinated and truly infected animals.[125]

Control of heartwater through discovery and development of improved vaccines remains the target for future research.[124] The success of inactivated vaccines in protecting against field challenge supports the concept that protective antigens can be identified. The genome sequences of 2 strains of E ruminantium provide the opportunity for comparative genomics and the prediction and identification of conserved vaccine antigen candidates. To develop an improved heartwater recombinant vaccine, it is necessary to understand the heterologous immunity and cross-protective mechanisms.[114] Once protective antigens have been identified the main challenge will be to design a recombinant vaccine, which induces cross-protective immune responses between strains.

SUMMARY

Chlamydial and rickettsial infections are a significant challenge to the small ruminant industry in several geographic areas. This review focuses on the treatment and control methods that are available. Different strategies should be implemented to control these infections. It is hoped that development of new recombinant vaccines using comparative genomics and proteomics will continue to progress.

REFERENCES

1. Longbottom D, Coulter LJ. Animal chlamydioses and zoonotic implications. J Comp Pathol 2003;128:217–44.
2. Aitken ID, Longbottom D. Chlamydial abortion. In: Aitken ID, editor. Diseases of sheep. 4th edition. Oxford (UK): Blackwell; 2007. p. 105–12.

3. Rodolakis A, Boullet C, Souriau A. *Chlamydia psittaci* experimental abortion in goats. Am J Vet Res 1984;45:2086–9.
4. Wittenbrink MM, Schoon HA, Bisping W, et al. Infection of the bovine female genital tract with *Chlamydia psittaci* as a possible cause of infertility. Reprod Domest Anim 1993;28:129–36.
5. Hyde SR, Benirschke K. Gestational psittacosis: case report and literature review. Mod Pathol 1997;10:602–7.
6. Buxton D. Potential danger to pregnant women of *Chlamydia psittaci* from sheep. Vet Rec 1986;118:510–1.
7. Bloodworth DL, Howard AJ, Davies A, et al. Infection in pregnancy caused by *Chlamydia psittaci* of ovine origin. Commun Dis Rep 1987;10:3–4.
8. Winter AC, Charnley JG. The sheep keeper's veterinary handbook. Ramsbury (UK): Crowood Press; 1999. p. 208.
9. Sachse K, Vretou E, Livingstone M, et al. Recent developments in the laboratory diagnosis of chlamydial infections. Vet Microbiol 2009;135:2–21.
10. Longbottom D. Enzootic abortion of ewes (ovine chlamydiosis). In: Manual of diagnostic tests and vaccines for terrestrial animals. 6th edition. Paris: World Organisation for Animal Health (OIE); 2008. p. 1013–20.
11. Stamp JT, Watt JA, Cockburn RB. Enzootic abortion in ewes; complement fixation test. J Comp Pathol 1952;62:93–101.
12. McCauley LME, Lancaster MJ, Young P, et al. Comparison of ELISA and CFT assays for *Chlamydophila abortus* antibodies in ovine sera. Aust Vet J 2007; 85:325–8.
13. Wilson K, Livingstone M, Longbottom D. Comparative evaluation of eight serological assays for diagnosing *Chlamydophila abortus* infection in sheep. Vet Microbiol 2009;135:38–45.
14. Laroucau K, Vorimore F, Sachse K, et al. Differential identification of *Chlamydophila abortus* live vaccine strain 1B by PCR-RFLP. Vaccine 2010;28:5653–8.
15. Wheelhouse N, Aitchison KD, Laroucau K, et al. Evidence of *Chlamydophila abortus* vaccine strain 1B as a possible cause of ovine enzootic abortion. Vaccine 2010;28:5857–63.
16. Sillis M, Longbottom D. Chlamydiosis. In: Palmer S, Soulsby L, Torgerson P, et al, editors. Zoonoses. 2nd edition. Oxford (UK): Oxford University Press, in press.
17. Papp JR, Shewen PE, Gartley CJ. Abortion and subsequent excretion of chlamydiae from the reproductive tract of sheep during estrus. Infect Immun 1994;62:3786–92.
18. Papp JR, Shewen PE. Pregnancy failure following vaginal infection of sheep with *Chlamydia psittaci* prior to breeding. Infect Immun 1996;64:1116–25.
19. Livingstone M, Wheelhouse N, Maley SW, et al. Molecular detection of *Chlamydophila abortus* in post-abortion sheep at oestrus and subsequent lambing. Vet Microbiol 2009;135:134–41.
20. Entrican G, Buxton D, Longbottom D. Chlamydial abortion: a brief overview. J R Soc Med 2001;94:273–7.
21. Rodolakis A. In vitro and in vivo properties of chemically induced temperature-sensitive mutants of *Chlamydia psittaci* var. ovis: screening in a murine model. Infect Immun 1983;42:525–30.
22. Foggie A. Preparation of vaccines against enzootic abortion of ewes. A review of the research work at the Moredun Institute. Vet Bull 1973;43:587–90.
23. Waldhalm DG, DeLong WJ, Hall RF. Efficacy of a bacterin prepared from *Chlamydia psittaci* grown in cell culture for experimental immunization of ewes. Vet Microbiol 1982;7:493–8.

24. Anderson IE, Tan TW, Jones GE, et al. Efficacy against ovine enzootic abortion of an experimental vaccine containing purified elementary bodies of *Chlamydia psittaci*. Vet Microbiol 1990;24:21–7.

25. Jones GE, Jones KA, Machell J, et al. Efficacy trials with tissue-culture grown, inactivated vaccines against chlamydial abortion in sheep. Vaccine 1995;13: 715–23.

26. Longbottom D, Livingstone M. Vaccination against chlamydial infections of man and animals. Vet J 2006;171:263–75.

27. Seshadri R, Paulsen IT, Eisen JA, et al. Complete genome sequence of the Q-fever pathogen *Coxiella burnetii*. Proc Natl Acad Sci U S A 2003;100: 5455–60.

28. Quevedo Diaz MA, Lukacova M. Immunological consequences of *Coxiella burnetii* phase variant. Acta Virol 1998;42:181–5.

29. McCaul TF, Williams JC. Developmental cycle of *Coxiella burnetii*: structure and morphogenesis of vegetative and sporogenic differentiations. J Bacteriol 1981; 147:1063–76.

30. Mearns R. Other infectious causes of abortion. In: Aitken ID, editor. Diseases of sheep. 4th edition. Oxford (UK): Blackwell; 2007. p. 126–36.

31. Maurin M, Raoult D. Q fever. Clin Microbiol Rev 1999;12:518–53.

32. Hilbink F, Penrose M, Kovacova E, et al. Q fever is absent from New Zealand. Int J Epidemiol 1993;22:945–9.

33. Arricau-Bouvery N, Rodolakis A. Is Q fever an emerging or re-emerging zoonosis? Vet Res 2005;36:327–49.

34. Palmer NC, Kierstead M, Key DW, et al. Placentitis and abortion in goats and sheep in Ontario caused by *Coxiella burnetii*. Can Vet J 1983;24:60–1.

35. Zeman DH, Kirkbride CA, Leslie-Steen P, et al. Ovine abortion due to *Coxiella burnetii* infection. J Vet Diagn Invest 1989;1:178–80.

36. Berri M, Souriau S, Crosby M, et al. Relationships between the shedding of *Coxiella burnetii*, clinical signs and serological responses of 34 sheep. Vet Rec 2001;148:502–5.

37. Sanford SE, Josephson GKA, MacDonald A. *Coxiella burnetii* (Q fever) abortion storms in goat herds after attendance at an annual fair. Can Vet J 1994;35: 376–8.

38. Crowther RW, Spicer AJ. Abortion in sheep and goats in Cyprus caused by *Coxiella burnetii* (sic). Vet Rec 1976;99:29–30.

39. Moore JD, Barr BC, Daft BM, et al. Pathology and diagnosis of *Coxiella burnetii* infection in a goat herd. Vet Pathol 1991;28:81–4.

40. Fournier PE, Marrie TJ, Raoult D. Diagnosis of Q fever. J Clin Microbiol 1998;36: 1823–34.

41. Barlow J, Rauch B, Welcome F, et al. Association between *Coxiella burnetii* shedding in milk and subclinical mastitis in dairy cattle. Vet Res 2008;39:23.

42. Berri M, Laroucau K, Rodolakis A. The detection of *Coxiella burnetii* from ovine genital swabs, milk and fecal samples by use of a single touchdown chain reaction. Vet Microbiol 2000;72:285–93.

43. Lang GH. Coxiellosis (Q fever) in animals. In: Marrie TJ, editor, Q fever: the disease, vol. 1. Boca Raton (FL): CRC Press; 1990. p. 24–42.

44. Hatchette T, Hudson R, Schezch WF, et al. Goat-associated Q fever: a new disease in Newfoundland. Emerg Infect Dis 2001;7:413–9.

45. Kovacova E, Kazar J, Spanelova D. Suitability of various *Coxiella burnetii* antigen preparations for detection of serum antibodies by various tests. Acta Virol 1998;42:365–8.

46. Smith MC, Sherman DM. Goat medicine. 2nd edition. Ames (IA): Wiley-Blackwell; 2009. p. 871.
47. Arricau Bouvery N, Souriau A, Lechopier P, et al. Experimental *Coxiella burnetii* infection in pregnant goats: excretion routes. Vet Res 2003;34:423–33.
48. Berri M, Crochet D, Santiago S, et al. Spread of *Coxiella burnetii* infection in a flock of sheep after an episode of Q fever. Vet Rec 2005;157:737–40.
49. Kazar J. Q fever - current concept. In: Raoult D, Brouqui P, editors. Rickettsiae and rickettsial diseases at the turn of the third millennium. Paris: Elsevier; 1999. p. 304–19.
50. Van den Brom R, Vellema P. Q fever outbreaks in small ruminants and people in the Netherlands. Small Rumin Res 2009;86:74–89.
51. Enserink M. Questions abound to Q-fever explosion in the Netherlands. Science 2010;327:266–7.
52. Behymer D, Ruppaner R, Riemann HP. Observations on chemotherapy in cows chronically infected with *Coxiella burnetii* (Q fever). Folia Vet Lat 1977;7:64–70.
53. Rodolakis A. Q fever, state of art: epidemiology, diagnosis and prophylaxis. In: Proceedings of the 6th International Sheep Veterinary Congress. Hersonissos (Greece); 2005. p. 96–8.
54. Babudieri B. Q fever: a zoonosis. Adv Vet Sci 1959;5:181–2.
55. Sawyer LA, Fishbein DB, McDade JE. Q fever: current concepts. Rev Infect Dis 1987;9:935–46.
56. Arricau-Bouvry N, Souriau A, Bodir C, et al. Effect of vaccination with phase I and phase II *Coxiella burnetii* vaccines in pregnant goats. Vaccine 2005;23:4392–402.
57. Rodolakis A, Berri M, Héchard C, et al. Comparison of *Coxiella burnetii* shedding in milk of dairy bovine, caprine and ovine herds. J. Dairy Sci 2007;90: 5352–60.
58. Rodolakis A. Q fever in dairy animals. Ann N Y Acad Sci 2009;1166:90–3.
59. Berri M, Souriau A, Crosby M, et al. Shedding of *Coxiella burnetii* in ewes in two pregnancies following an episode of *Coxiella* abortion in a sheep flock. Vet Microbiol 2002;85:55–60.
60. Hatchette T, Campbell N, Hudson R, et al. Natural history of Q fever in goats. Vector Borne Zoonotic Dis 2003;3:11–5.
61. Welsh HH, Lennette EH, Abinanti FR, et al. Airborne transmission of Q fever: the role of parturition in generation of infective aerosol. Ann N Y Acad Sci 1957;70: 528–40.
62. Tissot-Dupont H, Torres S, Nezri M, et al. Hyperendemic focus of Q fever related to sheep and wind. Am J Epidemiol 1999;150:67–74.
63. Tigertt WD, Benenson AS, Gochenour WS. Airborne Q fever. Bacteriol Rev 1961; 25:285–93.
64. Scott GH, Williams JC. Susceptibility of *Coxiella burnetii* to chemical disinfectants. Rickettsiology: current issues and perspectives. Ann N Y Acad Sci 1990;590:291–6.
65. Berri M, Rousset E, Champion JL, et al. Ovine manure used as a garden fertiliser is suspected to be a contamination source of two human Q fever cases. Vet Rec 2003;153:269–70.
66. Tissot-Dupont H, Amadei M-A, Nezri M, et al. Wind in November, Q fever in December. Emerg Infect Dis 2004;10:1264–9.
67. Sadecky E, Brezina R. Vaccination of naturally infected ewes against Q-fever. Acta Virol 1977;21:89.
68. Brooks DL, Ermel RW, Franti CE, et al. Q fever vaccination of sheep: challenge and immunity in ewes. Am J Vet Res 1986;47:1235–8.

69. Sampere M, Font B, Font J, et al. Q fever in adults: review of 66 clinical cases. Eur J Clin Microbiol Infect Dis 2003;22:108–10.

70. Souriau A, Arricau-Bouvery N, Bodier C, et al. Comparison of the efficacy of Q fever vaccines against *Coxiella burnetii* experimental challenge in pregnant goats. Ann N Y Acad Sci 2003;990:521–3.

71. Schmeer N, Muller P, Langel J, et al. Q fever vaccines for animals. Zentralbl Bakteriol Mikrobiol Hyg A 1987;267:79–88.

72. Dupuis G, Petite J, Petr O, et al. An important outbreak of human Q fever in a Swiss Alpine valley. Int J Epidemiol 1987;16:282–7.

73. Dumler JS, Barbet AF, Bekker CPJ, et al. Reorganization of genera in the families *Rickettsiaceae* and *Anaplasmataceae* in the order *Rickettsiales*; unification of some species of *Ehrlichia* with *Anaplasma*, *Cowdria* with *Ehrlichia* and *Ehrlichia* with *Neorickettsia*, descriptions of six new species combinations and designation of *Ehrlichia equi* and "HGE agent" as subjective synonyms of *Ehrlichia phagocytophila*. Int J Syst Evol Microbiol 2001;51:2145–65.

74. Uilenberg G, Van Vorstenbosch CJAH, Perié CJ. Blood parasites in sheep in the Netherlands. I. *Anaplasma mesaeterum* sp.n. (Rickettsiales, Anaplasmataceae). Vet Q 1979;1:14–22.

75. Friedhoff KT. Tick-borne diseases in sheep and goats caused by *Babesia*, *Theileria* or *Anaplasma* spp. Parasitologia 1997;39:99–109.

76. Splitter EJ, Anthony HD, Twiehaus MJ. *Anaplasma ovis* in the United States. Am J Vet Res 1956;17:487–91.

77. Zwart D, Buys J. Studies on *Anaplasma ovis* infection. II. Pathogenicity of a Nigerian goat strain for Dutch sheep and goats. Bull Epizoot Dis Afr 1968;16: 73–80.

78. Ilemobade AA. Blood parasites of African goats. In: Proceedings of the 3rd International Conference on Goat Production and Disease. Tucson (Arizona); 1982. p. 68–71.

79. Palmer GH, Abbott JR, French DM, et al. Persistence of *Anaplasma ovis* infection and conservation of the msp-2 and msp-3 multigene families within the genus *Anaplasma*. Infect Immun 1998;66:6035–9.

80. Barry DM, Van-Niekerk CH. Anaplasmosis in improved Boer goats in South Africa artificially infected with *Anaplasma ovis*. Small Rumin Res 1990;3:191–7.

81. Mallick KP, Dwivedi SK, Malhotra MN. Anaplasmosis in goats: report of clinical cases. Indian Vet J 1979;56:693–4.

82. Ndungú LW, Aguirre C, Rurangirwa FR, et al. Detection of *Anaplasma ovis* infection in goats by major surface protein 5 competitive inhibition enzyme-linked immunosorbent assay. J Clin Microbiol 1995;33:675–9.

83. Stuen S, Moum T, Petrovec M, et al. Genetic variants of *Anaplasma phagocytophilum* in Norway. Int J Med Microbiol 2006;296:164–6.

84. Ladbury GAF, Stuen S, Thomas R, et al. Dynamic transmission of numerous *Anaplasma phagocytophilum* genotypes among lambs in an infected sheep flock in an area of anaplasmosis endemicity. J Clin Microbiol 2008;46: 1686–91.

85. Stuen S. *Anaplasma phagocytophilum*—the most widespread tick-borne infection in animals in Europe. Vet Res Commun 2007;31(Suppl 1):79–84.

86. Bakken JS, Dumler JS, Chen S-M, et al. Human granulocytic ehrlichiosis in the upper Midwest United States. A new species emerging? J Am Med Assoc 1994; 272:212–8.

87. Foggie A. Studies on the infectious agent of tick-borne fever in sheep. J Pathol Bacteriol 1951;63:1–15.

88. Stuen S. In: *Anaplasma phagocytophilum* (formerly *Ehrlichia phagocytophila*) infection in sheep and wild ruminants in Norway. A study on clinical manifestation, distribution and persistence [Dr Phil thesis]. University of Oslo; 2003.

89. Øverås J, Lund A, Ulvund MJ, et al. Tick-borne fever as a possible predisposing factor in septicaemic pasteurellosis in lambs. Vet Rec 1993;133:398.

90. Stuen S. Tick-borne fever (TBF) and secondary infections in sheep. In: Kazar J, Toman R, editors. Rickettsiae and rickettsial diseases. Bratislava (Slovakia): Veda; 1996. p. 347–9.

91. Jamieson S. Tick-borne fever as a cause of abortion in sheep—part II. Vet Rec 1950;62:468–70.

92. Watson WA. Infertility in the ram associated with tick-borne fever infection. Vet Rec 1964;76:1131–6.

93. Tuomi J. Studies in epidemiology of bovine of tick-borne fever in Finland and a clinical description of field cases. Ann Med Exp Biol Fenn 1966;44(Suppl 6): 1–62.

94. Bakken JS, Dumler JS. Clinical diagnosis and treatment of human granulocytic anaplasmosis. Ann N Y Acad Sci 2006;1078:236–47.

95. Chen S-M, Dumler JS, Bakken JS, et al. Identification of a granulocytic *Ehrlichia* species as the etiologic agent of human disease. J Clin Microbiol 1994;32: 589–95.

96. Goodman JL, Nelson C, Vitale B, et al. Direct cultivation of the causative agent of human granulocytic ehrlichiosis. N Engl J Med 1996;334:209–15.

97. Paxton EA, Scott GR. Detection of antibodies to the agent of tick-borne fever by indirect immunofluorescence. Vet Microbiol 1989;21:133–8.

98. Gordon WS, Brownlee A, Wilson DR, et al. "Tick-borne fever" (A hitherto undescribed disease of sheep.). J Comp Pathol 1932;45:301–7.

99. Campbell RSF, Rowland AC, Scott GR. Sequential pathology of tick-borne fever. J Comp Pathol 1994;111:303–13.

100. Brodie TA, Holmes PH, Urquhart GM. Some aspects of tick-borne diseases of British sheep. Vet Rec 1986;118:415–8.

101. Woldehiwet Z, Scott GR. Tick-borne (pasture) fever. In: Woldehiwet Z, Ristic M, editors. Rickettsial and chlamydial diseases of domestic animals. Oxford (UK): Pergamon Press; 1993. p. 233–54.

102. Stuen S, Bergström K. The effect of two different oxytetracycline treatments in experimental *Ehrlichia phagocytophila* infected lambs. Acta Vet Scand 2001; 42:339–46.

103. Horowitz HW, Hsieh T-C, Aguero-Rosenfeld ME, et al. Antimicrobial susceptibility of *Ehrlichia phagocytophila*. Antimicrob Agents Chemother 2001;45:786–8.

104. Woldehiwet Z. Tick-borne diseases. In: Aitken ID, editor. Diseases of sheep. 4th edition. Oxford (UK): Blackwell; 2007. p. 347–55.

105. Stuen S, Bergström K. Serological investigation of granulocytic *Ehrlichia* infection in sheep in Norway. Acta Vet Scand 2001;42:331–8.

106. Scott GR. Tick-associated infections. In: Martin WB, Aitken ID, editors. Diseases of sheep. 1st edition. Oxford (UK): Blackwell; 1983. p. 209–13.

107. Stuen S, Bergström K, Petrovec M, et al. Differences in clinical manifestations and hematological and serological responses after experimental infection with genetic variants of *Anaplasma phagocytophilum* in sheep. Clin Diagn Lab Immunol 2003;10:692–5.

108. Brodie TA, Holmes PH, Urquhart GM. Prophylactic use of long-acting tetracycline against tick-borne fever (*Cytoecetes phagocytophila*) in sheep. Vet Rec 1988;122:43–4.

109. Samish M, Ginsberg H, Glazer I. Biological control of ticks. Parasitology 2004; 129:S389–403.
110. Stuen S, Hardeng F, Larsen HJ. Resistance to tick-borne fever in young lambs. Res Vet Sci 1992;52:211–6.
111. Sonenshine DE. Biology of ticks, vol. 2. New York: Oxford University Press; 1993. p. 465.
112. Bown K, Lambin X, Ogden NH, et al. Delineating Anaplasma phagocytophilum ecotypes in coexisting, discrete enzootic cycles. Emerg Infect Dis 2009;15: 1948–54.
113. Zhi N, Ohashi N, Rikihisa Y. Multiple p44 genes encoding major outer membrane proteins are expressed in the human granulocytic ehrlichiosis agent. J Biol Chem 1999;274:17828–36.
114. Barbet AF, Byrom B, Mahan SM. Diversity of Ehrlichia ruminantium major antigenic protein 1-2 in field isolates and infected sheep. Infect Immun 2009;77: 2304–10.
115. Willardsen P. Anti-tick vaccines. Parasitology 2004;129:S367–87.
116. de la Fuente J, Kocan KM. Strategies for development of vaccines for control of ixodid ticks species. Parasite Immunol 2006;28:275–83.
117. Titus RG, Bishop JV, Mejla JS. The immunomodulatory factors of arthropod saliva and the potential for these factors to serve as vaccine targets to prevent pathogen transmission. Parasite Immunol 2006;28:131–41.
118. Jongejan F, Uilenberg G. The global importance of ticks. Parasitology 2004;129: S3–14.
119. Uilenberg G. Heartwater (Cowdria ruminantium infection): current status. Adv Vet Sci Comp Med 1983;27:427–80.
120. Jongejan F, Uilenberg G, Franssen FF, et al. Antigenic differences between stocks of Cowdria ruminantium. Res Vet Sci 1988;44:186–9.
121. Allsopp MT, Van Strijp MF, Faber E, et al. Ehrlichia ruminantium variants which do not cause heartwater in South Africa. Vet Microbiol 2007;120:158–66.
122. Uilenberg G, Camus E. Heartwater (cowdriosis). In: Woldehiwet Z, Ristic M, editors. Rickettsial and chlamydial diseases of domestic animals. Oxford (UK): Pergamon Press; 1993. p. 293–332.
123. Maillard JC, Maillard N. Historique du peuplement bovin et de l'introduction de la tique Amblyomma variegatum dans les iles francaises des Antilles. Synthèse bibliographique Ethnozootechnie 1998;1:19–26.
124. Allsopp BA. Trend in control of heartwater. Onderstepoort J Vet Res 2009;76: 81–8.
125. Mahan SM. Diagnosis and control of heartwater, Ehrlichia ruminantium infection: an update. CAB Reviews: Perspectives in Agriculture, Veterinary Science, Nutrition and Natural Resources 2006;1(055):12.
126. Martinez D, Maillard JC, Coisne S, et al. Protection of goats against heartwater acquired by immunisation with inactivated elementary bodies of Cowdria ruminantium. Vet Immunol Immunopathol 1994;41:153–63.
127. Prozesky L, Du Plessis JL. The pathology of heartwater. II. A study of the lung lesions in sheep and goats infected with the Ball, strain of Cowdria ruminantium. Onderstepoort J Vet Res 1985;52:81–5.
128. Provost A, Bezuidenhout JD. The historical background and global importance of heartwater. Onderstepoort J Vet Res 1987;54:165–9.
129. Walker JB, Olwage A. The tick vectors of Cowdria ruminantium (Ixodoidea, Ixodidae, genus Amblyomma) and their distribution. Onderstepoort J Vet Res 1987;54:353–79.

130. Andrew HR, Norval RAI. The carrier status of sheep, cattle and African buffalo recovered from heartwater. Vet Parasitol 1989;34:295–308.
131. Peregrine AS. Chemotherapy and delivery systems: haemoparasites. Vet Parasitol 1994;54:223–48.
132. Van der Merwe L. The infection and treatment method of vaccination against heartwater. Onderstepoort J Vet Res 1987;54:489–91.
133. Camus E, Maillard JC, Ruff G, et al. Genetic resistance of Creole goats to cowdriosis in Guadeloupe. Status in 1995. Ann N Y Acad Sci 1996;791:46–53.
134. Tice GA, Bryson NR, Stewart CG, et al. The absence of clinical disease in cattle in communal grazing areas where farmers are changing from an intensive dipping programme to one of endemic stability to tick-borne diseases. Onderstepoort J Vet Res 1998;65:169–75.
135. Nyika A, Mahan SM, Burridge MJ, et al. A DNA vaccine protects mice against rickettsial agent *Cowdria ruminantium*. Parasite Immunol 1998;20:111–9.
136. Mahan SM, Allsopp B, Kocan KM, et al. Vaccine strategies for *Cowdria ruminantium* infections and their application to other ehrlichial infections. Parasitol Today 1999;15:290–4.
137. Collins NE, Pretorius A, Van Kleef M, et al. Development of improved attenuated and nucleic acid vaccines for heartwater. Dev Biol (Basel) 2003;1154:121–36.
138. Zweygarth E, Josemans AI, Van Strijp MF, et al. An attenuated *Ehrlichia ruminantium* (Welgevonden stock) vaccine protects small ruminants against virulent heartwater challenge. Vaccine 2005;23:1695–702.
139. Faburay B, Geysen D, Ceesay A, et al. Immunisation of sheep against heartwater in the Gambia using inactivated and attenuated *Ehrlichia ruminantium* vaccines. Vaccine 2007;25:7939–47.
140. Shkap V, de Vos AJ, Zweygarth E, et al. Attenuated vaccines for tropical theileriosis, babesiosis and heartwater: the continuing necessary. Trends Parasitol 2007;23:420–6.
141. Zweygarth E, Josemans AI, Steyn HC. Experimental use of the attenuated *Ehrlichia ruminantium* (Welgevonden) vaccine in Merino sheep and Angora goats. Vaccine 2008;265:G34–9.

Index

Note: Page numbers of articles titles are in **boldface** type.

Moving?

Make sure your subscription moves with you!

To notify us of your new address, find your **Clinics Account Number** (located on your mailing label above your name), and contact customer service at:

Email: journalscustomerservice-usa@elsevier.com

800-654-2452 (subscribers in the U.S. & Canada)
314-447-8871 (subscribers outside of the U.S. & Canada)

Fax number: 314-447-8029

Elsevier Health Sciences Division
Subscription Customer Service
3251 Riverport Lane
Maryland Heights, MO 63043

*To ensure uninterrupted delivery of your subscription, please notify us at least 4 weeks in advance of move.

Printed and bound by CPI Group (UK) Ltd, Croydon, CR0 4YY

03/10/2024

01040457-0009